BEST CARE EVERYWHERE

by
VA Professionals Across the Nation

edited by
THE SECRETARY OF THE DEPARTMENT OF VETERANS AFFAIRS
David Shulkin, MD

with Shereef Elnahal, MD, MBA, Ellen Maddock, MBA, *and* Megan Shaheen, MPH

U.S. Department of Veterans Affairs
June 2017 | P96877 | IB 10-1009

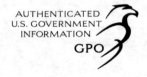

This is the official U.S. Government edition of this publication and is herein identified to certify its authenticity. ISBN 978–0–16–093958–7 is for U.S. Government Publishing Office official editions only. The Superintendent of Documents of the U.S. Government Publishing Office requests that any reprinted edition be labeled clearly as a copy of the authentic work, and that a new ISBN be assigned.

For sale by the Superintendent of Documents, U.S. Government Publishing Office
Internet: bookstore.gpo.gov   Phone: toll free (866) 512-1800;   DC area (202) 512-1800
Fax: (202) 512-2104   Mail: Stop IDCC, Washington, DC 20402-0001

ISBN 978-0-16-093958-7

Dedication

For the men and women in uniform who have served our country and preserved our freedom. For all of the health care professionals in VA who have dedicated their careers to keeping them healthy.

And finally, for Phillip Longman, who over a decade ago showed us that VA provides some of the best healthcare anywhere, and who inspired us to disseminate our best practices and pursue the audacious goal of delivering the best care everywhere to our Veterans.

Recognition

The Editors would like to recognize the following contributors, without whom this book would not have been possible:

Forest Plourde-Cole, Hillary Peabody, Elissa Hannam, Megan Willig, Megan Weibye, Thalia Sirjuie, Tiana Bouma, Jessica Adams, and the Atlas Research team; Eliza Spencer and the ERPi team; Andrea Ippolito and the VA Center for Innovation; Sankalpa Subbu and the Office of Strategic Integration team; Brian Mano and the Office of Acquisitions and Logistics team; Suzana Iveljic, David Jones, and the VHA Communications team; Vivieca Wright-Simpson, Edward Ledford, and all of the VA employees who supported this process.

Contents

Frequently Used Acronyms

Acronym	Definition
CBOC	Community Based Outpatient Clinic
CDC	Centers for Disease Control and Prevention
CPRS	Computerized Patient Record System
CPS	Clinical Pharmacy Specialist
DoD	Department of Defense
ED	Emergency Department
EHR	Electronic Health Record
FTE	Full Time Employee
FY	Fiscal Year
IT	Information Technology
LCSW	Licensed Clinical Social Worker
LPN	Licensed Practical Nurse
MD	Medical Doctor
NP	Nurse Practitioner
OEF/OIF	Operation Enduring Freedom-Operation Iraqi Freedom
ORH	Office of Rural Health
PACT	Patient Aligned Care Team
PC	Primary Care
PCP	Primary Care Physician/Provider
PTSD	Post-Traumatic Stress Disorder
RN	Registered Nurse
VA	Veterans Affairs
VACI	VA Center for Innovation
VACO	VA Central Office
VAMC	VA Medical Center
VBA	Veterans Benefits Administration
VHA	Veterans Health Administration
VISN	Veterans Integrated Service Network
VistA	Veterans Health Information Systems and Technology Architecture

Introduction — Secretary of the Department of Veterans Affairs, Dr. David J. Shulkin

As the Secretary of Veterans Affairs, it is my honor to work so closely and so routinely with the Veterans and their families whom we serve. I meet and consult with Veterans using their VA health care, benefits, and services here in Washington, DC. I meet and consult with Veterans when I travel to VA facilities around the country. I meet and consult Veterans when we talk about the Veteran experience and exchange ideas and observations at large conferences and at more modest town hall meetings. Since I still practice medicine with Veterans, I even listen to what Veterans tell me about their experiences with VA in examining rooms and, thanks to telehealth technology, in my office overlooking the White House. And consulting with Veterans who are leaders and members of Veterans Service Organizations is an important part of my weekly rounds as Secretary. All of these encounters are valuable opportunities to make sure that my priorities for improving VA for Veterans are precisely aligned with the needs and expectations of our most important stakeholders: the men and women who have served in uniform, the men and women to whom we and the entire nation owe the greatest debt.

Over the course of many conversations, a common theme emerged. That theme is about consistency. It is about an understandable expectation Veterans have for a consistent, seamless care experience at any VA facility across the country. Like many Americans, Veterans travel a good deal. That means they may also get sick on the road. For Veterans enrolled in VA health care, a natural response is to seek care in the nearest VA hospital or clinic. With over 1,700 sites of care, there is a good chance that one of our VA facilities is within driving distance of traveling Veterans. And Veterans naturally expect that one VA facility operates similarly to another VA facility. Too often, however, that's not been the case. Veterans have found that their experiences with VA vary, often widely, from site to site. And when I first arrived at VA as the Undersecretary of Health (USH), there was no guarantee that Veterans could even access every facility in the system with the VA card we gave them. Registration for care was site specific.

That significant problem of a consistent, predictable experience was one of the first challenges I directed the Veterans Health Administration to solve when I was USH. And for good reason. For Veterans, VA is their brand, and brands are about trust. If you are a member of Costco or Sam's Club, you expect access to those businesses no matter which location you visit. Consistently gaining access builds trust. The good experience of consistently receiving excellent customer service no matter where you find yourself builds trust. We have solved significant aspects of the access issue at VA, and we have a lot more to do in terms of access. But in terms of broad consistency of an excellent care experience, we have only scratched the surface. When I visit VA facilities across the country to meet Veterans and staff, I recognize the immense scale of this particular and very, very important challenge.

Before becoming Secretary, before coming to VA as USH, I led several hospitals and health systems in the private sector. So I know that achieving consistency in the care experience—for both clinical and administrative practices—is a sizable challenge for all of American health care, not just VA. Studies, most notably a report from the Institute of Medicine in 2001 called Crossing the Quality Chasm, have shown that it takes an average of 17 years for new medical evidence to reach patients in clinic or at the bedside. VA, the largest health system in the United States, is not exempt from this problem. But VA is leading American health care in fixing it.

Recognizing and embracing these challenges during my first months as the Under Secretary, I prioritized our organizational efforts. My five priorities for transformation were:

1. Improving access to our clinical care services.

2. Improving the morale and engagement of our employees.

3. Establishing consistency and spread of best practices across the system.

4. Building a high-performing network of care with our private sector and community partners.

5. Restoring trust in the VA health system.

In October of 2015, VA launched the Diffusion of Excellence Initiative primarily to address the priority focused on the third priority, best practices. With the advantage of hindsight, I can say that the Diffusion of Excellence process has addressed all five priorities in important ways.

VA's Innovation Ecosystem

By way of the Diffusion of Excellence Initiative, we have built a process, business rules, and a governing structure that works to promote consistency in our best practices and to function in earnest as an integrated enterprise. The Initiative incorporates all organization efforts that design and discover best practices. It offers a standardized path for frontline caregivers to learn about what is already being done well in many parts of the country. Through the Diffusion of Excellence Initiative, dedicated frontline employees are influencing VA health care far beyond their individual workspace. The goal is to identify clinical and administrative best practices, disseminate them to other sites of care, and deliver consistent, standardized, positive outcomes for Veterans.

We are changing culture. The Diffusion of Excellence governance structure collapses organizational silos, reforms the bureaucracy to enable and encourage progress, and allows resources to be targeted to the front lines in places where they are most needed. We are also breaking down cultural barriers by creating systematic incentives to share what has worked with others in the system. Within one year after the Diffusion of Excellence team began their work, we saw over 80 completed best practice replications, hundreds of ongoing projects, and over 100 facilities participating in this Initiative.

We are changing culture by elevating the people who have dedicated their careers to serving Veterans. Their energy, their enthusiasm, and their dedication have been the rocket fuel enabling this Diffusion of Excellence Initiative to take off. Best practice fellows—the very same innovators who have put our VA system among top systems in terms of innovation—have taken it upon themselves to improve the system around them. These employees represent the very best of American health care, and it is an honor to propagate their accomplishments.

The Diffusion of Excellence Initiative identifies the best projects and prototypes that we can replicate. With the support of the Innovator's Network, frontline employees are designing new practices with Veterans and other stakeholders. We have also leveraged the Diffusion Hub to enable frontline employees to keep track of their progress as they implement new practices and to achieve transparency and national oversight into that progress. Altogether, those three mutually reinforcing elements represent VA's Innovation Ecosystem.

The result has been employees empowered to impact the care system nationwide. Here are three examples of best practices and their implementing fellows that highlight the culture change that we have undertaken with this Initiative. You will find more details in the next chapters.

In Little Rock, AR, Dr. Kimberly Garner gathered Veterans in groups to teach them about advance care planning and to discuss their goals of care. This model empowers Veterans to decide how they would like to be cared for in the future, should they be too ill to communicate their wishes. By teaching Veterans in groups, this practice provides Veterans with the tools they need to discuss their wishes with family and caregivers in an efficient manner that increases access to this valuable service. With Dr. Garner's help, this practice was successfully replicated in Bedford, MA, is being adopted rapidly across VISN 1, and was selected for national standardization.

In Chillicothe, OH, Mr. Scott Bryant is a champion for the reapplication of a best practice developed at the VA San Diego Healthcare System through an Innovators Network grant. By simply using an iPad questionnaire that Veterans complete in the waiting room, this best practice decreased by half the time to document suicide risk and increased by 21 percent same-day access to mental health care and triage for urgent services. These electronic questionnaires allow clinicians to see responses to questions before walking into the Veteran's room, helping clinicians make appropriate referrals. This practice has been replicated successfully in six other facilities, and it's in demand at another 50 sites. We have a clear path to delivery.

In Madison, WI, clinical pharmacist Dr. Ellina Seckel not only provides high-quality medication management for her own patients, but also takes it upon herself to redesign the way clinical pharmacists interact with primary care teams. Now, clinical pharmacists are at the table with the rest of the care team, independently taking on patients with chronic conditions and long-term medications. Because these skilled pharmacists are equipped to take on patients who are coming in for medication issues only, Primary Care Physicians or Providers are free to see more patients with new problems. This practice improves overall access to primary care, and that's one of my top priorities for the organization. One example is the deployment of CPSs who independently see patients for medication management issues. Overall, PCPs increased access by 28 percent as pharmacists independently managed more patients. Twenty-one additional sites in VA are replicating this practice. If it is expanded VA-wide, 2 million more VA primary care appointments per year are achievable. With that kind of inherent untapped potential, leveraging our scope and scale is not just smart. It is our duty.

We are on the way to providing consistency in the care delivery experience and a highly-reliable system. We have created a path to the standardization of best practices developed by the front line, for the front line. We hope that this is restoring trust in our system. We believe that this is not only an Initiative that can benefit millions of Veterans across the nation, but also a model that any health system facing similar challenges can use.

In the meantime, we'll continue to work to empower frontline employees to impact countless more Veterans than they otherwise could have.

Introduction — Assistant Deputy Under Secretary for Health and Chief of Quality, Safety, and Value, Dr. Shereef M. Elnahal

One of Secretary Shulkin's top priorities for Veterans is "a consistent, seamless care experience at any VA facility across the country." That's a big challenge for VA, and it's a big challenge for other health care systems.

VA has a solution. VA's Diffusion of Excellence Initiative is achieving the kind of consistency in care Secretary Shulkin describes, and it's improving Veterans' lives. Indeed, the Diffusion of Excellence model could well serve all American health care.

With more than 1,700 sites of care and 300,000 employees, delivering a consistent health care experience is inherently challenging. For VA, decentralized leadership offers each facility the discretion—and opportunity for innovation—to address local issues in ways that best serve clients. That's an advantage for both providers and patients. Yet, that advantage carries with it a sizable challenge: standardizing the right best practices so we can consistently deliver value, no matter where those standardized practices are applied, all while preserving the valuable flexibility that answers local requirements. It's a great challenge for VHA health care, and it's a great challenge for US health care at large. At VA, we know we can answer that challenge for our Veterans with innovative, forward thinking, and there are many program offices at VA fueling innovation.

That's what **VA's Innovation Ecosystem** is all about. The goals of the Innovation Ecosystem are to identify clinical and administrative best practices, disseminate these practices to other sites of care, and encourage standardization of practices that deliver positive outcomes for Veterans and their families. Three mutually reinforcing elements of the VA Innovation Ecosystem—the **VA Center for Innovation, the Innovators Network**, and the **Diffusion of Excellence Initiative**—work together to achieve these goals. Each element in this precision ecosystem performs a vital function, and together they help VA innovation to thrive.

The **VACI** is an enterprise entity working with and across all lines of business. It focuses on delivering operational breakthroughs that answer strategic priorities, building innovation as a capability and culture at VA, and driving future thinking. And the VACI sponsors the **VA Innovators Network**, a collaboration of highly skilled change agents who lead and facilitate best practice implementation on VA's front lines. The Innovator's Network plays a key role in the first phase of innovation, and again in the second phase, implementation. The Network empowers frontline innovators with training, a tiered grant program that seeds and cultivates specific innovations, and ongoing integration into agency strategy. It helps diffuse best practices once they consistently prove to deliver positive outcomes for Veterans. Other offices, such as VHA's Office of Rural Health, play an important role, too, by driving field-based innovation and best practice standardization to priority groups of Veterans, rural Veterans among them.

Ultimately, identifying and propagating the best practices drives a consistent, predictable, and high-quality health care experience for Veterans, no matter where they find themselves. The **Diffusion of Excellence** team has built the framework that leverages our health care system's significant scope and scale to deliver positive outcomes to Veterans across the United States. Diffusion of Excellence begins, of course, with great innovations. The process then advances innovations to implementation.

And only after careful analysis and testing, the Diffusion process defines pathways to standardization. By way of the Diffusion of Excellence Initiative process, dedicated frontline employees are shaping health care delivery in positive ways that reach far beyond their own local facilities.

The Diffusion of Excellence Initiative plays a critical role in the Innovation Ecosystem by identifying, prioritizing, and disseminating top innovations and best practices across VHA. The Diffusion of Excellence Initiative governs without bureaucratic hurdles and allows deployment of resources to the front lines in locations where they are needed the most. Here's how it works. With support from the VA Innovators Network, frontline employees working with Veterans and other stakeholders are co-designing innovative new practices and pilot programs that rapidly respond to Veterans' needs. The Diffusion Hub, our technology platform, promotes national-level oversight and transparency and helps frontline employees as they begin implementation. Then, the Diffusion of Excellence Initiative packages successful innovation pilots as best practices, prototypes that can be replicated across the health care system—it gets best practices to rise to the top, and then spread. In 2016 alone, this model generated over 380 innovations across 100 facilities, including over 80 completed replications of 13 Under Secretary for Health (USH) Gold Status Best Practices (described in full below).

The Diffusion of Excellence Initiative is a permanent and sustainable process that not only allows us, but also encourages us to continually innovate, identify, and diffuse best practices across the system so we can provide consistent, seamless care experience at any VA facility across the country and change Veterans lives for the better.

Changing Veterans Lives

In just the few sites where some best practice innovations originated, the results have been impressive. For instance, Mr. Scott Bryant of Chillicothe, OH, is implementing a bike-sharing program that helps Veterans and employees quickly commute across the large Chillicothe campus. While the program facilitates travel across campus, the real goal of the program is to help support Veterans in vocational rehabilitation, provide an opportunity for Veterans to learn an employable skill, and start their own businesses. Through a partnership with the Small Business Administration (SBA), this bike-sharing program is giving Veterans entrepreneurial experience. Mr. Bryant completed most of his program as an Innovation Specialist within the Innovators Network. There is great potential to provide better health care to many more Veterans when best practices are scaled across the system. For example, if CPSs direct patient care is instituted nationally, this practice alone could free up two million primary care appointments each year.

VA also learns from the best academic and private sector medical centers. To that end, VA is partnering with the American College of Physicians (ACP) to exchange ideas. ACP will appoint clinicians and systems improvement experts to a Diffusion External Advisory Board, consisting also of Veterans and Veterans Service Organization (VSO) representatives. Likewise, VA Innovators looking to improve the VA health care system for Veterans will serve on regional advisory panels to guide ACP best practice infrastructure. This exchange is designed to diffuse VA best practices into the private sector and to enable VA to learn what some of the highest-performing and most prestigious institutions are doing to address their emerging operational challenges in health care.

VA's partnership with the YMCA is another example of how VA is learning from the private sector. Thanks to a YMCA and VHA Office of Community Engagement Memorandum of Understanding, VA facility staff are partnering with local YMCAs to expand and enhance services for Veterans in their communities. These services include wellness and fitness programs, sports, recreation, and other activities that respond to Veterans' holistic needs. In less than a year, 36 facilities have developed or are in the process of developing these kinds of local partnerships. Other partnerships are being fostered to achieve the same objectives: educate private sector medicine about VA best practices and learn best practices that will improve our performance in VA from American medicine.

No matter the source of the innovations, VA's **Diffusion of Excellence Initiative** is about identifying, selecting, and diffusing the best practices that change Veterans' lives.

5-Step Process for Identifying and Diffusing Best Practices

VHA has achieved success in implementing this model by leveraging three principles: **Process** (a consistent framework for evaluation and reapplication of practices, with clearly defined roles); **Governance** (vertical accountability to agency priorities, with regular engagement to achieve consistency and sustainment of high performance); and **Technology** (enables rapid, transparent information flow across organizational boundaries and regions). These three foundational principles inform five steps to achieving a high performance, learning health system.

Here's the five-step process we developed and some explanation of how we're leveraging these five steps to drive organizational improvement, enabling VHA to serve Veterans better.

Step 1: Identify Promising Practices

We sought to identify promising practices by launching a national solicitation through an internal social media platform. This solicitation initially attracted over 250 submissions from frontline employees, employees who changed their own local environments to improve Veteran care. Selection criteria for promising practices included 1) sustained high performance or improvement along strategic priorities, 2) efficient resource utilization, 3) applicability to different care environments, and 4) a 6–12-month implementation timeline.

Subject matter experts and senior leaders, as well as other frontline employee stakeholders across the system, reviewed the submissions to assess feasibility for wide application. The selection process leveraged both technology and effective governance: evaluations occurred at every level of the organization, but in a structured way.

To assure both alignment with leadership priorities and value assessment at the point of care when identifying the 13 USH Gold Status Best Practices that would be diffused across the health care system, three groups shared an equal stake in the selection: a frontline provider **community of practice**, a **Governance Board** of senior VHA leaders, and a group of mid-level managers and subject matter experts called a **Diffusion Council**. The Diffusion Council is composed of different operating units that span from central program offices to local leadership. The Council recommends to the Governance Board any necessary policy changes or resource allocations that would facilitate USH Gold Status Best Practice implementation. This structure provides ongoing operational support to Action Teams, but also accountability for progress at each level.

The Integrated Operations Platform (IOP), an online tool, allowed both innovators and local implementing champions to conduct lean implementation against milestones useful for local project execution. The IOP also serves as a knowledge hub that is searchable by any employee in the system. This kind of access allows champions to find projects that have worked at other sites of care for similar challenges they may be experiencing. In addition, milestone registration generates structured data that allows the Diffusion Council and Governance Board to track progress (or lack thereof) when data is aggregated for national review. Systemic barriers are therefore identified and addressed proactively with resources or policy changes. We used the same internal social media platform to quickly collect data from hundreds of employee evaluators. Today, every regional service network uses similar criteria to identify promising practices in their own forums.

Step 2: Find the Champions

Local champions, or "early adopters," are crucial for frontline implementation of best practices. VHA held a competition to identify locations where USH Gold Status Best Practices would initially be replicated. Nineteen innovators pitched best practices to 28 VAMC directors, and the directors bid resources—including employee time, space, and funding—required for implementation. Most importantly, directors had to identify a champion at their facility to own the initial phase of implementation. This approach solidified leadership commitment at field sites, ensuring alignment to local priorities and the resources necessary to inculcate the practice. Because participating facilities spanned the entire Nation, the competition was virtual, which enabled efficient information transfer and communication at no cost. As previously noted, 13 of 19 finalists were selected as USH Gold Status Best Practices based on bids from the VAMC directors and national leadership endorsement.

Step 3: Adapt and Replicate

Before national deployment, the Diffusion model calls for "Phase 1" implementation of each practice in at least one other location. That way, we can identify implementation challenges in different contexts. To achieve this end, we brought local implementing champions together with innovators (who initially developed the practices) for an in-person summit of intensive project planning. The two-day session promoted rapid-fire planning that minimized staff's time away from clinics. Along with a Lean-trained project manager, these implementing champions and innovators constituted Action Teams who conference regularly and track implementation. Four Action Teams defined by strategic priority (access, care coordination, quality and safety, and employee engagement) report to the Diffusion Council, the operational governance body.

Step 4: Establish Consistency and Standardize

After successful initial replication, certain USH Gold Status Best Practices were chosen for national standardization based on two criteria: 1) relative success with initial implementation and, 2) similar outcomes achieved when replicated in a reasonable timeframe. Within just five months of identification as a Gold Status Best Practice, 12 of 13 practices have been replicated at more than 14 sites (and the 13th site is in process).

With this success, Action Teams have begun developing national rollout plans for several of the practices that leverage shared resources (e.g., central IT servers for applications) and system-wide channels of communication (e.g., national communities of practice for clinicians or social workers). Because the Diffusion Council is composed of representatives from many program offices, national rollout can be supported for most practices.

To enable operationally consistent execution, champions must be identified in both regional service networks and individual facilities to ensure consistency. These champions use roadmaps generated by the Action Teams during the first phase of implementation. Standardization is measured by the consistency of Veteran or employee outcomes rather than strict adherence to a defined process. In this way, facility and network champions can apply human-centered design and tailor practices to local requirements.

Finally, because the IOP cumulatively records every facility's experience with implementation and barriers, data about system-wide resource requirements allow the Governance Board to make targeted investments accordingly.

Step 5: Sustain and Improve

Even before a best practice is scaled nationally, Diffusion of Excellence engages staff, resources, and technology to ensure sustainment once the practice is scaled. "Practice-based service lines" will pair the original innovators with an appropriate, national-level executive partner for ongoing validation and monitoring. This method combines content knowledge of the practices with the operational expertise required to monitor variation or changes in performance. VISN and facility champions in every site of care will continue to monitor the sustainment of implemented practices and adapt to changing needs. To ensure sustainment, lagging indicators (outcome data) must be tied to and correlated with already-established implementation metrics in the IOP. This technique allows for proactive assessments of performance shortfalls, now incorporated into a centralized operations center that will be replicated at every level of the organization.

In addition to a diffusion process based on implementation and dissemination science best practices, a fail-safe governance process and a technology platform that promote information sharing are key to success.

Gold Status Practice Summaries

Here are some brief descriptions of the 13 Gold Status Practices, information about fellows who designed the practices, their facilities, and facilities replicating the practices.

Improving Same-Day Access Using Registered Nurse Care Manager Chair Visits.

The Boise VAMC primary care team created a process by which same-day appointment requests are triaged and scribed by RN Care Managers. This process saves PCPs' time when they see patients between appointments to assess and confirm the care plan. The originators, Dr. Henry Elzinga and Debra Hendricks Lee, a PCP and nurse duo, took this practice on the road, providing real-time coaching to their peers to support implementation. Together, these facilities serve many rural Veteran patients.

- Gold Status Fellows: Dr. Henry Elzinga and Debra Hendricks Lee, Boise VAMC (Boise, ID)
- Implementing Facilities: Central Alabama Veterans Health Care System (Montgomery, AL), Carl Vinson VAMC (Dublin, GA), Albany CBOC (Albany, GA)

Access Data Dashboard to Improve Clinic Management

VA staff remains dedicated to VA's I-CARE values, to transparency, and a to a "we can fix that" attitude. That's why the data analysis team at Harry S. Truman Memorial Veterans' Hospital implemented a dashboard for clinic access metrics (no-shows, completed appointment wait times, clinic utilization, etc.). These metrics are posted monthly on an accessible dashboard that staff can use to solve problems and make key decisions that help Veterans get timely access to care. The dashboard encourages thoughtful discussion on ways to improve measures and mutual accountability for results. For example, clinic teams use the no-show data to actively engage in preventing future no-shows. No-show rates, wait times, and other access metrics improve when staff use the dashboard. The Harry S. Truman VA team helped Kansas City VAMC design a similar dashboard, and VHA's clinical analytics and reporting team have been working closely with Truman VA's data analysis team to integrate the model into the national Health Care Operations Dashboard.

- Gold Status Fellow: Michelle Pruitt, Harry S. Truman Memorial Veterans' Hospital (Columbia, MO)

- Implementing Facility: Kansas City VAMC (Kansas City, MO)

Planning for Future Medical Decision via Group Visits

When a patient is critically ill or mentally incapacitated, it may fall on family members or even staff to make difficult, life-altering decisions on behalf of the patient. Interactive and patient-centered group visits that engage Veterans in planning for future medical decisions allow patients' wishes to be known and, when the time may come, honored while reducing unwanted treatments. Now, thanks to Dr. Kimberly Garner and a team led by Bedford VAMC social workers, Veterans are having those important discussions early. This brings Veterans, their families, and those who care for Veterans peace of mind. This team has also been working tirelessly with VHA's Social Work Office and the National Center for Ethics to develop a toolkit for implementing this smart, compassionate practice across VA.

- Gold Status Fellow: Dr. Kimberly Garner, Central Arkansas Veterans Healthcare System (Little Rock, AR)

- Implementing Facility: Edith Nourse Rogers Memorial Veterans' Hospital (Bedford, MA)

Increasing Access to Primary Care with Pharmacists

At the William S. Middleton Memorial Veterans' Hospital, CPS Dr. Ellina Seckel and her colleagues knew that VA's CPSs authorized by their scope of practice may prescribe medications and monitor patients with diabetes and other chronic diseases. They also knew that CPSs are key members of the Patient Aligned Care Team (PACT). So, Dr. Seckel and her team matched CPS with multiple PACTs to conduct New Patient Intake calls one week before new patients have their first appointment with a provider. During New Patient Intake calls, the team collects information on medications, noting any formulary conversions, and orients the patient to VA. This effort has saved providers an average of 20 minutes during initial appointments. Thanks to this process, the team was also able to convert 28 percent of appointments from the PCP to the CPS, opening up hours of access for acute care patients. The facility's true team-based care practice has shifted the chronic disease workload from the PCPs to CPSs, and the CPSs can work at the top of their scope of practice as pharmacist providers. Now, PCPs have more time to spend with patients, and Veterans can get the care they need more quickly. With the support of the Middleton VA implementing team, the El Paso VA Health Care System (HCS) has started integrating CPS into PACTs to practice true team-based care. In just four months of implementation with one CPS paired with three PACTs, El Paso VA HCS has already seen improved access to care for Veterans. Now, they are expanding the practice to include all PACTs. This true team-based practice has also received significant recognition in the private sector: Health systems in the US and the United

Kingdom are looking for opportunities to shadow and learn from the William S. Middleton Memorial Veterans' Hospital team.

- Gold Status Fellow: Dr. Ellina Seckel, William S. Middleton Memorial Veterans' Hospital (Madison, WI)
- Implementing Facility: El Paso VA Health Care System (El Paso, TX)

Unit Tracking Board

Michael Finch, a clinical nurse leader at the C.W. Bill Young VAMC saw that key clinical unit data were not being effectively presented and shared with nursing staff. So he developed a simple and accessible Unit Tracking Board to post on floor units. Now, all staff involved in care can quickly see important data about patient trends. Staff is empowered to use that information to make the best decisions that will improve Veterans' care experiences. Since the board is posted publicly, the practice also supports VA's mission to foster a culture of transparency. Michael helped a nurse-led team at the White River Junction VAMC develop a similar board for the Intensive Care Unit. All inpatient units at the facility are soon to follow. The Young VAMC team is also working with VHA's national nursing leadership to standardize a model for all medical centers.

- Gold Status Fellow: Michael Finch, C.W. Bill Young VAMC (Bay Pines, FL)
- Implementing Facility: White River Junction VAMC (White River Junction, VT)

Journey to Open Access in Primary Care

Dr. Michael Tom, Chief of Primary Care Services at the VA Central California HCS is using VA's PACT model and system redesign principles to implement new protocols that increase same-day access opportunities for Veterans. Dr. Tom has worked hand-in-hand with the team at Gulf Coast Veterans HCS, a facility with significant access to care challenges, to mentor and help with this significant advance.

- Gold Status Fellow: Dr. Michael Tom, VA Central California HCS (Fresno, CA)
- Implementing Facility: Gulf Coast Veterans HCS (Biloxi, MS)

eScreening

The eScreening Program was developed to facilitate the screening process and improve care coordination and measurement-based care for Veterans. eScreening is a mobile technology that significantly improves care coordination and business processes. eScreening offers Veteran-directed screening, real-time scoring, individualized patient feedback, instantaneous medical record clinical documentation, immediate alerts to clinicians for evaluation and triage, and treatment outcome monitoring. And it's simple. Staff hand the Veterans an iPad when they check in for an appointment. Veterans complete required screening on the iPad. The information is then transferred directly from the waiting room to the patient's medical record. The tool can be used in any clinical setting, from primary care to urgent care to mental health. This best practice has already spread to three facilities organically and to three other facilities by way of the Diffusion of Excellence Initiative. There are 40 more facilities "on deck" and ready to implement.

- Gold Status Fellows: Dr. Niloofar Afari, and Liz Floto, VA San Diego HCS (San Diego, CA)
- Implementing Facilities: Lebanon VAMC (Lebanon, PA), Ann Arbor VAMC (Ann Arbor, MI), Edith Nourse Rogers Memorial Veterans' Hospital (Bedford, MA)

Code Tray Redesign

Certified Pharmacy Technician Kristine Gherardi at VA Boston HCS noticed that the code tray was not set up in a way that made it easy to find life-saving drugs in an emergency. So she created a simple and compelling solution to reduce the time it takes to find the right drugs during a code. This easy-to-implement, low-cost strategy reduces medication distribution errors and improves outcomes for Veterans. The Loma Linda HCS is already implementing this code tray, and more facilities are following quickly.

- Gold Status Fellow: Kristine Gherardi, VA Boston HCS (Boston, MA)
- Implementing Facility: VA Loma Linda HCS (Loma Linda, CA)

Regional Liver Tumor Board

The hepatology team at the Philadelphia VAMC combined a regional telehealth-supported Liver Cancer Tumor Board model, a web-based submission process, and a consolidated database to manage and track communications for patients with liver cancer. This practice has decreased the time it takes for Veterans with liver cancer to receive evaluations and first treatments. And it has reduced unnecessary biopsies, easing patients' and their families' minds and experiences during an intensely stressful time. Jackson VAMC, a facility without a dedicated hepatologist, is now implementing the practice in partnership with the Central Arkansas VA HCS, giving Veterans faster access to top notch clinical care.

- Gold Status Fellow: Dr. David Kaplan, Corporal Michael J. Crescenz VAMC (Philadelphia, PA)
- Implementing Facility: G.V. (Sonny) Montgomery VAMC (Jackson, MS)

Using External (Non-VA) Comparative Data to Achieve Excellence and Engage Employees

To do a better job of comparing outcomes—not only against the VA average, but also against "the best"—the Mountain Home VAMC expanded non-VA benchmark data to provide indicators of how Veteran and caregiver stakeholders view VA care and services in relation to other health care choices in their region. This expanded context results in higher performance and greater employee engagement. And staff can seize opportunities to improve while also instilling pride in the fact that VA truly provides world-class care for our Nation's Veterans. Using this model, the San Francisco VA HCS is replicating the practice for its Engineering service, ensuring that top-notch support services are provided at the facility.

- Gold Status Fellow: Jill Stephens, James H. Quillen VAMC (Mountain Home, TN)
- Implementing Facility: San Francisco VA HCS (San Francisco, CA)

WAKE© Score for Recovery from Anesthesia/Sedation

The WAKE© Score replaces a previous anesthesia recovery scoring system that often left patients with nausea, vomiting, lightheadedness, and pain. The WAKE© Score takes a "zero tolerance" approach to anesthesia side effects, improving patient experience and outcomes. Developed by anesthesiologist Dr. Brian Williams, the WAKE© Score has been evaluated and the results have been published in several peer-reviewed academic journals. To improve post-surgery outcomes at the Martinsburg VAMC, the anesthesia team adapted this model. VHA surgery senior leadership is currently assessing options based on this replication and other models to determine the best standardized model that will optimize improved Veteran outcomes post-surgery.

- Gold Status Fellow: Dr. Brian Williams, VA Pittsburgh HCS (Pittsburgh, PA)
- Implementing Facility: Martinsburg VAMC (Martinsburg, WV)

Direct Scheduling for Audiology and Optometry Services

Previously, Veterans had to see their PCP to receive a referral for simple audiology and optometry services, such as new eyeglass fitting. This new model, piloted first at Bay Pines VA HCS, allows direct scheduling for certain types of appointments. This direct scheduling process eliminates redundant consultations, consolidates clinic profiles, and standardizes communications. Altogether, the process means significantly reduced wait times for Audiology and Optometry. The direct scheduling model was rolled out at several VA facilities in 2016. Today, all facilities have direct scheduling for simple audiology and optometry service. Now, VA is looking to implement a similar policy and process for other services.

- Gold Status Fellow: Michelle Menendez, Bay Pines VA HCS (Bay Pines, FL)
- Implementing Facility: All VAMCs

Flu Self-Reporting Desktop Icon to Capture Employee Vaccinations Received Outside VA

The VA Boston HCS occupational health team devised the Flu Self-Reporting Desktop Icon. Now, with the click of a button, staff can quickly report on their computer's desktop when they've received the flu vaccine outside VA. Capturing an average of 500 vaccinations annually, this simple tool not only encourages staff to take care of themselves, but also protects patient's and families' health. The Boston VA HCS team worked closely with the Mountain Home VAMC and VISN 12 teams to replicate this practice and develop a national standardized model for rolling out this best practice at every medical center. Seeing the potential, more than 40 leaders at other facilities took the initiative over the last several months to roll out this capability in their own facilities.

- Gold Status Fellow: Vanessa Coronel, VA Boston HCS (Boston, MA)
- Implementing Facility: VA Great Lakes HCS (Westchester, IL), Mountain Home VAMC (Mountain Home, TN)

Conclusion

It's difficult to exaggerate VA employees' excitement and burst of energy when they see their great ideas translated into better access and outcomes for the Veterans they proudly serve. Giving frontline employees the opportunity, resources, guidance, leadership support, and—where needed—some relief from bureaucracy so they can apply best practices is crucial for standardizing top quality health care. Success requires striking a balance that not only creates a path to standardization, but also rewards and elevates innovation at the point of care. Dr. Garner (Little Rock, AR) and Mr. Bryant (Chillicothe, OH) exemplify our health care system's Innovation Ecosystem that we're now leveraging to Veterans' advantage.

VHA's decentralized model has created fertile ground for innovation—the decentralized model is one reason VA was recently recognized as a top innovator. With VA's Innovation Ecosystem, we're transforming the way we deliver health care to Veterans. While VA historically operated as a siloed system, we are moving beyond that restrictive culture. The Diffusion of Excellence Initiative is harnessing the ingenuity of that innovative environment to deliver better and better outcomes for Veterans. And it represents a new, critical capability for VA's Innovation Ecosystem that identifies, prioritizes, and disseminates best practices across VHA. The Diffusion of Excellence Initiative will continue to play a vital role in ensuring that Veterans get the best care that the nation has to offer.

Many large health care systems face similar challenges, especially as they acquire smaller hospitals and sites of care. Yet, no operational system to our knowledge has achieved diffusion or consistency of best practices on a scale comparable to what we're seeing at VA. Moving forward, VHA will continue to refine the Diffusion model to meet VHA needs while encouraging innovation and best practice development to meet both the constant and emerging needs of Veterans across the nation. In the meantime, we will continue to empower our frontline employees so they can improve the experiences of countless more Veterans than they otherwise might.

The Diffusion of Excellence Initiative will benefit not only millions of Veterans across the nation, but also patients of any health care system facing similar challenges in providing consistent care.

PATIENT EXPERIENCE

Mobile Veterans Program:
Aging as an Amazing Process

Karen Elechko, MSN, RN, Golden Memory Clinic Coordinator

Coatesville VA Medical Center, Coatesville, PA

karen.elechko@va.gov

The VA Mobile Veteran Program (MVP) is a partnership and collaborative effort between VAMCs and local Veteran Service Organizations (VSOs). The MVP dispatches a health care team to a local VSO site to provide support services to Veterans. This care-based mobile health strategy reduces barriers to access, allowing Veterans to benefit from structured, high-quality care at a local site closer to their home.

Introduction

A 65-year-old Vietnam Veteran, with a history of numerous medical problems, including two suicide attempts, was referred to the VA Mobile Veteran Program (MVP) by his VA PCP through his Mental Health Intensive Care Manager. The Veteran, who lives by himself, spent a day observing the Program and was then asked about his satisfaction. The Veteran shared, "A few months ago, I had plans. The plans failed. I'm very happy I failed in my plans because I now have a meaning for living. Yes, I love the Program and will return." Since enrollment, the Veteran has been more motivated and socially active. One month after he entered the Program, one of his friends committed suicide. The MVP team and participating Veterans offered him comfort and support. Since these interventions, the Veteran reports that he feels supported by the program, enjoys the camaraderie of other enrolled Veterans, and no longer has suicidal thoughts.

The preliminary impact of this program includes increased Veteran and caregiver satisfaction, decreased caregiver burden and stress, prevention or delay of institutionalized care, improved function and cognition, and suicide prevention.

The Coatesville VA MVP achieved the distinction of a Joint Commission Leading Practice, has been nominated for the Rosalinde Gilbert Innovations in Alzheimer's Disease Caregiving Legacy Award and the Hearst Health Prize for Excellence in Population Health. It also received Honorable Mention from VHA's Pulse Promising Practice Consortium.

Key Information

VA MVP is an innovative patient-centered program that was first implemented at the Canandaigua VAMC in Canandaigua, NY, through the New Models of Care Transformation to the 21st Century Non-Institutional Long-Term Care (T21 NILTC) sub-initiative. Mobile Adult Day Health Care (ADHC) brings VA care providers to Veteran Service Organizations (VSO) sites to offer ADHC closer to Veterans' homes. This program received the 2011 New York Organization of Nurse Executives Best Practice Award. Through expansion of T21 NILTC, the Coatesville VAMC in Coatesville, PA, implemented MVP in FY 2014. Coatesville VAMC sent a team of VA care clinicians to eight local American Legion and Veteran of Foreign War sites. This cost-effective and self-sustaining approach allows elderly and injured Veterans to benefit from structured care in an informal environment. This community-care-based mobile health strategy reduces distance barriers, improves access to and compliance with care, and provides support as well as respite care to family caregivers. The program empowers Veterans to remain independent and home-based, increases their quality of life, and helps them stay where they want to be, happily living in their homes.

Context

Coatesville VAMC is a Joint Commission-accredited complexity level 3 facility that serves Veterans in Pennsylvania, Delaware, and Maryland. Coatesville VAMC is located in Coatesville, PA, with outpatient clinics located in Springfield and Spring City, PA. Coatesville VAMC is an integrated health care system that provides high-quality care and service to Veterans. The 42-building facility, which sits on 128 acres, celebrated its 85th anniversary in November 2014. The medical center served 19,477 Veterans and completed 222,871 outpatient visits in FY 2014. The VA MVP assists Veterans transitioning into the community and prevents institutionalization.

Practice Description

Operating as a partnership, VA MVP is a collaborative effort between VAMCs and local VSOs. The program opens access to care by providing services in the community near the Veterans' home. This partnership strengthens the pledges between VA and VSOs to support and advocate for Veterans' health and well-being.

The VSO host provides a safe environment, with safety surveys performed by the VAMC. VA sends a team of health care professionals to the VSO site to provide an array of meaningful activities and supportive services designed to help with physical, social, and cognitive functioning. Examples include therapeutic exercise, memory-focused brain exercises, current event discussions, nail care, hand hygiene, music, art, trivia, social time, and other leisure activities. VA and VSO sites also provide a nutritious lunch to participating Veterans.

Replicability

The practice was adopted at the Coatesville VAMC in anticipation of offering a new option for VA care and services through partnership in the community. Effective communication with leadership, VSO groups, providers, and other services was an essential factor for success. Expanding this program to other VAMCs would be of tremendous benefit as a growing population of aging Veterans enter the system.

The impact of the VA MVP includes:

- Increased access to care
  - Brings care to the Veteran, thereby reducing distance barriers
- Increased Veteran and caregiver satisfaction
  - Satisfaction with services reported as very good to outstanding
  - Reduction of perceived caregiving burden, as measured by reductions of scores on the Zarit Caregiving Burden Inventory
  - Improvement of Veterans' cognition as perceived by caregivers
- Increased quality of care

- – Promotes high-quality, Veteran-centered care
- – Veterans' and primary caregivers' likes and dislikes of meaningful activities captured through a survey; the information is incorporated in the plan through structured activities for each Veteran
- Lower cost of care
  - – Increases the delivery of Long-Term Services and Supports (LTSS) in the community, reducing preventable hospital and nursing home stays

Recognition

Nina Mottern, Mandy Tramell, Lyn Ordonez, Nancy Schmidt, Karen Massey, Susan Lanen, Kenneth Shay, Richard Allman

Promoting Proactive Use of Secure Messaging Using Promising Practices

Jolie Haun PhD, EdS, Margeaux Chavez, MA, MPH; Wendy Hathaway, MA; Nicole Antinori, MBA; Brian Vetter, RD; Brian Miller, BA; Tracey Martin, RN, MSN; Terri Ruggerie; Lisa Kendziora; Kim Nazi, PhD

James A. Haley Veterans' Hospital, Tampa, FL
jolie.haun@va.gov

This collaborative project demonstrates opportunities and best practices in the use of secure messaging as an efficient method of providing clinical care to Veterans to improve access and workflow.

Introduction

Secure messaging, an asynchronous communication tool within My Health*e*Vet, provides an easy, convenient, and secure way for VA patients to communicate electronically with their VA health care teams. Secure messaging is a national transformation initiative and an integral part of VA's Blueprint for Excellence. It promotes new models of care in support of enhanced patient-provider communication. Electronic communication, such as secure messaging, is an effective tool for supporting increased access, patient engagement, self-management, and efficient utilization of health services and resources. For example, a systematic literature review conducted within VA suggests that the use of secure messaging improves glucose outcomes and increases patient satisfaction. The objective of this field-initiated collaborative was to improve integration of My Health*e*Vet secure messaging into the fabric of VA health care. The project aimed to do this by soliciting and disseminating opportunities and local best practices in the use of secure messaging as an efficient method of providing clinical care to Veterans to improve access and enhance workflow. This objective was assessed through a field-based national questionnaire that asked, "Please explain how you are using secure messaging to improve communication, efficiency, patient access, or workflow in your practice."

Key Information

My Health*e*Vet representatives implemented a simple questionnaire to collect best practices from clinical care teams throughout VA. A total of 171 entries were collected from nursing staff (n=55), providers (n=37), behavioral health (n=4), My Health*e*Vet Coordinators (n=3), and other care team members (n=72), representing PC (n=85), Specialty Care (n=61), Behavioral Health (n=16), Health Promotion and Disease Prevention (n=6), and Women's Health (n=3) across 15 VISNs within VA.

Context

The use of secure messaging supports increased access to care, enhanced patient-provider communication, efficient utilization of services, and improved patient outcomes. VA clinical team members in facilities across the nation are working to integrate secure messaging into care delivery and identify innovative uses. The proactive use of secure messaging is a key factor in its successful implementation and sustained use by VA care team members and Veterans.

Practice Description

Providers can use secure messaging to create an integrated culture. Facilities have created such by integrating it into clinical practice and service provision; before, at, and after the point of care. Establishing this culture enhances provider buy-in, utilization, and promotion. Secure messaging transcends the traditional brick and mortar clinical setting because it is available 24/7, from any location. Clinical team members create a culture of secure messaging by:

- Regularly educating staff and patients about the tool
- Integrating it within the enrollment process
- Integrating it into daily practice
- Endorsing proactive use
- Acknowledging that it crosses all VA services
- Integrating it into providers' workflow
- Managing population health and reaching patients broadly to alert them to seasonal health promotion activities, such as flu shots and wellness efforts

Replicability

The proper use of secure messaging can improve Veteran care and clinical team workflow and support the efficient use of VA's health resources. However, knowing how to effectively use the tool is a key factor in its usefulness. Clinical team members across the nation who are invested in the successful implementation of this tool have learned to integrate it into their daily practice to provide Veteran-centered care and improve workflow. With adequate knowledge and motivation, efforts to use secure messaging can be replicated by all VA clinical team members within the VA system.

Recognition

Brian Vetter, Brian Miller, Tracey Martin, Terri Ruggerie, Lisa Kendziora, Kim Nazi, Center of Innovation on Disability and Rehabilitation Research

Annie: Piloting Automated Texting to Promote Self-Care

Susan Woods, MD, Director of Patient Experience
VACO, Washington, DC
susan.woods@va.gov

The Annie App (Annie), an innovative automated texting mobile application that promotes patient self-care, is being piloted at four VA locations.

Introduction

In February 2016, Dr. Lynn Kataria, Chief of Neurology Education at the Washington, DC, VAMC enrolled the first VA patient in "Annie," VA's new mobile messaging system that promotes Veteran self-care.

With Annie, VA care teams can set protocols that send scheduled, automated reminders to their patients to do things like check their blood pressure, or remember to take their medication. Dr. Kataria is using Annie as part of a randomized single-blind trial research study on improving outcomes for Traumatic Brain Injury (TBI) and Obstructive Sleep Apnea (OSA) patients by helping them improve their use of Continuous Positive Airway Pressure (CPAP) machines.

Memory problems, which can lead to poor compliance with medication and treatment protocols, are a significant challenge for patients with co-morbid TBI and OSA. Dr. Kataria describes the ability of her patients to get regular text message reminders to wear their CPAP machine as a "game changer," and the system overall as something that makes them feel connected with their health. "It was powerful," she says, "When they got that first text message after pressing 'Start' they felt they were part of something bigger."

Though Dr. Kataria's study is still underway, very early on she began to see promising results in treatment adherence among study participants. She is looking forward to fully implementing Annie in her own practice, and also sees it as important for other disciplines. She is optimistic about how it allows for ongoing, regular tracking of health data to enable Veterans and their care teams to see how different issues connect and more easily identify patterns. "[Annie] allows us to reach our patients in ways we couldn't previously," she says. "All providers should use this. It can have an impact on the way we practice and ultimately we're going to see our outcomes improved."

Key Information

Annie was developed by VA's Office of Connected Care, which brings together digital health technologies from across VA, in partnership with the National Health Service (NHS) England. It is based on Simple Telehealth, more commonly called "Flo," a technology that has been used successfully by NHS England for several years. Phil O'Connell, the developer of Flo, describes it as "a health care system that comes to patients on their terms," giving them a clearer picture of their day-to-day health and empowering them to take control of their own care.

Flo, named for Florence Nightingale, was originally piloted with a limited patient population with Chronic Obstructive Pulmonary Disease (COPD) and heart failure. Flo now reaches over 35,000 patients across the United Kingdom with a wide variety of health issues and needs, including diabetes, pregnancy, mental health and more. It has proven successful in helping patients adhere to medications and treatment plans. Through Flo, NHS England has found that boosting patient self-management yields significant improvement in patient satisfaction and control over chronic conditions.

Like Flo, Annie is designed to help patients establish and stick to a personalized care plan. VA hopes to make Annie available to Veterans across the country this year, and anticipates that it will increase both patient autonomy and satisfaction.

Context

One marker of Flo's success has been the ability of clinicians to innovate—they see a problem in their practice and adapt Flo to meet that need. The goal of Annie is to serve the same purpose, meeting both clinicians and patients where they are, and giving them a holistic view of a patient's health over time.

In its first iteration, Annie was designed with protocols to help Veterans track blood pressure, pulse oximetry, blood glucose, weight loss, calories, and exercise. However, as with Dr. Kataria's study, that is already being expanded to reach other patient populations. Annie is a flexible and versatile system that can help patients with a wide range of health concerns.

Veterans can receive text messages from Annie on either a smartphone or a basic cell phone, making it an ideal system to reach elderly Veterans or those without access to a smartphone. Because it facilitates the collection and transmission of data, VA also anticipates that Annie will be particularly helpful for rural Veterans and others who, because of distance or mobility concerns, may not easily be able to come into a clinic or VAMC.

Practice Description

Annie works like this: Veterans works with their VA care team to establish a personalized care plan to help them track their own health data and meet health goals. The Veterans' doctor enters protocols into Annie that determine what information Veterans should be tracking, such as blood pressure or glucose readings. VA care teams are able to view the information their patients submit on an as-needed basis.

Annie texts patients on a regular schedule to ask them to report their readings, and lets them know right away if something is wrong. Annie can also send medication and appointment reminders and educational and motivational messages to help patients manage their care or learn more about their health. In addition to being able to receive text messages through any phone with a texting plan, Veteran users also have access to a smartphone app, computer, or any device with an Internet connection, allowing them to see their data over time, graph their readings, and track their information.

Replicability

Research has demonstrated the potential for text messaging to increase access to health care, enhance the delivery of health care services, and improve patient attitudes and behaviors. Evidence supports texting to improve attendance at appointments, promote quitting smoking, improve medication adherence for chronic conditions, and increase self-efficacy for some conditions. For NHS England, Flo has been a success because of the way it has been seamlessly integrated into existing patient care. Most patients who use Flo were already tasked with tracking certain information and reporting it back to their care team. Flo gives them a simpler way to do that, as well as creating a clear record and repository of their readings over time, helping them better understand what their readings mean, and identifying if there may be an issue with their health. Care teams were allowed flexibility to create the protocols they needed and use the system in the best way for their patients and their individual facility, which turned Flo into an extension of the existing care team and allowed all parties to access the health information they needed at a glance and incorporate it into overall care.

As is the case with Flo, VA does not expect that VA care teams will regularly monitor the data patients send to Annie. Rather, Annie gives patients a clear way to see their information, and helps them identify problems so they can contact their care teams if necessary. This helps to streamline provider workflow by only alerting them to issues that need their attention, and helps put Veterans in the driver's seat of their own care, increasing their autonomy, confidence, and control over their own health.

Recognition

Annie Fox, Neil Evans, Kathy Frisbee, Sue Woods, Ralph Strenglein, Beth Powell, Mary Lou Glazer, Erica Bilek, Carly Noreen, Phil O'Connell

Shared Decision Making for Aging Veterans

Sheri Reder, PhD, MSPH, Director, Shared Decision Making

VA Puget Sound Health Care System, Seattle, WA
sheri.reder@va.gov

Shared Decision Making (SDM) for aging Veterans is a national implementation project designed to encourage our Veterans to make patient-directed decisions that are in alignment with their goals, priorities and needs, and support independence as they age.

Introduction

Korean War Veteran Bob researched SDM online: "From the Geriatrics and Extended Care (GEC) website, I learned about long-term care options that might work for me both in my home and in my community near Tacoma, WA. I especially liked the section on Shared Decision Making. I printed off the Worksheet for Veterans and filled it out. I'm old enough to know what I want, but the Worksheet prompted me to consider a few things I hadn't thought about. My wife, Mary, filled out the Caregiver Self-Assessment. We know our situation could change based on my health or hers. But, I've watched what's happened with my friends and neighbors—heart failure, falls, all kinds of cancer and Parkinson's. I may not be able to avoid a health crisis, but I can avoid planning on the fly in the midst of a crisis. I want to stay in my own home, if at all possible, and I want to be prepared for the future."

Vietnam Veteran Larry lived in Salem, OR and often traveled to the Portland VAMC to receive care for his diabetes, vascular degeneration, neuropathy, and a few other ailments. Before his liver cancer diagnosis, he was featured in a VHA online article: "I went to VA's website, www.va.gov/geriatrics, to check out my options for long-term services and support. Nobody is ever ready to deal with this stuff, but the doctors have told me what I'll likely have to deal with. I know VA can provide palliative care, which is what I want to help deal with my symptoms and whatever it can do for my quality of life. I liked having a say in choosing where I wanted to be and what services I could get as my cancer gets worse."

Key Information

SDM is a patient-directed process for preference-sensitive choices, such as Long-Term Services and Supports (LTSS). SDM supports the Veteran, and their family/caregiver, in: 1) clarifying their goals and preferences; 2) participating in collaborative discussions with providers, social workers, and others; and 3) making a Veteran-directed choice. We have focused on SDM for aging Veterans because those 65+ years of age represent 46 percent of Veterans and are the fastest growing cohort we serve. Of note, two-thirds of people in this age group require LTSS at some point in time.

Successful implementation of SDM for aging Veterans supports them at the highest level of independence by encouraging exploration of home and community-based care options that address their health conditions, values and preferences, as well as the needs and level of support available from their family/caregiver(s). SDM, by definition, can help VHA achieve collaborative, patient-directed care.

Implementation of the project for aging Veterans was started in FY 2013 with T21 Non-Institutional Long-Term Care (NILTC) funding. Since that time, this work has also received funding from the ORH and the Office of Patient Centered Care and Cultural Transformation. In addition, it has been supported by close collaborations with many offices, including Care Management and Social Work Services and the National Ethics Office. The project was initially activated in a few sites, primarily in VISN 20, and has expanded to include most PACT, Geriatric Patient Aligned Care Team (GeriPACT), and Home Based Primary Care (HBPC) sites in VISN 9, and the Houston VAMC and its CBOCs in VISN 16. It is now expanding to include many rural CBOCs and PACT teams, funded by ORH-Social Work, around the country.

Context

Research on older people has documented preferences, gaps, and needs that are similar for aging Veterans and that can be addressed by SDM:

- Older people and their families lack information about LTSS, especially home and community-based services, and are not planning for long-term care needs.

- People prefer to remain in their own home, living as independently as possible.

- People want to be asked their preferences. Discussions are as important as goals, and priorities may change.

- While research has documented the effectiveness of decision aids in general, there is a need for decision aids and SDM processes specific to aging Veterans.

The Guide to LTSS, a core component of the Geriatrics and Extended Care (GEC) website, www.va.gov/geriatrics, was developed to provide information, and the SDM process, including the decision aids, were developed to facilitate Veteran-directed decision making about LTSS.

Practice Description

Implementation of SDM for aging Veterans requires an educational and ecological approach to behavior change. Our implementation includes:

- Orientation and training for providers/administrators: a 45-minute orientation/training for all staff of a participating clinic; and a 1.5-hour follow-up training for those most involved in facilitating SDM discussions (social workers).

- Information and tools for Veterans and family caregivers: the GEC website provides comprehensive information on LTSS and other preference-sensitive decisions (e.g., advance care planning); decision aids, including a Veteran and caregiver SDM worksheet; and hard copy folders that include complete LTSS information and decision-making tools.

- Policy and program changes: collaboration and dissemination of programs and policies that address provider/administrator concerns, such as using electronic wait lists to advocate for needed services, and ensuring that community-based as well as VA services are used to address Veterans' LTSS needs.

This SDM work is led by a small group located at VA Puget Sound, which includes a national SDM project director, health educator, evaluation consultant, and support staff. The project team also includes a webmaster for the GEC website, and field coordinators at Houston, TX, and Louisville, KY.

Of great importance, we work closely with VACO leadership, particularly Geriatrics and Extended Care, Care Management and Social Work Services, the National Ethics Office, and Rural Health.

Replicability

Conducting quality improvement assessments with Veterans, caregivers, leadership, and staff is an ongoing piece of the implementation of SDM for aging Veterans. From these assessments we continually enhance our understanding of what works most effectively. The practice description above indicates many of the factors that we have found most important for successful SDM implementation. They include:

- Quality, comprehensive information for Veterans, caregivers, and staff
- A process for making Veteran-directed, collaborative decisions
- Orientation for the entire clinic/program team, including management
- Training for those most involved with facilitating SDM discussions
- Addressing policy and program barriers to service availability
- Leadership support for implementation of SDM

The SDM project now has the above components in place, and is moving forward with ways to deliver them to a national audience. For example, we are planning to increase the number of trainers available for SDM orientation and training, and to make SDM orientation available online. We are also exploring avenues for making the hardcopy SDM materials easily replicable by clinic/program sites. We are also integrating SDM into programs, such as transitional care planning.

Recognition

Richard Allman, Kenneth Shay, Laura Taylor

Home Coaching Program

Jason Wilcox, Health Behavior Coordinator

VA Roseburg Healthcare System, Roseburg, OR

jason.wilcox2@va.gov

The Home Coaching Program is an interactive and patient-centered approach for bringing patient education to Veterans when and where they want it. The Program helps Veterans with chronic disease management, pain management, or weight management.

Introduction

The Home Coaching Program (HCP) was originally developed in VA Montana, where Helen Williams and Jason Wilcox felt there was a need to increase access to chronic disease programs. The aim was to develop a library of coaching programs that Veterans are able to use in their own home and at their own convenience. They were being developed for uses like chronic pain self-management, weight management, and chronic disease self-management.

Key Information

Home Coaching Programs are chronic disease management classes put into DVD format and combined with a workbook for at-home adult learning. The suggested way to implement the program is to have follow-up health coaching in between each class.

At Veterans' requests, a hypertension class was redesigned for video and workbook format. This Project (2014–2015) included the education department, ambulatory care teams, nutrition, physical therapy, and pharmacy. Over 200 Veterans participated. The program resulted in behavior changes, lowered blood pressure, and rapidly expanded to include Type 2 Diabetes and Congestive Heart Failure (CHF) home videos.

Context

Montana has one of the largest per-capita Veteran populations. The VA Montana Health Care System provides a VA presence in every major city in the state through a series of CBOCs, a Community Living Center, and an acute care medical center.

The VA Roseburg Healthcare System (VARHS) consists of one VHA facility located in Roseburg, OR, and three CBOCs. VARHS offers PC and hospital services in medicine, surgery, and mental health for the 62,000 Veterans who reside in central and southern Oregon and northern California.

Practice Description

In the first hypertension pilot, 90 percent of the Veterans brought their hypertension to normal levels. The Veterans and staff reported they really enjoyed using the program. One Veteran reported he was mildly cautious, feeling he already knew about hypertension, but reported back after watching that he really enjoyed the DVD classes and learned a lot from them.

Jason Wilcox moved to Roseburg VAMC in 2014 and through a rural grant purchased the equipment to replicate the program and continue making a library of various topics for PACT teams. The library impacts access to care for rural Veterans, Veterans without Internet access, those who live a significant distance from the facility or CBOCs, or Veterans who work during the day. This library creates access so that Veterans can improve their chronic disease management, chronic pain management, or weight management. After receiving the equipment in Roseburg, Jason worked with his prevention and wellness team to select a program for the first video series. Finally, they decided to make a weight management HCP based off the MOVE! curriculum.

Presently, the Prevention and Wellness program at Roseburg VA is in the pre-production phase of making the latest HCP with support and guidance from the National Center for Health Promotion and Disease Prevention. The steps we have taken and will take to produce the program start with:

1. Buying or having the equipment
2. Developing the content and the scripts
3. Filming the content
4. Editing the content
5. Developing the workbook
6. Creating the DVD
7. Marketing and producing the workbook with DVD
8. Working with Veterans over the phone after they watch a class each week

Replicability

In Montana, many Veterans are spread across the state in rural areas. It was difficult for many rural Veterans to drive far distances for weekly group medical appointments. We surveyed Veterans before we started the Hypertension HCP, and 95 percent of the Veterans were interested. With program funding, we purchased the equipment and organized a team to film and develop the classes. Other facilities may have a difficult time producing films unless they have a medical media department. However, if the program is adopted for use at all facilities, it would be easy to adopt.

Recognition

Hellen Williams, NCP Office, James Hay, James Johansen, Fletcher Watson, Jessica Kovarik, Kayla Allen

Integrative Medicine Patient Aligned Care Team for Pain

Henri Roca, MD, Chief, Integrative Medicine, Program Director, IMPACT; Matthew Jennings, MD, ACOS PC; Wendy Parent, RN, BFA; Brooke Giaccio, RD Functional Nutrition; Ken Mayo, RN, BFA; Catherine Hampton, LPN; Mira Lelovic, PT, RYT; Mark Heiland, Clinical Psychologist; Thomas Webb, Clinical Pharmacist; Cecil DuPriest, DC; Trina Gantt, MSA

Eugene J. Towbin Healthcare Center, Little Rock, AR
henri.roca@va.gov

This personalized, patient-centered pathway supports self-care behaviors in an interdisciplinary primary care setting for pain patients. The team coaches Veterans in enhancing wellness behaviors, reversing chronic disease, and engaging in life using and reinforcing integrated Personalized Health Plans.

Introduction

The Integrative Medicine Patient Aligned Care Team (IMPACT) for Pain was designed to help Central Arkansas Veterans Healthcare System (CAVHS) support Veterans as they work to live more effective and fulfilling lives with chronic pain. IMPACT is a hybrid service combining both PACT concepts and pain rehabilitation concepts. Our results to date indicate that Veterans have become more active in their own self-care practices. Veterans attend an introductory class and then choose among a series of five foundational life skills classes. Veterans who are "stuck," engaged but not improving, receive more intensive support and services. IMPACT serves Veterans from every CBOC region as well as all of central Arkansas. While within IMPACT, the team takes over PC responsibilities for the Veterans and may order, adjust, coordinate, and plan any or all aspects of care. We do this because "pain" cannot be separated from any other disease process or mental health state experienced by the Veteran.

IMPACT's practice of medicine is done exclusively from a Health Coaching perspective utilizing the Personal Health Inventory and Personalized Health Planning process. We work to have Veterans create their own path forward with support and guidance from the team. Our focus is not on numbers (labs, radiology); rather, we focus on the quality of life of each individual Veteran. Our care is highly personalized and patient-centered, and it is also highly proactive and preventive. We utilize Functional Medicine as the medical construct that informs our treatment plans. This medical perspective includes taking a thorough history over the course of the person's entire life, including family history, uterine history, early life history, and adult history. The symptoms noticed in the individual represent the sum total of exposures and interactions between a person's environment and their genes. Utilizing Functional Medicine, we work to unwind and untangle the complexities involved in pain. By working to determine all the potential triggers, drivers, and mediators of pain, we change the conversation with the Veteran and allow them to see additional pathways through their symptoms to a more fulfilling life. Functional Medicine also informs our approach to nutrition. In IMPACT, nutrition is more than just the energy required to live; it provides information that turns healing genes on and illness-producing genes off.

Veterans who participate in IMPACT assess that:

- When all is said and done, I am the person who is responsible for managing my health care: 95 percent.

- Taking an active role in my health care is the most important factor in determining my health and ability to function: 97 percent.

- I am confident that I can take actions that will help prevent or decrease some problems associated with my health condition: 91 percent.

- I am confident that I can maintain lifestyle changes like diet and exercise even during times of stress: 83 percent.

Veterans within IMPACT commonly volunteer to wean themselves off their narcotic medications. A Veteran arrived to IMPACT threatening to commit suicide if his methadone was not refilled. After an initial visit, the Veteran was provided steps to improve his nutrition, stretch his body, and shown effective ways to address stress management, and acting out behaviors, as well as steps to improve his relationship. Returning one month later, the Veteran reported he felt happy, had no suicidal intention, and had voluntarily weaned himself off methadone after many years of use. These stories are common—significant weight loss without dieting, improvement in flexibility and pain through stretching, improvements in sleep and mood, reduction of medication burden, and re-engagement in life.

IMPACT has been so successful that administration granted approval for expansion to a whole wing of our hospital. Three other PACT teams have been trained toward this type of care.

Key Information

IMPACT began as a single PACT Team within PC designed to help Veterans successfully live with pain. Our partners included Food and Nutrition services that provided our RN. Later, Physical Medicine and Rehabilitation provided our physical therapist/yoga teacher; Mental Health provided our health behavior psychologist and Pharmacy provided our clinical pharmacist. With the advent of our Integrative Medicine and Wellness Center (IMWC), the three trained PACT Teams will join us. Funding has come from CAVHS operating budget. A small amount of funding originated from the ORH early in the process.

Our IMWC is equipped with a training room designed to educate IMPACT teams from other facilities. During such training, teams will be able to shadow providers and learn the nuts and bolts of how IMPACT works and how Functional Medicine can be implemented.

Context

Pain is a multi-modal illness with many drivers and mediators. Rarely is pain a single entity and rarely does an MRI or other radiologic finding explain the preponderance of symptoms. Combined with the fact that the primary treatment option has been narcotics for all and every type of pain, Veterans often found themselves stuck in pain and addicted to pain medications. Among other drivers of pain are insomnia, diabetes, nutritional deficiencies, alcohol consumption, smoking, PTSD, hormone deficiencies, and inflammation. Lifestyle factors, such as obesity, a sedentary lifestyle, stress, poor coping skills, and anger also contribute to pain. Support of healthy lifestyle skills helps to unwind and resolve pain. Such information must be presented in a way Veterans can easily grasp, because behavior change is difficult and requires support to achieve action over time.

Practice Description

Veterans attend our Introduction to IMPACT Class and then choose one of the following core skills training groups: Reducing Pain through Flexibility (movement class); Reducing Inflammation through Diet; Stress Management; Rest, Relax, Revive (sleep class); or Creating a Plan for a Healthy Life (health coaching). After they are engaged, participants or providers can request/offer individual services to assist Veterans in reaching higher functioning. These include our Pain Rehabilitation Group; PTSD/IMPACT combined Group; Elimination Diet Nutrition Class; Yoga I/II/III/IV classes; and Battlefield Acupuncture Group, as well as individual appointments. Each class or group is an opportunity for Veterans to explore their edge *thoughts, feelings, memories, or sensations) and to learn how to adapt or address them. Veterans can continue any of our foundational classes until they are engaged and activated. Health Coaching is used to help them along.

Replicability

Our success is attributed to both Whole Health Coaching and Functional Medicine. Both are teachable, and CAVHS has a system in pace to accomplish this. We have trained three additional PACT teams and are preparing to train three others. These approaches can be implemented at any facility either in whole or in part. Our providers listen carefully to Veterans and translate the medical outcomes desired into goals and activities that Veterans care deeply about. Hence the discussion is not focused on pain or HbA1c but rather on walking and vitality. A manual will be disseminated to PACT teams at our onsite training.

Recognition

Matthew Jennings

Warriors Walk

Andrea Boyd, PhD, RN, Associate Nurse Executive Research and Education
William Jennings Bryan Dorn VA Medical Center, Columbia, SC
andrea.boyd@va.gov

Using a VA grant, Dorn VAMC was able to expand the hospice unit to a 14-bed, home-like environment and establish an experienced hospice team. Collaborating with Bay Pines VAMC and the Opus Peace Project, Warriors Walk developed a unique, evidence-based, Veteran-centric approach to hospice care.

Introduction

It is our mission to fulfill President Lincoln's promise "To care for him who shall have borne the battle and for his widow, and his orphan" by serving and honoring the men and women who are America's Veterans. When a Veteran finds him or herself facing their final days, the Dorn VA Warriors Walk hospice program allows the Veteran to die with dignity, respect, and with peace. Having treated over 800 Veterans and their families since the unit opened in 2009, Warriors Walk provides inpatient hospice care setting in a home-like environment with a Veteran-centric approach to the hospice experience.

The staff of Warriors Walk not only treats the Veteran, but also supports the family, understanding that loved ones are an integral part of the Veteran's death experience. An example of this was a dying Veteran who wanted to reconnect with his estranged family. With extensive research using social media and limited information from the Veteran, the staff was ultimately able to locate his brother. The Veteran's brother, who lived out-of-state, asked to come to Warriors Walk to meet the staff who provided support and care during his brother's last stage of life. During his visit, the staff conducted the Ceremony of Remembrance, a ceremony aimed at healing the family, while honoring the deceased Veteran. After a Veteran has died, a gold footprint with the Veteran's name is placed on a pair of white gloves on a table in front of a mural. The staff and family are encouraged to share memories of the Veteran, and a memory book is presented to the family. The family is then asked to hang the footprint on the mural where they feel the Veteran would wish to be (e.g., on the beach, in the mountains). Bereavement support for the family continues through the first year following a Veteran's death. The Ceremony of Remembrance and subsequent support often brings much needed support and remembrance to a Veteran's grieving family.

Key Information

The Dorn VAMC evaluated the need for an inpatient hospice program, and a proposal for three years of VA funding was submitted to create an inpatient hospice unit. A LCSW and Nurse Manager were hired, and they began seeking evidence-based practices, educating staff, and creating policies and procedures for the new Warriors Walk hospice unit. The group collaborated with VISN 8, Bay Pines hospice program, and VA nurses via the Opus Peace Project. Additionally, a physician with extensive hospice experience was hired, and the core Warriors Walk team was solidified. In 2013, Warriors Walk was expanded from the original unit created in 2009 into the newly renovated 14-bed unit.

Context

The Dorn VAMC opened in Columbia, SC, in 1932 at its current location. Today, it consists of seven CBOCs serving the upstate, Midlands, and Pee Dee areas of South Carolina. Dorn VAMC is a level 1C, tertiary care teaching hospital providing a full range of patient care services, with state-of-the-art technology, education, and research. Comprehensive health care is provided from PC through hospice care in areas of medicine, surgery, psychiatry, physical medicine and rehabilitation, cardiology, neurology, oncology, dentistry, geriatrics, and extended care. As one of the Teague-Cranston Act medical schools, University of South Carolina (USC) School of Medicine is located on the campus of Dorn VAMC with 48 residency positions between USC/VA. Dorn VAMC is growing rapidly, with an increasing number of military and Veterans moving into the area. In FY 2014, Dorn processed the highest number of Compensation & Pension (C&P) examination requests in the nation. For FY 2013, Dorn VAMC had 2.8 percent growth in enrolled patients, and it has continued to increase in enrolled patients every year since.

Prior to the creation of the Warriors Walk inpatient hospice unit, the Dorn VAMC determined that Veterans were dying without a peaceful, symptom-controlled, emotionally supportive environment that was unique to provision of end-of-life care. After the creation of the Warriors Walk unit, the Warriors Walk team began an initiative to educate all hospital providers regarding end-of-life care that included the hospice philosophy, role of medication, and the selection of patients who would benefit from the service.

Practice Description

Warriors Walk is a Veteran-centric, 14-bed, inpatient, hospice care unit that allows for the honorable death of Veterans and enables the staff and volunteers to recognize the Veteran and the entire family for the Veteran's service. It is staffed by a multi-disciplinary team that includes medicine, nursing, social work, chaplain services, dietary and nutrition, pharmacy, and recreation therapy.

Warriors Walk applies Veteran-centric practices to achieve the best quality of life for the Veteran at end of life through the relief of suffering and control of symptoms, while remaining sensitive to the unique needs of each Veteran and their family. One of these practices includes the Life Review where the Veteran is able to address his or her unique life journey as a military member and any aspects that have been left unacknowledged. Another unique aspect of Warriors Walk is the Ceremony of Remembrance (previously described) and the Holiday Tree Gathering, aimed at providing healing for the family while honoring the Veteran. During the Holiday Tree Gathering, held at the end of each calendar year, each Veteran's name is called and a family member is given the footprint that was originally placed by the family on the hospice mural. This ceremony helps many families deal with a first holiday without their loved one.

Replicability

Warriors Walk was successfully implemented at the Dorn VAMC due to support from upper level leadership and leadership within the affected service lines. Additionally, the core team (MD, NP, LCSW, NM) had previous hospice experience which helped facilitate the creation and implementation of Warriors Walk. The team knew what criteria were needed to produce the desired experience in an inpatient setting. Finally, each of the staff had the commitment, passion, and drive that made Warriors Walk a success. These factors make it possible to reproduce this practice in other facilities.

Recognition

John Frutchey, Debra Layer, Diane Gatling, Susan Zourzoukis, Effson Bryant, Heather Marquette, Brett Jones, Rosemary Riles, Michelle McFadden, Shelia Brown, Angie Overton, Deidra Willis, Lisa Peterson, Tonette Neal, Roxanne Major, Sandra Talley, Tonya Moore, Herman Allen

Actively Dying Veteran Signage

Martha Burns, RN, BAN, CHPN Clinical Resource Leader

Fargo VA Health Care System, Fargo, ND
martha.burns@va.gov

The Actively Dying Veteran Signage is placed outside the room of any actively dying Veteran, allowing all those entering to establish an environment of honor and respect. This is something that can only be created once in the life of the Veteran.

Introduction

A Veteran was actively dying with family at the bedside, and the Actively Dying Veteran Signage was placed outside the room. Each staff member who entered was able to show honor, dignity, and respect to the Veteran and his or her family.

Upon the death of the Veteran, the family chose to participate in the Honor Escort, another practice used at the Fargo VA HCS to honor a deceased Veteran.

The Veteran's family sent a card thanking us for the end-of-life care, honor, and respect we showed their loved one. This Veteran had chosen not to have a funeral or service. Our care for him through the Actively Dying Veteran Signage and the Honor Escort practice served as his family's service and helped them with their closure.

Key Information

The Fargo VA implemented Patient-Centered Care and has a committee focused on this topic. A staff suggestion came from one of the Patient-Centered Care Engagement Sessions to create some form of communication for all staff working with the inpatient Veterans to alert them when a Veteran is actively dying. This suggestion was the trigger for us to adopt the Actively Dying Veteran Signage. The idea was initially started by the Community Living Center (CLC) Nurse Manager, Nicole Ueckert. The sign and implementation process was established collaboratively by both of us. We presented the idea to the Patient-Centered Care Committee and the practice was implemented in September 2015. Through this new signage practice, we at the Fargo VA are able to provide end-of-life care allowing the staff to create an environment only generated once in the Veteran's life. The environment provides them the honor, dignity, and respect deserved in the last stage of life.

Context

The Fargo VA has an outpatient clinical setting as well as an inpatient setting. We have a four-bed ICU ward, a 25-bed Medical-Surgical ward, and a 38-bed CLC ward. In FY 2015, 112 Veterans received their end-of-life care at the Fargo VA. Veterans receiving care have a wide range of diagnoses, which often makes it difficult for the frontline staff to know when a Veteran being cared for in a room is actively dying. Staff felt it was difficult to display the appropriate demeanor if they were unaware of the situation before entering the room.

Practice Description

After the signage was created, a process to educate employees on the practice was implemented. A document with the signage attached was sent to all unit managers and chiefs to share with their staff at upcoming meetings. It was also determined that for new staff members, the signage would be explained at the new employee orientation, which is held the first week of every month. Because the majority of the Veterans that die are on the CLC ward, the team decided that the manager and the clinical resource leader would be responsible for the ongoing education and awareness around the signage.

Replicability

At Fargo VA, we consider it an honor and privilege to care for dying Veterans. This practice of placing Actively Dying Veteran Signage outside the Veteran's room is one of the many practices that help us provide the best patient-centered care possible.

This practice would be very easy to replicate in any VA health care system. It entails creating and laminating the signs, and educating staff on the meaning of the signage.

Recognition

Fargo VA staff

Outpatient Palliative Medicine Program

Elizabeth Cobbs, MD, Chief, Geriatrics, Extended Care and Palliative Care
Washington DC VAMC, Washington, DC
elizabeth.cobbs@va.gov

The development of outpatient palliative care has filled the gap of services that face many Veterans living with serious illness. Interdisciplinary palliative providers team up to provide the right balance of VA and community-based services to honor personal preferences throughout the life span.

Introduction

An outside hospital diagnosed with advanced colon cancer a female Veteran in her 50s who had struggled with depression and homelessness. Subsequently, she was admitted to the Washington, DC VAMC for a colonoscopy because she had no one to take her home after the procedure. She returned to the VA hospital for mediport placement and initiation of chemotherapy, at which time her VA oncologist entered a consult for outpatient palliative care. She had pain, weakness, fatigue, and anorexia. She was confused about her treatment options and prognosis. She lived alone and lacked a support system.

The VA palliative care physician arranged for a VA oncology appointment and a VA Transitional Coach NP home visit. The VA palliative physician also documented advance care planning, arranged for a massage therapy session, and referred her for home hospice services. The patient wanted all possible disease-modifying therapy, including chemotherapy, but did not desire any attempt at cardiopulmonary resuscitation or mechanical intubation. Six weeks later, the community hospice nurse found the patient confused and unable to care for herself. The community hospice nurse contacted the VA palliative care team who arranged for admission to the Palliative Unit of the VA Community Living Center (CLC). Symptoms of pain, constipation, bowel obstruction, weakness, and fatigue were alleviated with medical and integrative treatments. Under the direction of the patient, the community social worker cleared out her apartment and designated possessions and books to give away to needy community organizations. Two friends visited and provided support for her and each other. After three months in the CLC, she died peacefully. In response to the patient's request, the VA NP arranged for the donation of the patient's body to a medical school.

This story illustrates the partnership between VA and community organizations and significant others in the care of Veterans throughout the life span. VA has implemented an integrated and comprehensive program for Veterans with serious illness and advancing age. In Washington, DC, the VA team of physicians, nurses, therapists, administrators, and healing artists is embedded in a full-service urban medical center. The goal is to provide "person-centered care" for each Veteran and their family. The full spectrum of VA programs is in place with a CLC, Home Based PC (HBPC), Geriatrics Clinic, Inpatient Geriatrics and Palliative Consults, and Transitional Coaching. Our latest program is Outpatient Palliative Medicine Consult and follow-up service.

Key Information

The elements of experience of living a long life or living with serious illness are often predictable, although the timing of decline may not be. VA is designed to support Veterans to live the best possible life while coping with the functional decline and symptoms that frequently accompany trajectories of serious illness. By creating a cascade of clinical services that meet the needs of Veterans at every stage and integrating these services effectively with other programs (e.g., PC, specialty care, hospital care), our Geriatrics and Extended Care (GEC) program has facilitated early identification and education of patients and families about options for care. We honor Veterans' preferences for care at the end of life, and improve well-being and quality of life even in the face of dying. Outpatient palliative care provides a dimension of continuity that was previously lacking. The collaboration between VA and the community is of fundamental importance because VA alone cannot provide all that patients need when living with advanced illness. Outpatient palliative care maintains a focus on the preferences of each patient and family and forges connections to both VA and community resources as best fits needs and preferences.

Context

The Washington, DC, VAMC serves 72,000 unique Veterans and is located in the nation's capital. It collaborates with four medical schools, four nursing schools, and multiple other educational institutions around the training of inter-professional health teams. Washington, DC VAMC has a growing enrollment due to the closure of nearby hospitals and the growing population of older Veterans seeking comprehensive services.

Practice Description

Outpatient Palliative Medicine joins the spectrum of GEC services designed to promote wellness and honor preferences in Veterans living with advanced age or serious illness. These include the Outpatient Geriatrics Clinic, which provides consultations, and the Geriatric Patient Aligned Care Team (GeriPACT); Inpatient Geriatric Medicine and Palliative Medicine consultations; and the Community Living Center (CLC), which provides hospice, palliative, rehabilitation, and long-term care. Other services include: HBPC; the Amyotrophic Lateral Sclerosis (ALS) Clinic and its Home Care; non-institutional care services to help functionally impaired Veterans remain in their homes; Transitional Coaching, which provides assessment, home visits and education; and vesting for home bound patients, which targets Veterans having difficulty coping with their health challenges and who are at risk for hospital and ED usage. The new Outpatient Palliative Medicine program provides enhanced access to assessment, symptom relief, education, and referral to other resources when Veterans and families are ready (e.g., community hospices, activities of daily living assistance, and medical management of symptoms, such as pain).

Replicability

The GEC programs of the DC VAMC depend on fluidity and connectivity between inter-professional provider communities to created person-centered assessments and care plans. Honoring Veterans' preferences defines the care. GEC services balance the acute and specialty services by supporting patients, families, and providers to achieve more than disease-modification. In-hospital admissions and deaths have been reduced. Expected death occurs more often at home. Patients, family, and providers are more pleased. Outcomes of care are improved.

This practice has been successful in our facility due to the critical mass of GEC services and providers, the shared campus that allows cooperative relationships to grow, and the additional resources from VACO (T21 project for Transitional Coaching). Facilities that lack a critical mass of GEC providers or split them into separate campuses face obstacles to building a seamless care continuum and high functioning inter-professional collaboration.

Recognition

Karen Blackstone, Shabir Dard, Anca Dinescu, Nadine Dubowitz, Flo Etienne, Robert Kaiser, Joy Laramie, Nickie Lepcha, Carol Ramsey Lucas, Sonika Pandey, Rachel Stewart

The Health*e*Living Assessment

Jane Kim, MD, MPH, Acting Chief Consultant for Preventive Medicine
VACO, Washington, DC
jane.kim3@va.gov

The Health*e*Living Assessment (HLA), VA's health risk assessment, is available 24/7 through My Health*e*Vet (www.myhealth.va.gov) and provides Veterans with an online assessment of the impacts of their health habits and lifestyle choices. This tool provides personalized health recommendations for Veterans.

Introduction

A number of facility staff noted the positive impact that the Health*e*Living Assessment (HLA) has had on Veteran patients. A nurse from a CBOC in VISN 23 said, "One of the CBOC RN care managers…told me a story about a Veteran who took the HLA only to find that his 'health age' was lower than his actual age. He was so excited at what he felt he had been able to accomplish…It really meant something to him. This tool also helps keep people motivated to continue to practice healthy behaviors. They don't just feel it in their bodies—they see it on paper." A former Health Promotion Disease Prevention Program Manager in VISN 21 said, "It helped Veterans visualize the toll that poor health was taking on their well-being… Many thought they were powerless to really change their health, but the HLA has shown them they are much more in control than they originally thought… Patients see their health age and say things like, 'Whoa, I better do something about my health!' Some sense that they need to change, but may not know how unhealthy their lifestyles are. Both the HLA and health age give them specific guidance to get healthier."

According to a 2015 survey of HLA users, this online tool is helping individuals understand and lower their health risks and improve their overall health. Of the 1,699 respondents who completed the HLA, 79 percent agreed or strongly agreed that the questions and response choices in the HLA were easy to understand. The survey revealed that about one-third had already made changes to their health behaviors, and almost a quarter were working on changing at least one health behavior. About 73 percent said they would recommend it to others, and 76 percent thought it was a useful tool.

Key Information

The HLA is VA's health risk assessment. It is an online tool available on My Health*e*Vet and is a set of questions that asks about health behaviors, family and personal history, and other health information. It provides each individual with a personalized "health age," which is an age that takes into account the effect that an individual's health behaviors and habits have on their risk of mortality. The HLA is available to any registered user of My Health*e*Vet. Since its launch in March 2013, HLA completed over 42,000 assessments.

Context

The VHA National Center for Health Promotion and Disease Prevention (NCP) (10P4N) is a VACO Program Office within Patient Care Services (10P4). NCP is VA's primary source for healthy living, prevention, and health education. It provides evidence-based programs, resources, and policy guidance to engage Veterans in healthy living. NCP programs and resources work to empower health, reduce chronic disease, and improve VA health care. With the high proportion of overweight and obese VHA-enrolled Veterans, as well as the continual challenge of addressing smoking, problem alcohol use, and other health behaviors that contribute to increased morbidity and mortality, the HLA is a unique tool that provides immediate feedback to Veterans. They receive their health age and a summary report with information and links to programs and resources to improve their health. The HLA can be taken at a time and location that is convenient for the Veteran, allowing access to immediate feedback on health habits and behaviors that is tailored for the individual.

Practice Description

The HLA was developed in a joint effort between the NCP and Office of Information & Technology (OI&T), working closely with Connected Care staff and key stakeholders and subject matter experts from throughout VHA. A clinical content governance workgroup comprised of individuals from VHA Central Office as well as field-based staff reviewed and gave input into the questions in the HLA during its design. The HLA successfully launched in March 2013 on My HealtheVet and is available for use by any registered user of My HealtheVet.

There are a number of new features for the HLA that are currently in development. These include the development of a clinical summary report for VHA-enrolled Veterans that will be transmitted to VHA clinical teams via secure messaging, an analytics portal that will allow data from the HLA to be analyzed to assess trends and perform analyses on specific subgroups, and updates to the clinical content of the HLA to ensure that it is up to date with current VA guidelines and evidence-based practice.

Replicability

The HLA's success may be due to a number of various factors. The ability to access this tool 24/7 by any registered My HealtheVet user allows the HLA to be taken at a time and place of the Veteran's choosing. The HLA is customized for Veterans and contains questions that are specific to them, such as screening for PTSD, military sexual trauma, and environmental exposures. The HLA is already available nationwide, but there continue to be efforts to promote the use of the HLA to Veterans and to incorporate the results into clinical care.

Recognition

Theresa Hancock, Neil Evans, Kathy Frisbee

Veterans Voices: Capturing Customer Experience Analytics to Drive Innovation

Kim Nazi, PhD, FACHE, Management and Program Analyst
VACO, Washington, DC
kim.nazi@va.gov

My HealtheVet has used an industry standard survey tool since 2007 to capture Veteran's voices, assess needs and preferences, and elicit direct feedback on important topics to ensure that My HealtheVet meets current and future needs.

Introduction

Capturing Veteran voices has been an effective strategy to ensure that My HealtheVet meets the current and future needs of our nation's Veterans. When Veterans were asked about additional services that were important to them in 2007, VA listened. Veteran feedback was used to identify and develop significant enhancements and to prioritize additional services. For example, early data collected using the Customer Experience Analytics survey tool on My HealtheVet showed that Veteran's priorities for additional services were the ability to view their upcoming appointments (87 percent), schedule or change their VA appointments (74 percent), view information from their VA medical record (73 percent), and use online secure communication with their provider (64 percent). Three of these features were subsequently delivered to Veterans as high priority initiatives. The ability to schedule VA appointments is anticipated as part of VA's Veteran Appointment Request mobile application, currently in pilot testing. Eliciting Veterans voices to identify top priorities and align resources to improve the Veteran experience has increased access to VA services and increased satisfaction.

Key Information

As a major Veteran-focused initiative, the Veterans and Consumers Health Informatics Office of the Office of Connected Care has utilized the Customer Experience Analytics (CXA) Survey since October 2007 to measure and monitor customer satisfaction with VA's My HealtheVet Patient Portal, assess user needs and preferences, and elicit direct feedback from Veterans on important topics. The survey allows for continuous input from Veterans and is based on the industry standard American Customer Satisfaction Index (ACSI) for assessing the "voice of the customer" to produce actionable results. A 4 percent random selection of site visitors who have navigated four or more pages on the site during their visit are invited to participate in a brief voluntary and anonymous online survey. Model questions are used to quantify specific drivers of satisfaction, along with creating an overall satisfaction index. Top priorities for improvements are identified based on current score and anticipated impact of change. In addition to model questions, the survey also uses custom questions to collect additional feedback on specific areas (e.g., experience in accessing visit notes, preferences for delegation features, use of mobile devices, interest in various health topics, main improvement suggestions, etc.). The office also conducts Quarterly Satisfaction Insight Reviews with key stakeholders and workgroups to monitor customer satisfaction, examine specific segments of the user population, and explore various customer satisfaction drivers in order to identify actionable improvements based on data-driven evidence.

Context

The Veterans and Consumers Health Informatics Office of VHA's Office of Connected Care is responsible for VA's My HealtheVet Program. My HealtheVet (www.myhealth.va.gov) is a suite of tools that enables Veterans to create a web-based Personal Health Record (PHR), access health education resources, and refill VA prescriptions. VA patients who complete authentication can also import data extracted from the VA EHR, and communicate electronically with their health care team using secure messaging. The VA Blue Button, added in August 2010, allows Veterans to view, print, and download a single electronic file that contains all their personal health information available in My HealtheVet. As of February 2016, My HealtheVet serves more than 3.5 million registered users.

Practice Description

The goals of the My HealtheVet Evaluation Program are to optimize the My HealtheVet program to improve Veterans' health care, generate evidence-based knowledge to support clinical adoption, meet agency requirements, engage, and inform external partnerships, and contribute to the field of health care informatics. The CXA survey represents an effective and innovative Office of Management and Budget (OMB) approved method for accomplishing these goals. The CXA survey represents an important tool in the program evaluation toolbox. Leveraging custom question capability to gather direct feedback from Veterans generates important insights.

Replicability

Measuring customer satisfaction is a key component of any evaluation program. Given federal requirements for OMB approval of public surveys, our use of the CXA tool has been effective and efficient, resulting in crucial insights that have driven innovation. This practice may be replicated by other program offices that offer Veteran-facing products and services.

Recognition

ForeSee Results

My Life, My Story

Thor Ringler, Writer and Editor

William S. Middleton Memorial Veterans Hospital, Madison, WI
thor.ringler@va.gov

My Life, My Story is a program that interviews Veterans about their life stories. With Veteran approval, the story is added to the VA medical record and shared with the Veteran's care team. The goal of the project is to foster a closer connection between VA providers and the Veterans in their care.

Introduction

I first met Mr. X in a VA hospital room. I sat by his bed for an hour and asked him what he wanted his VA care team to know about him. I recorded our interview and took notes as he told me his story. After the interview, I printed the story for his family and entered it into the CPRS. I notified his inpatient and PC teams that the story was there. This is how it starts:

"My mother was a high school mathematics teacher and my father worked for the Union News Company as a supplier for railroad concession stands. I have one older sister who lives in Alabama now. My sister and I were, as she puts it, 'Arch-enemies as children, and best friends today.' Life does have a way of changing people and their opinions. At a tender age my dad developed mastoiditis, which almost killed him, and he never recovered from it. He was in the hospital for over a year and lost his job. He and I sort of split trails because he was being very hard on my mother, and they ended up getting divorced. Being loyal to my mother, I dropped him—somewhat to my regret in later years.

"Uncle Sam put a collar on me and I went into the US Army in April 1943... In 1944 we sailed to Bournemouth, England, on a converted luxury liner. We kept training in Bournemouth until we got new orders: 'No more training. Keep your equipment shiny and bright.' One night we were smuggled out of town at 2 a.m. and taken to a seaport. We were not told a damn thing but there was row upon row of LSTs [Landing Ship Tanks] stretched along the beach. I was assigned to a service battery. Our job was to keep the gun batteries supplied and the crews fed and clothed. We were bundled into a Mack truck with all our supplies and loaded onto an LST. I was the lead truck in the LST. Later on I was not so happy about that. We set off at 3 a.m.—it was the morning after D-Day.

"We were heading for a coastal area that had several landing sites, they were sand dunes really. I don't remember the name of it, but what I do remember is significant. Careful...I break down every time I try to tell it [choking up]. As we neared the coast, all we could see was bodies, floating in the surf. And then above that on the sand—bodies—scattered all the way up to the cliffs. And they were all our newly dedicated Soldiers. The Germans were not surprised. They had zeroed in with their machine guns on every square inch of sand. The next day it was a lot clearer. Our planes had done their job and knocked out most of the anti-aircraft. We were led up a steep trail to the top of the cliffs... and I wasn't shot at once. That came later [crying]. I've never even been able to tell my wife this story."

Key Information

My Life, My Story is a program that interviews Veterans about their life stories. Since April of 2013, the team at the Madison VAMC has interviewed over 900 Veterans and shared their stories with thousands of providers and family members. We have also reached out to the wider community, recruiting and training over 30 community volunteers to interview and write Veteran stories. A poll of VA providers found that 68 percent of them agreed that, "Reading the 'My Story' note (in CPRS) will help me provide better treatment." When we surveyed Veterans who were interviewed for the project, 79 percent of them "felt that my story was a helpful part of my care."

Context

Veteran stories are a powerful way to engage Veterans, providers, family members and the larger community in the mission of VA. A Veteran wrote, "It was nice having someone listen to my story and even better when I see it in print. Sharing stories or thoughts can be very healing. Many vets don't have anyone to listen." A provider wrote, "The My Story note was wonderful. I truly feel it has helped me to understand my patients better and to know where they are coming from. This is invaluable to VA where experiences shape our patients in such a profound way." Another Veteran said, "It is programs like this that give me confidence in the VA system."

Practice Description

In FY 2015, the program expanded to pilot sites at VAMCs in Vermont, New York, North Carolina, Iowa, Kansas, and Nevada. The Madison team visited each site and hosted a two-day training workshop for program staff. The practice received a Strong Practice Designation from the Office of Mental Health Operations (OMHO). In FY 2016, the Madison team will conduct training workshops at other VA facilities interested in starting their own programs.

Replicability

My Life, My Story is a flexible program that can be implemented at any VAMC. The Madison team has developed extensive training materials (video, toolkit, and workshops) for sites that are interested in piloting the program. Please contact our program office directly on vhamadmystory@va.gov or call 608-256-1901 Ext. 11962 for more information.

Food Service Operations: Room Service

Ellen Bosley, National Director, Nutrition and Food Services; Anne Utech, Deputy National Director, Nutrition and Food Services

VACO, Washington, DC
ellen.bosley@va.gov

Room Service is a food service operation that features made-to-order, freshly-prepared food. Veterans order what they want, when they want it, from a fixed restaurant-style menu.

Introduction

Contemporary Veteran-centric food service operations improve Nutrition & Food Service Departments' customer service by offering Veterans food service experiences like Room Service. Veterans are able to make choices regarding the foods they eat while under VA care. This flexibility vastly improves patient satisfaction scores. In fact, according to Don Miller and Associates (DM&A), customer satisfaction scores tend to skyrocket to the 90th to 99th percentile with the Room Service Model.

A good example of this took place at the Iowa City VAMC, which currently operates with Room Service. They received a letter that stated "I know that you all may not remember me, but I wanted to write a small note to tell you what superb food and staff you have. The food that I was served was better than any restaurant I have been in. I want to take this time to thank each and every one of you for the superb food and care that I received while I was a patient. All of you will always have a special place in my heart. Thank you so very, very much for everything!"

Patients only order what they want to eat. In Room Service, food quality and presentation improve because food is made to order. Facilities experience a cost savings because so little food is held in storage. Therefore, there is much less plate waste. Additionally, Hazard Analysis Critical Control Points (HACCP) improve because food does not sit for long periods in storage or on a tray line. Instead, staff members make the food fresh. Nationally, those facilities that have transitioned to Room Service have experienced about an 8 percent increase in patient satisfaction scores.

Key Information

Room Service has been implemented in seven VAMCs across the country, including Des Moines, IA; Las Vegas, NV; Baltimore, MD; Chicago, IL; Iowa City, IA; and Detroit, MI. Each facility develops its own set of Nutrition & Food Services leaders to help implement Room Service. Room Service can be implemented at any time, but it does require support from upper leadership because kitchen changes (possibly construction) are necessary to support a food service operation change.

Context

The Clement J. Zablocki VAMC in Milwaukee, WI, has experienced barriers in starting up their Room Service. This facility serves about 150–180 acute care meals at each meal service. The cook-chill method favored employee schedules, not patients. Food was prepared in advance and often unpresentable due to the outdated equipment. This cook-chill method is utilized at many VAMCs across the country. As the Milwaukee VAMC waits for construction completion of the Room Service kitchen, our team has transitioned to a hotline service. Veterans are not yet able to choose what they want to eat. However, in Room Service, Veterans choose what they want to eat and when they want to eat it.

Practice Description

Room Service is a food service operation that features made-to-order, freshly-prepared food. Veterans order from a fixed restaurant-style menu within dietary restrictions. To promote Room Service as a gold-standard food service operation, the Veteran's Experience Food Service Operations team developed a toolkit available on its SharePoint site that provides VA facilities the tools they need to implement the program.

Transitioning a food service operation to Room Service requires position description updates, new hires, changes in policy and procedure, and support from various disciplines within the VAMC. All of these changes are outlined in the Room Service Toolkit, and each facility currently employing Room Service went through the processes in order to implement this contemporary, Veteran-centric operation.

Replicability

Room Service will be adopted at the Milwaukee VAMC because it improves the customer service we provide. Room Service allows for the most customized options, and patients can eat when they feel hungry. This operation will go live at the Milwaukee VAMC as soon as kitchen construction is complete. Specific factors that made this possible included support from our top management team and a food service administrative team dedicated to making our department more Veteran-centric.

Other facilities can easily reproduce or replicate this practice with support of their leadership team. Upon leadership's approval, utilization of the Room Service Toolkit will help facilities implement this "best practice" into medical centers.

Recognition

Kayleen Wichlinski, Valerie Adegunleye, Krista Arneson, Valerie Baker, Ellen Bosley, Erin Bouslaugh, Krista Jablonski, Emily Kohls, Julie Kurtz, Jolie Rubin-Lewis, Mark Morgan, Wendy Ottosen, Joy Petterson, Chelsea Skillman, Ellen Tolson, Anne Utech, Brandy Weber- Minor, Kayleen Wichlinsiki

Implementation of the Whole Health Partnership

Alyssa Adams, PsyD, CNS, Chief, Patient Centered Care Service and Director, Integrative Health & Wellness Program; Amanda Hull, PhD, Field Implementation Team Lead, Office of Patient Centered Care and Cultural Transformation; Christie Eickhoff, MS, Program Specialist

Washington DC VAMC, Washington, DC

alyssa.adams2@va.gov

The Whole Health Partnership builds a relationship with the Veteran upon entry into the VA system and provides a proactive, patient-centered framework for conceptualizing health as the Veteran engages in Whole Health programming, complementary and integrative health modalities, and clinical care.

Introduction

The Patient-Centered Care (PCC) Service at the Washington, DC VAMC is committed to offering innovative Whole Health programming for Veterans through the Whole Health Partnership model. This model will empower Veterans to explore their health goals as well as design and implement a health plan. This partnership will foster Veteran empowerment and underscore VA's commitment to a patient-centered, proactive approach to health.

The Whole Health Partnership presents a model for empowerment by identifying areas of self-care, discussing the interplay between values and health, and providing the roadmap for achieving self-identified health goals. The DC VAMC roadmap also includes entry into the Integrative Health & Wellness (IHW) program, a well-being center that offers a unique opportunity to access various integrative health modalities. Veterans also receive information on other hospital programs and community-based options in support of their health goals, including access to virtual well-being resources, such as experiential services (e.g., guided meditation and mindfulness recordings).

The IHW program is an example of a patient-centered well-being program that is designed to offer various integrative health services to Veterans in an outpatient setting. The IHW program operates in a dedicated space in the DC VAMC and offers integrative health programming five days per week. Veterans are referred by a provider and, after completing a program orientation, are able to attend various integrative health services at the frequency of their choosing. In FY 2015, providers from over 50 different departments at the DC VAMC referred Veterans to the IHW program for 1,508 consults. Regardless of referral source, pain or mental health symptoms were the primary health concern of Veterans participating in the program. The total number of newly enrolled Veterans has increased every year since inception, with the majority of referrals coming from PC. Preliminary findings suggest that after only eight weeks of program participation, Veterans reported improved physical and mental health symptoms, decreased medication use, and high satisfaction with the program. Additionally, Veterans participating in the IHW program made the following statements regarding their satisfaction with the program and their health improvements:

- "The IHW program contributed to my overall sense of well-being. Many times, I have come to the classroom anxious and tense. The music, pictures, and plants contributed greatly and the facilitator's calming demeanor helped make a soothing atmosphere. Thanks to your team for a good job."

- "Less pain, better sleep, overall relaxation."
- "I learned to be more focused on the importance of proper nutrition. The acupuncture services have taught me lots about the importance of mindfulness and self-healing. Can't say enough about the benefits of the IHW program to me."

Key Information

The Whole Health Partnership design includes three central components: pathway, well-being centers, and clinical care. The pathway partners with Veterans at the point of enrollment and creates an overarching personal health plan that integrates VA and non-VA care. Well-being centers provide an integrative health approach to optimizing health and well-being and offer services to all Veterans regardless of diagnosis. Clinical care represents the conventional clinical care with an enhanced emphasis on healing environments, healing relationships, and the integration of integrative health and personal health planning practices into treatment plans. The DC VAMC has been an early innovator, capitalizing on both leadership investment and grassroots movements to establish the components of the Whole Health Partnership. The PCC Service at the DC VAMC has implemented this multi-tiered approach to care. Representatives from multiple services, clinical providers, and executive leadership collaborated to implement this innovative approach to care. The IHW program, an example of a well-being center, opened in 2012, and the Whole Health pathway component opened in 2016. As Veterans navigate through PC clinics, specialty services, and the health and well-being program, they will be empowered self-advocates with their health care providers as they will have integrated the Whole Health principles and approach.

Context

The DC VAMC serves over 98,311 Veterans across several locations, including the main facility in downtown Washington, DC, and four CBOCs. This inner-city VA provides care to Veterans of various ages, demographic profiles, and socioeconomic statuses. Complementary and integrative health approaches were offered occasionally and throughout various departments at the DC VAMC since 2007. However, these services were difficult for Veterans to access, care was sporadic, and integrative health services were based on specific diagnoses. The PCC Service coordinated the integrative health programming in the facility and initiated a consult to house these services under one program (i.e., IHW Program). This effort allowed Veterans easier access to integrative health services through a well-being center and allowed Veterans to access these modalities regardless of diagnosis. Recently, the Pathway was initiated in order to provide a holistic, empowerment-based model of health education and self-management in which Veterans may enroll from the point of entry to the DC VAMC. This approach lays the foundation for their future care throughout the VA system.

Practice Description

The Whole Health Partnership offers a partnership with the Veteran upon entry into the DC VAMC and a proactive, patient-centered framework for conceptualizing health as the Veteran begins to interact with the hospital's departments, providers, and services. The Whole Health Partnership provides a model that transcends the bounds of VA, as this approach to health will reside with the Veteran as he or she navigates well-being services, community resources, and health care throughout his or her life.

The Pathway offers a brief overview to the Whole Health model immediately following new patient orientation at the facility. Veterans are offered immediate entry into a nine-week Whole Health Facilitation group during which Veterans complete the Personal Health Inventory (PHI), create a personal health plan, engage in health education focused on the Whole Health model, and receive information on facility, community, and virtual services available to them. Veterans receive a referral to a well-being center, the second component of the Whole Health Partnership. The IHW program organizes itself along two tracks: Integrative Medicine (IM), and well-being and education. Within the IM Track, an IM physician provides consultation services one day per week for outpatient Veterans at the DC VAMC. Veterans with fibromyalgia, chronic pain, chronic fatigue, and gastrointestinal issues are referred to this consult service by a medical provider. Within the well-being track, integrative health programming includes wellness massage, auricular acupuncture, yoga, meditation, iRest Yoga Nidra, biofeedback, qigong, Tai Chi, nutrition workshops, an integrative nutrition group, Mindfulness-Based Stress Reduction, and Whole Health education group.

Replicability

First, Veteran demand and interest were at the heart of these practices. Second, a grassroots movement of dedicated and passionate staff who believe that the Whole Health approach is key in the transformation of Veteran health care was imperative in the implementation process. Third, leadership support was important for the sustainability of this innovation. Additionally, funding, space, and a dedicated staff were essential for the expansion of this innovation.

Recognition

Brian Hawkins, Christine Merna, Lauren Roselli, Melane Rose-Boyce, Alaine Dunca

Telephone Lifestyle Coaching

Sophia Hurley, MSPT, Prevention Programs Coordinator

VACO, Washington, DC

sophia.hurley@va.gov

Telephone Lifestyle Coaching (TLC) supports health behavior change and improved health by providing care for Veterans when and where they want it. Using VHA Healthy Living messages delivered via telephone, this individualized health coaching empowers Veterans to make positive lifestyle changes, such as losing weight and being physically active.

Introduction

Ms. X smoked for 32 years, but always wanted to quit. "My husband recently passed away from the complications of emphysema and chronic obstructive pulmonary disease, and that was what finally motivated me to make the change." When Ms. X's PCP at the James E. Van Zandt VAMC in Altoona, PA, recommended Telephone Lifestyle Coaching (TLC), she knew it was a good fit. The coaching support and program convenience really appealed to her, in part because of her history of unsuccessful attempts to quit tobacco. "I'd had no success with cessation programs over the years… until I started TLC. TLC gave me the help and encouragement I needed to make such a big lifestyle change." Ms. X raves about the telephone support her health coach provided. "The number of calls was just right—not too many or too few—and it was really convenient being able to call from home. On each call, my coach provided the helpful tips and education I needed to keep moving toward my goal. It was nice to know that I could call back anytime I wanted and it was nice to feel like someone really cares about me and my goals." With the support of TLC program staff, and weekly appointments with a behavioral health social worker, Ms. X was able "to quit, and stay quit!"

TLC is also helping Ms. X address another long-standing health challenge: weight. "My weight has fluctuated since I was a teenager, and as with smoking, I've tried different weight-control programs without success. But with the help of my coach, I've also been able to achieve my goal of losing weight. Through TLC, I've gone from 252 pounds down to 206 pounds! I'm aiming for 189 pounds, and with the support of TLC and my health coach, I know I can do it!"

Key Information

Telephone-based health coaching is an effective way to promote health behavior change across a variety of behaviors. TLC is a patient-centered, convenient, and highly accessible pilot program focused on delivering individualized health coaching via telephone to assist Veterans who choose to make healthy lifestyle changes in six health behaviors. These behaviors follow the National Center for Health Promotion and Disease Prevention (NCP) healthy living messages: Be Tobacco Free, Eat Wisely, Be Physically Active, Strive for a Healthy Weight, Limit Alcohol, and Manage Stress. Coaching services were provided via an external contract that was competitively awarded to Alere Wellbeing Inc. Coaching was available outside typical medical facilities, six days a week, and 16 hours a day in all continental US time zones.

Context

The VHA NCP (10P4N) is a VACO Program Office within Patient Care Services (10P4). NCP is VA's primary source for healthy living, prevention, and health education. It provides evidence-based programs, resources, and policy guidance to engage Veterans in healthy living. NCP programs and resources work to empower health, reduce chronic disease, and improve VA health care. TLC provides a convenient, patient-centered option of care for Veterans who choose to make a health behavior change to improve their health and well-being.

Practice Description

The TLC intervention was developed based on several behavioral theories and approaches, including Social Cognitive Theory, Cognitive Behavioral Therapy (CBT), Motivational Interviewing (MI), and Mindfulness. Highly trained and skilled TLC coaches used a variety of strategies derived from these theoretical approaches, including relationship building, assessment of needs, values and motivation collaborative goal setting, self-monitoring, problem solving, and encouraging use of social support.

Supporting print materials were provided for each TLC participant. Content was based on the VA's MOVE! Weight Management Program (MOVE!), Alere's Quit For Life® Program, the Office of Public Health's Tobacco and Health Policy Program, the Dietary Approaches to Stop Hypertension Diet (DASH), the 2008 Physical Activity Guidelines for Americans, Mindfulness-Based Stress Reduction, and the National Institute on Alcohol Abuse and Alcoholism Guidelines. During a PC visit, Veterans who were ready to make a behavior change and interested in receiving telephone coaching were offered a referral to TLC. Alere's staff completed consult management and documentation in CPRS. Participants received individualized telephone coaching to support their goals over several months. Call schedules were collaboratively created by patient and coach to maximize success with identified goals.

Outcomes from TLC were impressive. At six months post-enrollment, 40 percent of smokers reported they had quit, and 895 Veterans received tobacco cessation pharmacotherapy from their VA providers through the program. Clinically significant weight loss (5 percent or more of body weight) was reported by 33 percent of those with a weight loss goal. Additionally, 12 percent of those without a weight loss goal reported clinically significant weight loss, and 18 percent of smokers who did not have a tobacco cessation goal had also quit.

Replicability

Twenty-four medical centers across VISNs 4, 8, 15, 16, and 21 implemented the pilot. At each pilot facility, the TLC point of contact managed educating PACT teams about TLC services and their facility implementation plan. As coaching services were provided by an outside vendor, resources required at participating sites were limited to a point of contact, Clinical Applications Coordinator (CAC) support to load the designated documentation templates into CPRS, and Information Security support to manage access for vendor staff to CPRS for consult management and documentation. Following the successful pilot outcomes, the VA's ORH agreed to provide funding to support implementation of TLC for the next four years with a focus on reaching VA's rural and highly rural Veterans.

Recognition

TLC Integrated Product Team, Elizabeth Gilbert, James Nicholson, ORH

Whole Health Education

Laura Krejci, Associate Director
VACO, Washington, DC
laura.krejci@va.gov

Empowering patient self-care is a critical core competency for VHA's future. The comprehensive Whole Health Education Program develops this through innovative offerings and diverse resources to advance Whole Health skills and expertise, supporting the systematic transformation of Veteran health care.

Introduction

Mr. X served in Iraq as a member of the US Marine Corps. After returning home, he began struggling with sleeplessness, alcohol abuse, and social isolation. Desperate to break the cycle, he visited his local VA facility where his care team recommended a Whole Health plan of action that included acupuncture and one-on-one therapy. Five years after returning home, Mr. X no longer had nightmares, he quit drinking, and he rediscovered the joy of social engagements. Thanks to a Whole Health approach, he was able to forge a new beginning.

Context

- Chronic conditions consume more than 75 percent of health care costs and are largely affected by patient choices and behaviors.

- Health care consumes 18 percent of our Gross National Product (GNP), and costs continue to rise with unsatisfactory results. This is unsustainable. The US will lose its ability to compete in the global market and the consequences are significant.

- The current health care model doesn't work because we do not have a core competency in engaging the patient to optimize their health and manage their disease.

Practice Description

Whole Health: Advancing Skills in the Delivery of Personalized, Proactive, Patient-Driven Care. "Whole Health" refers to patient-centered care that affirms the importance of the partnership between the provider and the patient. The focus is on the whole person and co-creating a personalized, proactive, and patient-driven experience. The Whole Health approach is informed by evidence and makes use of all appropriate therapeutic approaches and disciplines to achieve optimal health and healing.

The Office of Patient Centered Care and Cultural Transformation (OPCC&CT) currently provides the following educational offerings to support the expansion of this model across VHA:

- "Whole Health Foundation Toolkit": A selection of modules that a facility may use to advance patient-centered care concepts with any employee who works at a VA facility. It also includes an individual TMS course, Whole Health Foundation: A Personal Experience (VA 3871323).

- Whole Health: Change the Conversation Clinical Course: VHA's core course for clinicians in advancing skills in the delivery of personalized, proactive, patient-driven care.

- Whole Health Coaching Course: A six-day, intensive, in-person training on coaching and communication skills using the four-step coaching process model. This experiential course involves substantial practice and mentoring.

- Whole Health Group-Based Program: This program started as a pilot Program and it is now expanding to seven additional sites in 2016. This program is led by Veteran peer, volunteer, or other non-clinical facilitators to provide Veteran participants the opportunity to receive education in improving their self-care behaviors to support their personal mission for life and health. The main objective of this program is to provide Veteran participants the opportunity to think differently about their health. Along with thinking differently, the Whole Health Group-Based Program seeks to engage Veterans in improving their self-care behaviors to support their personal mission for life, health, and well-being. The group program is a nine-week program designed around the Components of Proactive Health and Well-being and will utilize the Personal Health Inventory.

- Whole Health Online Library: Includes educational overviews and clinical tools organized into modules that correspond to the "Circle of Health."

Replicability

To date, the courses have been replicated in 44 VA facilities:

- Nearly 2,588 VHA employees trained in Whole Health (number includes only those who completed full course; many more attended in part)
- 44 host facilities
- 63 total courses

OPCC&CT invited Army colleagues to participate in the Whole Health Clinical Course, and Army Surgeon General Move2Health classes have been held at 10 sites based on the Whole Health: Change the Conversation Clinical Course.

Recognition

Pacific Institute for Research and Development, University of Wisconsin

ACCESS

Increasing Access to Primary Care

Ellina Seckel, PharmD, PACT Program Manager, CPS

William S. Middleton Memorial Veterans Hospital, Madison, WI
ellina.seckel@va.gov

Clinical Pharmacy Specialists play a larger role in the care team, helping PCPs support patients and increase Veterans' access to care.

Introduction

Access is a key issue across all VA facilities, and, on average, PACT providers only have the capacity to schedule a patient 2.5 times per year, not nearly enough for aging Veteran patients on complex medication regimens. In addition, PACT providers often have inadequate support and feel the pressures of increased patient demand.

To address local access issues, pharmacy leadership at the William S. Middleton Memorial Veterans Hospital established a multi-modal approach to increase access to PC through use of CPSs.

Key Information

The pharmacy leadership team led interventions to increase access and advance pharmacy practice in the PC setting. Interdisciplinary involvement from the Chief of PC and PACT providers was crucial for success. The facility Chief of Staff also supported the project.

Context

The William S. Middleton Memorial Veterans Hospital is a 129-bed teaching facility. The hospital provides tertiary, surgical, neurological, and psychiatric care as well as a full range of outpatient services. In addition to the onsite PC clinic in Madison, there are five CBOCs providing care to Veterans in outlying areas of Wisconsin and Illinois. Implementation of the following interventions occurred at the main PC clinic, and later expanded to the CBOCs.

Methods involved were multi-modal. First, a strong educational campaign ensured PACT providers knew the disease states CPS could help them manage. At the same time, each PACT received CPS assignments. Additionally, the team created a New Patient Medication Intake Clinic to call new VA patients prior to their first appointment. During this initial phone session, an accurate medication list was obtained, reconciled, and interventions were made to optimize medication use and safety. Lastly, return to clinic orders for PACT providers were reviewed by a CPS in a newly created prospective appointment conversion program. Rescheduling appointments appropriate for CPS management, including PACT provider visits and CPS visits, came next. With the support of the PACTs, a proposal was written requesting additional CPS resources be allocated to PC.

Practice Description

In September 2014, the CPS Clinic Educational Campaign launched. Analysis from October through December 2014 revealed CPS Clinic utilization rates increased by an average of 13.8

percent (11.2 percent growth in face-to-face clinics and 20.2 percent growth in telephone clinics). In addition, the assignment of CPS to PACTs resulted in enhanced communication and improved team satisfaction. As a result of the New Patient Medication Intake Clinic, the CPS was able to save PACT providers 20 minutes, on average, on every new patient appointment. In addition to saving time, medication discrepancies identification and resolution became easier, which augmented medication safety. In the first three months of the appointment conversion program, 28 percent of PACT provider appointments were converted to CPS appointments. Commonly converted appointments included follow-ups for diabetes, hypertension, hyperlipidemia, pain, gout, thyroid, and vitamin D management. Each appointment conversion immediately opened an appointment slot in the PACT provider schedule.

Lastly, facility leadership approved four new positions to expand permanent CPS presence in PC. Through a multi-modal approach, CPS increased patient access to care and advanced practice in the PC setting.

Replicability

The expanded use of CPS to increase access to care is replicable in any primary or ambulatory care setting. Prospective review of upcoming provider appointments with conversion to CPS appointments can instantaneously open access in provider schedules for patients with more acute or diagnostic needs. Performing a New Patient Medication Intake Clinic also saves providers time that can be reallocated for other appointments or patient care services. Facilities looking to implement these practices should have strong clinical pharmacy leadership with a clear vision for team-based care. Support from the Chief of Staff and Chief of PC is integral.

Recognition

Andrew Wilcox, Janelle Vittetoe, Hilary Friedman, Jean Montgomery, Alan Bridges

Direct Scheduling for Audiology and Optometry

Joann Fenicchia, Supervisory Program Analyst for Systems Redesign and Accreditation; Michelle Menendez, Chief, Audiology and Speech Pathology Service
Bay Pines Healthcare System, Bay Pines, FL
joann.fenicchia@va.gov

Direct Scheduling of audiology and appointments bypasses the need for a PCP to enter a consult for routine ear and eye care, resulting in reduced wait times and increased patient satisfaction.

Introduction

Ms. Q, a Veteran and Bay Pines VA employee, found it cumbersome to visit her PCP to obtain regular consults to optometry and audiology. Her father, also a Veteran and former Bay Pines VA employee, shared that opinion. They believed that the process was time-consuming and outdated. Now, with Direct Scheduling, both Veterans can promptly contact optometry and audiology and receive immediate and convenient services. Overall, the feedback from the Direct Scheduling pilots echoed positive sentiments. The pilot reduced overall wait times for audiology and optometry appointments for new patients by 19.18 and 9.43 days, respectively, and the number of completed audiology and optometry appointments increased by an average of 5.83 percent and 4.54 percent. Direct Scheduling reduced the number of audiology and optometry consults by 143.03 percent. Conversely, participating health care systems experienced mixed results regarding specialty wait times: (Mountain Home audiology +1 day), (White River Junction audiology +10.19 days), (Bay Pines audiology -5.79 days), (Mountain Home optometry +3.96), (White River Junction optometry +6.41 days), and (Bay Pines optometry +3.96 days).

Key Information

Direct Scheduling of audiology and optometry's goal is to simplify Veterans' health care access. This pilot bypassed the need for a PCP to enter a consult for routine ear and eye care, while simultaneously reducing the burden on Patient-Centered Primary Care (PCPC) services. Implementation of a Direct Scheduling pilot occurred at three health care systems: Bay Pines, FL (March 30, 2015—Audiology and Optometry); Mountain Home, TN (April 6, 2015—Optometry, May 15, 2015—Audiology); White River Junction, VT (June 1, 2015—Audiology and Optometry). Health care system improvement practitioners, the Pittsburgh Veterans Engineering Resource Center (VERC), and MyVA Performance Improvement Team organized teams and local stakeholders to develop an implementation plan. As the Bay Pines team began their efforts, they easily determined why this project mattered, "Veterans deserve to be seen for audiometric and optometric services without bureaucratic barriers and should receive better PC access for complex issues."

Context

Bay Pines VA Healthcare System, is a complexity level 1a facility that provides comprehensive health care to more than 100,000 Veterans in East Central and Southwestern Coastal Florida. Services include primary and various specialty care services, inpatient (medical/surgical/psychiatric) care, inpatient nursing home and hospice care, inpatient domiciliary care, mental health services (inpatient and outpatient), and women's programs. We offer services through our Cape Coral outpatient clinic and seven CBOCs. The Direct Scheduling pilot had several key motivators that continue to simulate the transformation of this health care system: 1) the voice of the Veteran; 2) unencumbered access for Veterans; 3) increased patient satisfaction in self-scheduling; 4) increased PCP access; and 5) simplified scheduling and appointment process.

Practice Description

Simply put, the Direct Scheduling current state is patients with audiology or optometry needs telephone VHA service schedulers to request an audiology and/or optometry appointment (the PC gatekeeping step removed), and the patient receives his/her care appointment. Staff experienced an elimination of routine consults, saving the time required to review them. Importantly, Veterans are automatically vested in group two without a level three history and physical.

Replicability

Any site may adopt procedures to eliminate consults for uncomplicated hearing loss or non-medical vision deficiencies. As with any improvement activity, the practitioners must be motivated and positive. Notably, the direct scheduling process is elegant in its simplicity. The biggest challenge is growing a process that allows Veterans to approach specialty service directly for the scheduling of appointments. Moreover, Veteran notification of this new practice is paramount to its success. The second biggest task is having a mechanism to notify physicians should the patient's needs become non-routine or medically complicated in nature.

Processes for dealing with cerumen removal, traveling Veterans, and eligibility must be detailed prior to implementation. Notification of the obvious stakeholders, as well as the Clinical Applications Coordinators and Union partners, should occur as part of the planning practice to ensure a smooth and efficient transition.

Recognition

Shelly Wilt, Lawrence Diehl, Jenette Cantrell, Thomas Mattras, Joseph Miller, Rene Wilson, Colleen Hall, Deanne Adams-Boozer, Anthony Batill, Johnny Quinones

Harry S. Truman Memorial Veterans' Hospital Access Data Dashboard to Improve Clinic Management

Michelle Pruitt, Program Analyst

Harry S. Truman Memorial Veterans' Hospital, Columbia, MO
michelle.pruitt2@va.gov

The Access Dashboard tracks critical components of access, such as no-show rates and completed appointment wait times, helping staff solve problems and make key decisions.

Introduction

Incremental improvements in clinic access metrics represent positive impacts to thousands of Veterans who experience shorter wait times for appointments. For example, the Harry S. Truman Memorial Veterans' Hospital (Truman VA) completed over 3,000 new patient PC appointments in FY 2015, during which the percentage of appointments completed in fewer than 30 days from the "create date" increased from 81.9 percent in September 2014 to 97.3 percent in September 2015. Truman VA also completed over 69,000 established patient appointments in PC. The percentage of appointments completed in fewer than 30 days from the "patient preferred date" increased from 98.40 percent in September 2014 to 99.98 percent in September 2015. From the Veteran's perspective, that is an increase of 1,000 more PC patient visits within a 30-day period.

Key Information

To improve clinic management, clinic access metrics (no-shows, wait times, clinic utilization, etc.) are posted monthly on the Truman VA System's dashboard. The dashboard is accessible on SharePoint by all employees and is printed and displayed in a busy conference room. The facility director, Executive Leadership Team (ELT), service chiefs, systems redesign committee, data analyst, and visual information specialist cooperate to develop, review, and focus attention on the dashboard to drive improvement.

Context

Truman VA in Columbia, MO is one of seven medical center facilities in the VA Heartland Network (VISN 15). Truman VA's primary service area is within a 200-mile radius of Columbia and includes more than 26,000 square miles encompassing 45 rural and underserved counties with a Veteran population of approximately 113,000. The facility operates 110 beds and has CBOCs in eight communities. In FY 2015, Truman VA provided care for 37,097 Veterans with 444,245 outpatient visits through a full continuum of support services. Truman VA is also the open-heart referral center for VISN 15 facilities.

Practice Description

In 2014, Truman VA implemented an Access Dashboard to track critical components of access, such as no-show rates and completed appointment wait times. The dashboard is an Excel spreadsheet that combines multiple metrics on a single page, formatted and color-coded so it is easy to see trends and targets. It's accessible and understandable by all staff on the facility SharePoint site and it's printed and posted in a busy conference room.

VHA collects and analyzes an immense amount of data on a daily basis. The dashboard adds value by focusing on a limited number of critical metrics and making trends and targets easily understandable by all employees. Public display of metrics encourages transparency and a "we can fix that" attitude. If access metrics drop or fail to improve, the facility is alerted and can address any process issues. It also encourages thoughtful discussion and mutual accountability for results.

Replicability

The spreadsheet is supported by a data analyst with expertise in SQL, Excel, and Pyramid who prepares daily and weekly detail reports pushed to the services. The data analyst also responds to special requests for data drilldown on any operational or decision-making question. Partial update automation is possible; however, the ability to provide data drilldown is critical for process improvement efforts.

Most importantly, the dashboard serves as a focus for discussions in the normal workflow of the facility led by the director and ELT. The facility director, ELT, service chiefs, systems redesign committee, data analyst, and media specialist cooperate to develop, review, and focus attention on the dashboard to drive improvement.

Recognition

Wade Vlosich, Kelly Harris, Billy Cargile, Heather Brown, Sandi Pope, Joseph (Zeke) Rupnick

Improving Same-Day Access Using Nurse Care Manager "Chair" Visits

Henry Elzinga, MD, Section Chief, PC, MC

Boise VAMC, Boise, ID
henry.elzinga@va.gov

RN care managers triage and scribe same-day appointment requests, saving PCPs time when they see patients between appointments to assess and confirm the care plan.

Introduction

Great PC and specialty care access matters. It matters to any patient who is concerned about a symptom or health problem that could represent something serious. Clearly, the best people to help are the Veteran's own PC team because they already know the patient. In addition to being familiar with the patient's prior concerns and history, they often have an established relationship built on trust with the patient. This is where good patient care starts; with trust, with relationships, with knowing. Leveraging the understanding and experience of the PC team seems like the right thing to do. In addition, nursing staff and PCPs want to help. But how can they do this? Most of the time, their work schedules are already too long and demanding.

Simply extending provider work schedules with more traditional appointment slots may help improve same-day access but it also increases the risk of burnout and staff turnover, which in the end will likely worsen access and continuity of care. Is there a better solution than longer workdays?

Key Information

Approximately five years ago, VA understood that team care (sometimes called the "patient-centered medical home" or "PACT" within VA) could provide better, more consistent longitudinal care for patients. Key members of this team (in addition to the Veteran) include the clerical associate (or clerk), the clinical associate (often a health technician or LPN), the nurse care manager (usually a RN) and the PCP. Together this team can provide better care between visits. Can this expanded team somehow meet the challenge of providing consistent and reliable same-day care as well?

Practice Description

The clinic manager and staff devised a structured process for seeing Veterans who had unscheduled same-day care needs. Perhaps the team could "share the care" making the additional work seem manageable? Clerks would help identify the basic concern and assist with scheduling when needed. Next, Veterans with symptom-related concerns would undergo a simple triage followed by a more thorough assessment by nursing staff. Providers would leverage the detailed assessment and pre-work already done by nursing staff, add their own specialized assessment, when needed, and provide the decision-making and treatment plan. Finally, nursing staff would coordinate care after the visit and assist with documentation, when needed. Together, the entire team could efficiently provide a focused and meaningful care experience with little overall net increase in workload. Nursing staff and clerks didn't have to say, "No." Most importantly, everyone felt satisfied with the end-result.

Veterans could get care when they needed it from the team who knew them best, and together, the nursing staff and providers delivered meaningful, effective, patient-centric care.

Replicability

This promising practice in Caldwell, ID, continues to spread to other clinics and clinic areas in the Boise VAMC systems.

Recognition

Debra Hendricks, Caldwell clinic staff

The Journey to Open Access in Primary Care at VA Central California Health Care System: Achievement and Sustainment

Michael Tom, DO, FACP, Chief, PC Service

VA Central California Health Care System, Fresno, CA
michael.tom@va.gov

Using system redesign principles and VA's PACT model, this practice focuses on implementing new protocols that increase same-day access opportunities for Veterans.

Introduction

Our journey to same-day access started approximately five years ago. We were rooted in an indigenous doctor-centered culture with significant access challenges. Our new and established patients had long appointment wait times, and there was a limited ability to see patients when they wanted to be seen, especially for same-day requests. The ED had to see most of the walk-in patients, which had the downstream effect of even longer wait times and delays in care for both acute and non-acute visits. This resulted in poor satisfaction for both patients and staff. In particular, the staff felt they could not provide the continuity and same-day access that they wanted for their patients. At that time, staff could only see 21.6 percent of our same-day appointments with their assigned PCP, and the Third Next Available Appointment (TNAA) wait time averages were as high as 29 days.

Key Information

Utilizing system redesign principles and PACT philosophy, we proceeded to methodically analyze our current state and plan for a future state of open access, with a particular emphasis on creating a future where patient(s) would have a high likelihood of being able to see their provider and PACT as needed. Leadership in the PC service conceptualized the structure of this system and it was supported by executive leadership. Implementation required the participation from PC clinical nurse managers and the members of the core and extended PACT. Although this system had myriad steps to achieve fruition, it was well worth the result of open access to PC for Veterans when they needed it.

Context

VA Central California Health Care System (VACCHCS) is a medium complexity-level facility in the heart of California. The health care system provides PC to 26,232 Veterans at CBOCs in Oakhurst, Merced, and Tulare, as well as at a main facility in Fresno. Although the population is ethnically and economically diverse in nature, all patients had commonality in that they were seeking medical care that they could access at their convenience. Veterans and clinic staff wanted to have confidence in a system that could deliver that care in a timely, high-quality manner.

Practice Description

We realized that in our current practice model we were falling short of providing the type of experience that we wanted our Veterans to have. Veterans did not have the relationship with their care team, and they did not have the confidence that their team could see them when they had a medical concern. Fortunately, these realizations coincided with the adoption of the PACT model of care. We embraced the PACT philosophy and aggressively implemented plans to improve our system. There were numerous iterations of plans and Plan-Do-Study-Act (PDSA) cycles, but some of the most important steps included:

1. An analysis of clinic appointment supply and demand was conducted. Initially, backlogs had to be addressed so we could achieve open access.

2. Clinic schedule modifications were performed to balance the need for scheduled same-day access and non-face-to-face care for physicians and nurses.

3. Gains in efficiencies and increased employee and Veteran satisfaction were developed by utilizing nontraditional modalities of care, i.e., telephone encounters, secure messaging, and telehealth solutions.

4. PACT staff was educated about appropriate communication tools and processes to promote patient flow in the clinic and streamline individual visits.

5. Our culture changed from being provider-centered to patient-centered. Today, there is a practice pattern of performing today's work, which translates into seeing patients when they desire to be seen.

6. Definitions of the roles and responsibilities of all PACT members were defined so that team members worked at the top of their competencies and provided enhanced access to Veterans at the right time and the right place.

7. Buy-in from the providers focused on value-added appointments over routine appointments.

8. Routine review of the Pharmacy Benefits Management (PBM) Access to Care Dashboard to ensure that a patient's needs were addressed and that patients saw providers based on their desired timeframe.

9. Effective utilization of extended team members (pharmacist, PC-Mental Health Integration (PC-MHI) team, dietician, social worker, etc.) to get the patient to the appropriate staff member who can best assist them.

10. Discharge documentation was modified to clearly explain to patients the treatment plan, next steps in care, and follow-up. This also reduced unnecessary phone calls and/or appointments that were made for administrative reasons. Teams continued to use the recall system for notifying patients of upcoming appointments.

11. Creation of surrogate and back-up plans to continue open access for patients when team members took leave. Utilization of fee-basis or locum providers for long-term absences.

12. Continuous monitoring of access indices, including new patient appointment availability, so that interventions occur when needed.

These are some of the steps that have led us to an improvement in our access. In FY 2010, we were able to see 21.6 percent of our same-day appointments with the assigned PCP and by FY 2014 we were able to achieve 95.6 percent. We are currently able to offer a wait time for new and established patients, on average, of less than one day.

Replicability

This system has been successful at our facility because our staff is able to understand and embrace that this is beneficial to our patient's health care outcomes and enhances satisfaction rates. The dramatic effect that it has on patients' lives inspires staff and improves their own satisfaction as well. Taking the time to build infrastructure through process work was essential to maximize our chance for success. We were fortunate to have the leadership that could provide appropriate education to the staff, patience to persevere through the large upfront investment in time, and energies required to change decades of culture and past practices, all while weathering the cycles of change to get to our end goal. Any facility can achieve success if they are able to change their culture to a patient-centered culture and create processes that get the patient to the right person at the right time.

Recognition

Vishal Pall, Wei Gu, Mike Bethel, Pamela Many, Wessel Meyer, Vic Lumbad, Shannon Deen, Sabino Medina, Veronica Barragan, Debra Zamora, PC Fresno staff

Mobile Hearing Aid Distance Fitting Application

Allison Amrhein, Innovation Coordinator, Brian Stevenson, Innovation Coordinator

VHA Innovation Program, Washington, DC

allison.amrhein@va.gov

The Hearing Aid Distance Fitting Application (HADFA) practice allows the provider to communicate with the Veteran through video, utilizing either an Android or iOS smart phone, to help the Veteran adjust his/her hearing aids.

Introduction

Audiology clinics are the most overpopulated clinics in VA, with the longest wait times. Veterans often drive two hours each way for available audiology clinic times and then wait an hour for a 15-minute appointment. Several Veterans participating in the Hearing Aid Distance Fitting Application (HADFA) pilot enjoyed coming to VA and found the social aspect rewarding. However, most Veterans preferred to have the opportunity to conduct their 15-minute appointment at home. The impact of HADFA on Veterans in Phase 1 was extremely positive, even when technical obstacles existed. Increased access to audiology care not only affects a patient's hearing, but has the potential to affect other co-morbid conditions related to hearing loss.

Forty-four subjects (mean age = 64.5; min = 32; max = 83) were recruited by audiologists at the Louis Stokes Cleveland VAMC to participate in the Phase 1 HADFA pilot study from September 2013–May 2014. The following direct quotes from Veteran participants include:

- "Very educational, helped adjusting my left aid."
- "Very easy and comfortable process."
- "This cutting edge tech is a wonderful thing!"
- "Saves a lot of time."
- "The process could not have been easier. Only took a few minutes."
- "It was a clear and simple process. The aids I'm wearing are greatly improved. I'm happy to participate in studies that help with progress."
- "This is great. It saved me 100+ miles and three hours of my time. Very convenient and easy."

Key Information

In Phase 1 (completed in 2014), the pilot study prototype enabled audiologists to program a subject's hearing aids from the comfort of the subject's own home using an Android smartphone. The prototype was successful and the connections were robust. Three updates during the study period improved usability and robustness of HADFA. The audiologist successfully connected to the hearing aids in 95 percent of the appointments. The 5 percent of connections that were unsuccessful were due to a dexterity issue and a possible equipment issue (low battery).

In Phase 2 (start date of August 22, 2016), HADFA technology and patient reach expanded. Two prototypes were developed, one for Android operating systems and one for iOS. HADFA will integrate with any existing provider-facing fitting software, and enable video conferencing between Veterans/caregivers and VA medical staff over Wi-Fi. Phase 2 features a pilot at three VAMCs.

Context

Upon completion of Phase 2, HADFA will be available to all Veterans with hearing aids and a smartphone. Approximately 600,000 Veterans are issued new hearing aids per year; over half (336,000) of those Veterans currently have smartphones (56 percent of the total Veteran population). Given the 20 percent increase in general (not just Veteran) smartphone adoption rates from 2011–2014, an assumption can be made that by 2018 (when the application is fully developed) approximately 420,000 Veterans could potentially use the application.

Practice Description

In Phase 2, VACI is supporting further development of the Phase 1 technology to include the addition of video capability and the development of the Apple-compatible version of the application. At the completion of this effort, it is expected that ownership of the technology and process will be transferred to VHA Rehabilitation and Prosthetics Services and Telehealth.

The reach of this effort demonstrates the need for VA partners from both VACO and the field to work together to achieve the goal of increasing access for Veterans. Coordination and teamwork through innovation is itself a strong promising practice demonstrated by HADFA.

Replicability

This practice was selected for national deployment because of the audiology clinic back-up and patient access issues. After Phase 1, we know the technology works and Veterans want to use it. We also assume that Phase 2 will be equally successful, so by its completion, the application will be fully available (hence replicated) nationally.

Recognition

The audiology team at the Cleveland VAMC, Darlene Moenter-Rodriguez, Chris Galizio, Lu Beck, Chad Gladden, Rachel McArdle, Brian Stevenson

The Path to Primary Care Open Access

Timothy Dresselhaus, MD, MPH

VA San Diego Healthcare System, San Diego, CA
timothy.dresselhaus@va.gov

The Path to Primary Care Open Access practice describes a bundle of high-leverage, proven access changes that, implemented together, assure appointment supply exceeds patient demand, the necessary precondition for open access in PC.

Introduction

Dr. O started his VA career in another facility where he was proud to deliver quality care to his patients. He was passionate about his work and dedicated to the VA mission, but his clinic slots were often full and scheduled out into the future. He struggled to provide the kind of timely service he knew his Veterans deserved, and he worked long and late at the expense of his young family.

When he recently joined VA San Diego PC, he encountered a different approach called "open access." Though assigned a full panel of patients, he also had "open" appointments each day and into the future. Using open access, he was able to see patients with same-day needs as well as provide timely care for routine new or follow-up appointments. He was also able to address the administrative tasks in support of his panel during routine business hours. As a result, he started each day on time and left on time. His work satisfaction rose, and his wife and two sons were pleased with the restored family time.

As a result of open access, the majority of practices at VA San Diego have Third Next Availability Appointments (TNAA) of today or tomorrow. Staff satisfaction surveys demonstrate improved morale and reduced burnout, with corresponding reductions in provider turnover.

Key Information

The Path to Primary Care Open Access practice entails the bundled implementation of four high-leverage access changes that favorably impact the demand/supply relationship: 1) respect panels—contingency planning, 2) respect panels—build capacity ahead of demand, 3) reduce annual revisit rate, and 4) validate grids.

Facility-wide implementation of these changes took place at the VA San Diego Healthcare System. This effort was the result of collaborative leadership by the facility Director, the Chief of Staff, the PC Service, and the interdisciplinary PC management team. Implementation has been iterative, with achievement of open access in 2010 and sustainment of open access since that time. This has improved access for Veterans and increased staff satisfaction.

Context

VA San Diego PC serves approximately 65,000 Veterans living in an area extending from Camp Pendleton (to the north) to the border with Mexico (to the south). Delivery of PC occurs at six locations throughout this region. An interdisciplinary leadership triad (physician, nurse, and administrator) leads each site. The effort to achieve and sustain open access addresses the highest strategic priority of VA to provide timely care.

Practice Description

The relationship between access and the demand/supply ratio (utilization) is curvilinear (Erlang's Law); that is, high utilization leads to exponentially rising delays, while lower utilization (lower demand/supply ratio) results in open access. Maximizing utilization and achieving open access are mutually exclusive. Thus, the path to open access requires creating space such that demand is less than supply, with a ratio desirably in the 0.75 to 0.80 range. To achieve this, the determinants of demand (namely, panel size and annual visits per patient) and supply (appointment slots in schedule) are critical and point to four high-leverage access changes (implemented as an access-opening bundle):

1. Respect panels—contingency planning. Insofar as panel size is a key component of demand, respecting panels is a necessary and non-negotiable first step toward open access. Right sizing panels begins with applying VHA PC Management Module (PCMM) standards and determining not to exceed PCMM targets. It further requires that panel-holding positions cover all times. This is assured through robust contingency planning, whereby near- and long-term gaps are seamlessly covered through float/gap providers or locum tenens. Strategy has been successfully applied at VA San Diego to assure consistent panel coverage and respect of panels.

2. Respect panels—build capacity ahead of demand. Panel target might be threatened if capacity is not built ahead of demand, especially for growing practices. To build capacity ahead of demand, VA San Diego projects future capacity and demand to determine thresholds at which new teamlets should receive approval and recruiting to create supply ahead of anticipated demand. This strategy has been especially important to sustaining timely new patient access.

3. Reduce annual revisit rate. The frequency with which patients receive care is a key determinant of demand and is largely under the influence of the care team. This rate can be reduced, and access opened, by employing patient-centered approaches such as max-packing (doing today's work at each visit), extending the return clinic interval, and using alternatives to face-to-face visits (phone, secure messaging, care team).

4. Validate grids. On the supply side, grid validation is a strong practice to assure that panel size (based on time in PC) aligns with the actual clinic schedule. At VA San Diego, a business rule was established to make 85 to 90 percent of clinical time bookable for seeing patients in clinic. This effectively opens up capacity to create space for same-day visits.

Replicability

This bundle of high-leverage access change is rooted in the access dynamics of Erlang's Law and the fundamentals of the demand/supply relationship. The effective implementation of this bundle hinges on the commitment of executive leadership who make critical buy decisions to assure that panels are respected, capacity built, and contingency plans implemented. It requires collaborating with managers and frontline staff to apply business rules around grid validation, and it depends upon interdisciplinary collaboration at the team level to optimize revisit rates. This model can be generalized to any facility where executive leadership, PC managers, and frontline teams are similarly aligned and focused on access improvement.

Recognition

Stan Johnson, Jeff Gering, Robert Smith, Justin Sivill, the interdisciplinary PC leadership team and frontline staff at VA San Diego

Physical Therapy Direct Access for Rehabilitation Services

Mark Hayden, Physical Therapist

VA Central Iowa Health Care System, Des Moines, IA
mark.hayden@va.gov

A Physical Therapy (PT) clinic located within the PC clinic allows direct access to PT services, which improves access, reduces wait times for services, and improves quality of provided services. This practice embodies a team-centered focus to providing care to Veterans.

Introduction

Better health care outcomes come from early intervention, improved multi-disciplinary communication, and the development of an integrative, team approach rooted in patient-centric care planning. This affects all Veterans with acute and chronic health conditions who benefit from receiving the right treatment at the right time. This vision has led to embedding and utilizing direct access from physical therapists within the PACT. Direct access supports early intervention through a collaborative model of care that addresses initial concerns related to pain management, vestibular dysfunction, immediate Durable Medical Equipment (DME) needs, physical inactivity, and neuromuscular challenges, minimizing the risk of falls and further institutional care. Early access to Physical Therapy is associated with lower costs and fewer visits. Musculoskeletal ailments are the number one reason Veterans returning from OEF/OIF/Operation New Dawn (OND) seek VA care, which might increase further with the recent publication of CDC guidelines to reduce opiate use. Direct access is allowed in all 50 states and the District of Columbia, permitting physical therapists to work at height of license. One PC at VA Central Iowa commented:

"It is great! Veterans are getting treatment faster, and assistance with addressing safety issues, as well as decreasing complications from delay in care due to scheduling. No complaints at all and the Veterans are very appreciative!"

Key Information

The team consists of physical therapists and key stakeholders across service lines to include PC, medical support, and nursing staff. The team collaborates to strategically plan for available space, communications, and initiation of the project. This program assists in unburdening PC from evaluating conditions that normally refers to PT. This results in eliminating one patient visit and consult processing time, thus expediting the delivery of specialized rehabilitation care.

Context

This practice assists with proactive health care as well as the maintenance of well-being at the highest level practicable. The collaboration allows for enhanced continuum of care and open communication to facilitate direct access and patient-specific care plans. Additionally, choice and non-VA care utilization for therapy and rehabilitation services occur in a timely manner. This practice improves access and provides the right care at the right time.

Practice Description

The current process is to allow Veterans direct access to PT when they are visiting their PACT team for other functional deficits. The physical therapists currently have a room embedded within our PC PACT teamlets. This innovative strategy allows for walk-in capabilities, immediately taking care of the musculoskeletal, balance, and assistive device. If further treatment is required, it is set up within the PT clinic area for a future date. In both events, the Veteran will get an evaluation with increased access and a head start on treatment to reduce any continued decline in function that they might have had to wait for during a scheduled initial appointment.

Replicability

This has been a transformational program that requires teamwork of many disciplines. VA Central Iowa started implementation on July 1, 2015. In just the short time of initiation, PT evaluations in the surrounding nine counties, which were paid out of non-VA care in FY 2015, averaged 116 per month. So far, in the first quarter of FY 2016, the average has decreased to 55 per month, a 50 percent decrease. The FY 2015 All Fee Purpose of Visit report demonstrated an average cost of $568 dollars per referral. Therefore, the decrease has saved VA Central Iowa an approximate total of $93,720 in the first quarter of FY 2016 alone.

This practice has been part of a transformation that allows for working at the highest level of licensure. In previous national PT calls, the field has heard from other successful sites, which served to enhance the knowledge and spread: Salt Lake City VAMC, Coatesville VAMC, Tampa VAMC, White City VAMC, and Jacksonville Outpatient Clinic (OPC).

Recognition

Mark Hayden, Kathy Young, Lana Martinez, Kevin Quinn, Nisha Patel, Chaz Williamson, Ryan Spreitzer, Chris Rowedder, Mark Havran, Denise Behrends, Bobbi Karr, Glenace Shank, Kevin Massick, Maya Johnston, Angie Goodson, Christian Wyman, Ed Lyle, Jeremiah Moore, Greg Krautner, Curtis Ivins, Arthit Phomachan

Same-Day Clinics for Surgeons

Jennifer Lindsey, MD, Assistant Chief, Ophthalmology Section VA TVHS

Tennessee Valley Healthcare System, Nashville, TN
jennifer.lindsey@va.gov

The Same-Day Clinics for Surgeons program provides Veterans with same-day access for ophthalmology exams, and allows the ophthalmologist to hold open clinic on days when they do not have access to the Operating Room (OR).

Introduction

Mr. X served our country during three tours in Vietnam. He is the proud father of two daughters and even prouder grandfather of three. He is active in his community and helps provide financial support to his family. He earns his living as a long-haul truck driver. His last Department of Transportation (DOT) physical, however, brought bad news. Mr. X did not pass his eye test and couldn't legally do his job. He turned to his VA PCP for help. His PCP entered an eye consult for Mr. X, but warned him that the eye clinic is extremely busy with a significant backlog of patients. He might have to wait several months for an appointment or go outside VA via the Choice program. Mr. X needed this exam as soon as possible so he could get back to work. He considered going to a local pharmacy for an eye exam but was reluctant to pay out of pocket for a service for which he was eligible through VA.

Luckily for the Veteran, the Alvin C. York VA Eye Clinic in Murfreesboro, TN, had just instituted a new program. Thanks to the Same-Day Clinics for Surgeons program, Mr. X was able to get an appointment with an ophthalmologist on the same day that he saw his PCP. His PCP diagnosed him with cataracts and he received cataract surgery. Now, he has 20/20 vision and is able to pass his driver's test without glasses. He can see better now than ever before in his life. When he comes to see his eye surgeon for follow-up, he cannot say enough about how grateful he is to his VA clinic. He even gets a little tearful.

Since its implementation in May 2015, the program has provided timely access to approximately 80 patients per month for ophthalmology exams, over and above the usual clinic volume of 460+ exams per week. Many of these patients go on to have eye surgery or other treatments to help restore and preserve their vision. Though we still have a significant backlog of Veterans awaiting care, we have made an impact. Our patients in the program are grateful to get timely and often expedited care, and our ophthalmologists are gratified to provide much-needed services to our Veterans.

Key Information

The Same-Day Clinics for Surgeons program was implemented in May 2015 in the eye clinic at the Alvin C. York VA Hospital in Murfreesboro, TN. Thelisia Simmons, LPN, and Jennifer Lindsey, MD, led the practice. Collaboration between surgical service, the ophthalmology section, nursing, and business office was critical to the success of the program. The program, in keeping with VA True North key drivers of access, quality, and communication has significantly improved access for our Veterans who need eye care.

Context

The Alvin C. York VA Hospital in Murfreesboro, TN, is one of two facilities to offer eye care in the Tennessee Valley Healthcare System (TVHS), VISN 9. TVHS has approximately 90,000 Veterans who are eligible for eye care services. Of these, many have chronic eye disease, such as glaucoma or macular degeneration, and require multiple visits per year. As a result of the Accelerated Care Initiative (ACI), the Alvin C. York VA Hospital Eye Clinic has grown from two ophthalmologists, one optometrist, three technicians, and one nurse, to five ophthalmologists, one optometrist, nine technicians, and one nurse. Though this expansion has helped provide access to many more of our eligible Veterans, we still have a significant number of patients waiting to be seen. After referral by their PCP, many of these patients travel significant distances to our facility in one of our 11 CBOCs.

Practice Description

Most of our ophthalmologists at Alvin C. York VA Hospital have certain days of the week designated as clinic days, and one day a week for surgical cases. Due to anesthesia staffing and other issues, occasionally an ophthalmologist does not have access to the Operating Room (OR) on his or her designated day. Though there is plenty of administrative and educational work to keep our doctors busy, we knew we had numerous patients waiting, and wanted to offer as much clinic access as possible. This is where the "same-day clinic" idea was born. What if the ophthalmologist could have a clinic open on days when s/he did not have access to the OR? The concept required coordination and cooperation between surgical service, the business office, and the Central Scheduling Unit (CSU). Key people from each of these services had to step outside of their usual routine and perform extra work to make these Same-Day Clinics a reality.

Our clinic nurse and surgical scheduler, identified dates (due to OR unavailability) when ophthalmologists would be available (and have enough space and ancillary support in clinic) to staff same-day clinics. A clinic grid was developed that could be opened on short notice and only when needed for an available provider. The clinic grid was used for same-day clinics and is now accessible as determined necessary. When we see a date that will be available for a same-day clinic, we email the action group to initiate a request. When the appointment slots are opened, usually a few at a time as needed, the eye clinic front desk staff go to work calling in patients who have active ophthalmology consults. Our team directs efforts by highlighting the patients on the active consult list who: may be able to travel to our facility on short notice; have a more pressing issue; and are already in the building for another appointment on the same day (same day referrals from PC or other services at our hospital). The Veterans are offered same-day or near future (within 30 days) appointments and are seen in the clinic.

Replicability

The key factors that make this practice work in our facility are communication, a willingness to think "outside the box," flexibility, a strong work ethic on the part of our physicians, and a strong desire across departments to work together to serve our Veterans. Our colleagues are willing to take on the extra work of opening and scheduling a clinic that is outside of the usual routine. Our doctors have been willing to take on extra clinic loads and to tolerate a great deal of variability in their schedules to make sure we serve as many patients as possible. Other facilities could replicate this practice if they have similar open communication between departments and the willingness to try new things and take on extra work for the benefit of our Veterans.

Recognition

Thelisia Simmons, Kirk Bowles, Bina Patel, Amy Chomsky, Candi Howard, Kelly Shanks, Lola Posey, Linda Napier, Sciara Griffin, Tracie Dimitri, Erika Holsey, Donna Joplin

Sleep Study Access

Rosanna Powers, Program Specialist

North Florida/South Georgia Veterans Health System, Gainesville, FL

rosanna.powers@va.gov

Utilizing Lean tools and principles and working collaboratively allowed quicker access to sleep studies for Veterans.

Introduction

The process for getting patients into a sleep study was so full of bottlenecks that it sometimes took over a year. Our patients were tired and irritable, their spouses were tired and irritated, and they were all seeking answers to their sleep issues. We knew problems in the process existed, but getting results was going to take time, effort, and willingness to accept the necessary changes.

Our team efforts began in July 2014. The team was comprised of a Lean Six Sigma (LSS) group, a champion, process owner, facilitators, and those who touch the process. In the define phase of the project, we assessed the extent of the problem and learned there were over 3,000 patients on the electronic wait list for sleep studies, and that it was taking over 300 days from the day the consult was placed until the sleep study was scheduled. We had many patients waiting a very long time.

After further analyzing the data, we learned that as a result of such a long wait, there were many duplicate consults. After scrubbing for the duplicate consults, the team worked to accommodate some of the patients in the community and managed to decrease the number of patients waiting for a sleep study to 1,000. To improve the process, the team implemented solutions, such as home sleep studies, increased hospital appointments, and redesigned consult trees.

Home sleep studies were effective and more patient-friendly because they eliminated the need to travel and permitted patients to sleep at home in their own beds. The team effectively worked the waitlist and built in new error-proofing techniques to avoid a further backlog. The team recommended a future project on the process after the issuance of the Continuous Positive Airway Pressure (CPAP) treatment, relating to follow-up care where there are additional backlogs. Chartering of the team occurred and improvements are already underway.

Key Information

This promising practice involved breaking down broken processes and implementing improvements using LSS in the North Florida/South Georgia Veterans Health System. Two LSS Green Belt facilitators, with support from the project champion, process owners, and leadership led the team. The promising practice was chartered in January of 2014, with implementation through May 2015. The practice improves broken processes through LSS utilization and keeps the patient and their needs at the center of improvements.

Context

The North Florida/South Georgia Veterans Health System (NF/SGVHS) consists of two medical centers, three large multi-specialty outpatient clinics, eight CBOCs, and one rural health outpatient clinic. NF/SGVHS serves over 126,000 Veterans each year.

Practice Description

In April 2013, over 3,000 Veterans were waiting for a sleep study. The wait time from consult to treatment (CPAP) varied from two months to two years, and the sleep lab was underutilized at 76 percent. The practice entailed chartering an LSS Green Belt team and utilizing the Define, Measure, Analyze, Improve, Control (DMAIC) framework for project completion. The team set objectives to decrease cycle time to 90 days, reducing backlog by 50 percent and providing a means for dynamic/flexible capacity to supplement fixed capacity for sleep studies.

The team learns the intricacies of all pieces of the process through walking the GEMBA (a term used in LSS for direct observation) and process mapping. The team relied heavily on data to make decisions and identify necessary changes. The team worked to remove wastes in the process, implement quick hits, and make major changes in the program. All came together for a successful closeout with reductions in consult to treatment by 87 percent, zero Veterans waiting for a sleep study, a reduction of 93 percent in active/pending consults, and improvement in sleep-lab utilization.

Replicability

We had extraordinary leadership support and engaged staff willing to support a lean culture. Keeping the patient-centered focus and removing barriers were great successes in this practice. Any facility can remove waste from a poor process and implement practices for the betterment of their patients using lean tools, experienced lean facilitators, and top-down support with bottom level ideas and involvement.

Recognition

Naomi Nelson, Rosanna Powers, Chona Macalindong, Emily Beck, Richard Berry, Ashish Prasad, Daniel Harloff, Lorraine Mercier, Donna Stout, Luisa Wertz, Brandi Bearce, Tom Wisnieski, Nancy Reissener, Bradley Bender, Peggy Givens, Maureen Wilke

Increasing Hepatitis C Virus Treatment with Shared Medical Visits

Rachel Rogers, HIV/HCV CPS

South Texas Veterans Health Care System, San Antonio, TX
rachel.rogers@va.gov

A Shared Medical Visit (SMV) allows Veterans with chronic Hepatitis C Virus (HCV) to be treated in a group setting, making treatment more efficient, while maintaining a high level of care. The group visit fosters camaraderie among Veterans undergoing similar experiences, tailors care to meet the Veteran's needs, and promotes an environment of shared information and learning.

Introduction

In South Texas, there is a large population of Veterans with chronic Hepatitis C Virus infection. Due to recent treatment algorithm changes, our facility is now able to offer HCV treatment to all Veterans regardless of stage of liver disease. Previously, some motivated Veterans interested in treatment did not qualify for HCV treatment due to the prioritization of treatment of those patients with advanced liver disease. With this new change, providers were able to offer treatment to all patients, but then another issue arose in providing access to treatment with clinic visits. There were patients who qualified for treatment, but not enough providers to adequately treat in a timely manner.

As part of the HCV treatment process, the Veteran meets with a CPS trained in HCV. The HCV CPS is an integral member in determining which treatment regimens are chosen and if patients qualify for treatment. To increase throughput, the HCV CPS could lead a Shared Medical Visit for patients who did not have cirrhosis. After offering this service, the uptake was immediate and Veterans were grateful for an opportunity to receive care in a quicker fashion.

Key Information

A Shared Medical Visit is a group visit of eight Veterans all with chronic HCV. The patients may be on the same treatment or on a different medication. The commonalities are reviewed first and individual differences are addressed on a patient-by-patient basis. Minimal monitoring is required and no dosage adjustments are needed while on therapy. Patients only need three to four appointments while on treatment, based on duration of therapy. Seeing less complicated patients in a group setting allows the hepatology providers the time needed for patients that are more complicated. Implementation began in April 2016 at the South Texas Veterans Health Care System (STVHCS) at the Audie L Murphy Campus. The SMV is led by the HCV CPS, Rachel Rogers. Dr. Tera Moore, who collaborated with Dr. Rachel Rogers, nursing leadership, hepatology physicians, and logistical support, brought the SMV concept forward. HCV treatment is a national priority in VA. Improving access to care and providing treatment to all Veterans is paramount in the success of this mission.

Context

The STVHCS is comprised of two inpatient campuses: The Audie L. Murphy Memorial VA Hospital in San Antonio and the Kerrville VA Hospital in Kerrville, TX. Together, they act as one of the largest primary service areas in the nation. With over 3,100 employees, South Texas provides primary, secondary, and tertiary health care in medicine, surgery, psychiatry, rehabilitation medicine, and numerous satellite clinics to 93,000 Veterans. The number of Veterans with chronic HCV who needed treatment was not feasible through regular clinic visits; it was a significant challenge to treat all candidates needing treatment in a timely manner. The development of this SMV improved access to care and allowed more Veterans the opportunity to receive care quickly.

Practice Description

SMV meets weekly on Mondays. Veterans who are initiating treatment with HCV medications meet at 9:00 a.m. and follow-up patients meet at 10:00 a.m. At the initial visit, Veterans receive an overview of HCV and its treatment. Medication discussions take place in detail, to include briefly how medications work, anticipated side effects, duration of treatment, and important drug interactions. Veterans then meet individually with the HCV CPS to discuss patient-specific details prior to leaving to pick up the medication from the pharmacy. Follow-up appointments in the SMV review labs, any experienced side effects, the renewal process, and what to expect at the next visit. Finally, at the end-of-treatment visit, labs are again reviewed and the plan for the next 12 weeks is discussed; discussions address Sustained Virologic Response (SVR) or cure, which medications to restart, need for further follow up, and what happens if the patient should relapse. Veterans receive a reminder to return for lab draw to determine SVR.

Replicability

This practice was adopted to increase treatment of Veterans with chronic HCV. This adoption allowed the hepatology practitioners the ability to focus on patients who required closer follow-up in a clinic visit. Veterans were excited for the opportunity to have quicker treatment. Support from pharmacy, physicians, and nursing staff led to the success of this endeavor. Pharmacy leadership assisted greatly in the development of the SMV and coordinated with nursing staff to have the support of a light-duty nurse to assist in taking vitals of the Veterans at the beginning of the SMV. Physicians were available for discussion of patients, as needed. This easily replicable practice could be implemented in other facilities.

Recognition

Tera Moore, Jordan Nelson

Rural Hepatitis C Program

Becky Ashcraft, Rural Hep C Clinic Coordinator

VISN 19: Rocky Mountain Network, Glendale, OH

becky.ashcraft@va.gov

The Rural Telehealth Hepatitis C program allows Veterans access to specialty care and treatment of their chronic Hepatitis C Virus (HCV) at VA clinics within their communities.

Introduction

The Rural Hepatitis C program was Dr. Ken Berman's creation. With a three-year public health grant and support from Dr. Lithium Lin, the program became a reality in 2013. We serve Hepatitis C Virus Seropositive (HCV+) Veterans in rural Colorado, Wyoming, Montana, and Utah by using telehealth technology. The Rural Hep C team was comprised of one attending MD, one NP, and one RN Coordinator. We have service agreements with Grand Junction, Sheridan, Ft Harrison, and Denver to evaluate and treat in all the medical centers and CBOCs/Primary Care Telehealth Outpatient Clinics (PTOCs). In January 2014, we began telemedicine clinics in 15 CBOCs and two VAMCs. Clinical PharmDs in Denver-Grand Junction and Sheridan have been our support in the VAMC and we were the first in the country to mail our HCV medication to patient homes. We have treated over 140 patients and evaluated fewer than 250 rural patients with known HCV. Our program extends to assist with Hepatocellular Carcinoma surveillance and follow-up post Transarterial Chemoembolization/Radiofrequency Ablation (TACE/RFA) for patients in rural communities. We use the HCV-Clinical Case Registries and HCV-Dashboard for locating viremic patients and have the ability to self-consult with provider permission. This allows us to locate and communicate with patients, decreasing the burden on the PCP. The ordering of labs and imaging prior to evaluation helps decease the burden on PCPs and decreases the time between identification and evaluation of treatment candidates. Patients and families are pleased with our 99 percent compliancy rate with lab, medication, and follow-up results.

Key Information

The Census Bureau defines rural as 16 percent of the population living in 90 percent of the country, whereas urban is 84 percent of the population living in 10 percent of the country. VA studies show slightly more than 35 percent of the currently enrolled Veterans live in rural areas of Colorado, Wyoming, Utah, and Montana. The mission of ORH is to improve access to specialty and quality health care for all Veterans through a combination of community-based clinic expansion, increased partnerships with non-VA rural providers, increased use of telemedicine and IT, and a new effort to recruit and retain health care providers to rural areas.

Context

Both patients and providers are accepting telemedicine through use of telehealth technology. Telemedicine serves the large population of Veterans living in rural areas of the VISN, giving them access to specialty care not otherwise available without great burdens of travel and expense. It increases compliancy with recommended treatment regimens and allows patients to have relationships with specialty care providers and support staff. The greatest challenges were the amount of collaborating with the different entities in the VAMCs. PCP and support staff education was important to garner the needed buy-in and support. We traveled to Grand Junction and Pueblo for site visits and used Tandberg to educate staff in more remote areas by joining in staff meetings. Drs. Berman and Redington participated in the Specialty Care Access Network-Extension for Community Healthcare Outcomes (SCAN-ECHO) program, educating medical staff on HCV basics and reviewed case studies as a consulting program for rural physicians.

Practice Description

The Rural Hepatitis C program began in May of 2013 under Dr. Ken Berman as a self-consulting program. To build a patient population, I ran clinical case registry reports and located chronic HCV patients, conducted chart reviews, and selected patients that met criteria for evaluation for HCV treatment in the telemedicine clinic. This meant working with Clinical Application Coordinators (CACs) to set up consults, templated notes, and patient/provider letters. We worked with patient education staff to create a monthly Rural Hepatitis C Patient Education program via telehealth. We held monthly meetings with Dr. Lithium Lin and lab/path supervisor, Veterans Equitable Resource Allocation (VERA) staff, the pharmacy supervisor and clinical PharmDs in the treating facilities, VISN staff, the telehealth supervisor, and PCPs. We collaborated with the telehealth supervisor to schedule staffing and Telehealth Clinical Technicians (TCTs) time with providers. The Rural Hepatitis C program selection begins with a report run from the Clinical Case Registry for HCV. Reports are then categorized according to patients FIB4 and Geno-type. With this information, I review patient charts. Patient selection criteria determined by VA guidelines and American Association for the Study of Liver Diseases (AASLD) are: compliant with current medical regime and appointments, co-morbidities, current test results, age, and imaging that estimates the stage of advanced liver disease. Cost of medication and need for compliance and stage of liver disease have determined treatment needs. PCPs are notified by letter that their patients meet evaluation criteria.

Replicability

The program was adopted in VISN 19 as Dr. Berman understood the demographic and patient population needs as well as the advancing treatment of HCV that would allow patients treatment via telehealth. His initiative, my persistence, and ELT buy-in proved positive factors for VISN 19 rural Veterans. The National Hepatitis Innovative Team has a telehealth group that meets monthly to compose a written process that will help make it easier to create telehealth programs in the future.

Recognition

Kenneth Berman, Lithium Lin, Jay Redington, Marsha Costello, Heidi Cooper-Justus, Emily Oien, Yvette Tong, Katrina Campbell, Nancy Randazzo, Stephanie Welch

Hospital In Home

Andrew Grubbs, MD, Assistant Chief PC, Medical Director

Louis Stokes Cleveland VAMC, Cleveland, OH

andrew.grubbs@va.gov

The Hospital In Home (HIH) program provides an in-home alternative to inpatient hospital care for Veterans who are medically stable but require more advanced or intensive therapy than that provided by Home Based PC (HBPC) or other traditional outpatient care settings.

Introduction

Mr. X is a 31-year-old Veteran of the Gulf War. He received a referral to Hospital In Home from the ED for ongoing treatment of an abscess and cellulitis of the right posterior lower arm/elbow. He underwent a drainage of the abscess, had the wound packed, received the first dose of IntraVenous (IV) antibiotics in the ED, and was discharged to HIH. The HIH team arranged and delivered the IV antibiotics to the home and the HIH RNs made daily visits to repack and dress the wound, ensure that IV antibiotics administration was appropriate, and that the IV site was patent.

On day three of antibiotic therapy, the blood cultures obtained in the ED come back as positive for Staphylococcus Aureus. Clinically, the patient was stable. Placement of a Peripherally Inserted Central Catheter (PICC) line occurs as an outpatient to allow completion of a 14-day course of IV antibiotics at home. The HIH RN staff trained the patient to self-administer the IV antibiotics. This enabled the patient to continue to work each day after the IV antibiotics infused. The HIH program made it possible for the Veteran to avoid hospital admission for IV antibiotics and allowed him to continue to work during his treatment.

Key Information

The goal of the Hospital In Home program is to provide an in-home alternative to inpatient hospital care for Veterans who are medically stable but require more advanced and intensive therapy than provided by Home Based PC services or other traditional outpatient care settings. The pilot initially took place at the Portland VAMC in 1999 and now operates in the Cincinnati, Southeast Louisiana, Philadelphia, and Honolulu VAMCs. In 2015–16, three additional sites established a mentoring relationship with the Cincinnati program, including Providence, San Antonio, and Tampa VAMCs.

These programs used specific funding through the Office of Geriatrics and Extended Care Transition to the 21st Century (T-21) Non Institutional Long-Term Care initiative under the Innovative Models of Care: Patient-Centered Alternatives to Institutional Extended Care.

Context

In general, all the HIH programs were interested in addressing problems related to decreasing inpatient bed-days-of-care, decreasing ED visits, increasing access to care, increasing patient satisfaction, decreasing caregiver stress, and increasing support and education available to patients and caregivers.

A wide variety of VHA settings adopted the HIH model. For example, the Southeast Louisiana program helped fill the void of Veteran care after Hurricane Katrina destroyed their inpatient facility. The Honolulu HIH program helped in a setting of limited inpatient VHA beds in Hawaii. Because Hawaii does not have a VAMC, VA pays to have Veterans admitted to the Tripler Army Medical Center. Tampa adapted the HIH for the Spinal Cord Injury (SCI) patient population. The demand for acute SCI inpatient hospital beds often exceeds the number of beds available. The Cincinnati program was interested in the HIH program initially as a way to decrease the 30-day readmission rate for Congestive Heart Failure (CHF) patients, and it is now recognized as a leading practice by the Joint Commission.

Practice Description

HIH is an innovative patient-centered, cost-efficient program that provides high-quality care to patients that require treatment for acute episodes of illness but are stable enough to be treated in their homes. It offers Veterans more choice in how and where they receive their care, inherently providing a more patient-centric delivery approach. Related studies and Quality Improvement (QI) evaluations have indicated improved access to care, strong patient and provider satisfaction, and suggest greater cost effectiveness.

Veterans are referred from multiple sources, including the inpatient hospital service as early discharges, PC clinics, HBPC, surgical service, or cardiology service and directly from the ED. Veterans are admitted by an MD or NP and initially seen daily by RN staff in the acute HIH model. Veterans can then be seen as often as necessary (usually one to two times per week) for 30 days to allow for rapid interventions in the home setting to prevent ED visits, repeat hospitalizations, and 30-day readmissions. Depending on facility resources, the team consists of an MD and NP, three to six RNs, clinical pharmacist, social worker, dietitian and a program support specialist.

Replicability

There are many benefits to expanding the HIH program to other VHA facilities, including increasing access to care, increasing inpatient bed capacity by avoiding hospital admissions, and reducing inpatient days of care with early discharges. The result is increased Veteran and caregiver satisfaction and lower cost of care.

The single most important factor in the replication of the HIH program is the availability of start-up funding. It is difficult for new programs to develop when they have to compete for local limited funding. In addition, the success of the HIH program is maximally effective when there is local facility leadership support not only during initial implementation, but also in ongoing sustainment of these services. For the programs to flourish, the development of strong relationships with ED, inpatient services, pharmacy, and subspecialty services prior to and during the planning and implementation stages is essential. New programs should utilize a mentoring site to shorten the learning curve during implementation of the service. The program should be sustainable now that it has its own stop code and is included in the Veterans Equitable Resource Allocation (VERA) system.

Recognition

GEC Patient-Centered Alternatives to Institutional Extended Care, Richard Allman, Kenneth Shay, Karen Massey, Susan Lanen, the leaders of each VHA Hospital In Home program

Primary Care Mental Health Integration

Andrew Pomerantz, MD, National Mental Health Director for Integrated Services
VACO, Washington, DC
andrew.pomerantz@va.gov

This nationwide initiative has incorporated care for common mental health conditions into routine PC, increasing the number of Veterans identified with and treated for mental illness within the PC clinic.

Introduction

Mr. X is a Veteran having distressing dreams and daytime memories of his combat experience. His functioning at work has deteriorated, and he has gotten several unsatisfactory reviews. During his PC visit, he screens positive for possible PTSD, and reluctantly agrees to a mental health referral in two weeks. When the day arrives, he does not show up. A week later, his boss claims that he may have to fire him.

Imagine a different scenario: After screening positive for PTSD, Mr. X's PCP asks if he would be willing to meet same-day with a mental health professional that is part of his PC team. Mr. X is hesitant, but agrees. His PCP introduces him to a mental health professional, and it is clear that his PCP trusts this team member. He is pleased to be seen so rapidly without having to go to an unfamiliar clinic, and not have his problems "…blown out of proportion." Together, the three develop an initial plan for Mr. X to improve his functioning at work. Ultimately, he receives the care he needs in a setting he is comfortable with, allowing him to improve his performance at work.

Key Information

Open access Co-located Collaborative Care (CCC) resulted from a performance improvement project at the White River Junction VAMC in July 2004. By 2005, it had won a Gold Award for innovation from the American Psychiatric Association (APA) and later, the Secretary of Veterans Affairs National Champion Award for Advanced Clinical Access. The Office of Mental Health Services selected the program as a promising best practice in 2006. In 2007, the approach combined with another program, Depression Care Management, and became PC Mental Health Integration (PCMHI). The White River model and VA's care management initiatives developed by Mental Health Quality Enhancement Research Initiative (QUERI) and the VISN 4 Mental Illness Research, Education and Clinical Center (MIRECC) are now the gold standard for integrated PC in VA. The Uniform Mental Health Services Handbook mandated PCMHI in 2007 and national implementation began in 2008.

Context

PCMHI now exists in every VA facility and a growing number of CBOCs. Most individuals with mental illness in the US are undiagnosed and untreated. Most are seen only in PC and either decline referral to a specialist or do not engage in treatment after referral. National PCMHI program evaluation has demonstrated an increase in individuals identified and treated for mental illness in PC as well as an increased likelihood of engagement in more specialized care. In many successful programs, this has meant a reduction in the number of Veterans needing referral into specialty care and subsequent increased capacity in those programs. As of the first quarter of FY 2016, 7.3 percent of all PACT patients have been treated as PCMHI patients.

Practice Description

Embedded mental health clinicians are members of the discipline-specific PACT. They serve as expert consultants, providing recommendations to improve care and provide direct assessments and mental health treatment, as needed, for many patients with uncomplicated illness. They also serve to support care for individuals who have received mental health care in specialty clinics and return to PACT for ongoing care. Same-day access as part of a PC visit helps to overcome the stigma and ambivalence often associated with mental health referrals and avoids the attrition associated with referral delays. In addition to addressing mental illness in the PC population, these clinicians support PC efforts in managing other conditions. Care management provides follow-up for individuals undergoing treatment for depression, anxiety, and at-risk alcohol use. Veterans receive periodic calls from a nurse, psychologist, or social worker assessing symptoms and medication adherence and any side effects. Care managers link PCP and psychiatrists, providing medication recommendations to PC.

Replicability

Prior to the policy mandate and special purpose funding in FY 2008, a few facilities adopted PCMHI during a time of ongoing attrition of mental health staff, a rising mental health workload, and the inevitable increased waiting times for care. By reallocating a small percentage of staff to PC, early adopters found that many patients with uncomplicated conditions, who previously would have required the significant resource investment necessary in specialty clinics, could now be treated with a minimum of resource expenditure in PC. This increased capacity and reduced waiting times in specialty care. PCMHI has steadily spread throughout VA and VA is increasingly recognized as a national leader in integrated PC, often seen as a model for other systems. The keys to success include leadership understanding of the program and willingness to provide staffing and space in PACT, clear roles and responsibilities and clinical staff who understand and accept this approach to care and have the skills to work successfully as a member of an inter-professional team.

Recognition

Lisa Kearney, Laura Wray, Kathryn Dollar, John McCarthy, Edward Post, Maureen Metzger, Patricia Dumas

Clinical Pharmacist Reassignment Clinic

Jeff Clark, PharmD, BCPP, Mental Health CPS

VA Eastern Colorado Health Care System, Denver, CO
jeffrey.clark18@va.gov

In 2015, the Denver VAMC had a period of high prescriber turnover in the outpatient mental health clinic, leaving numerous Veterans without a prescriber for medications. The solution was a psychiatric clinical pharmacist-run medication management clinic that provided coverage until their new prescriber saw them.

Introduction

Finding ways to improve access to care has been a top priority for VA. However, access to mental health care has been challenging for many facilities. In 2015, the Denver VAMC experienced a period of high prescriber turnover in its outpatient mental health clinics. This left a considerable number of Veterans without a mental health prescriber and without medications. Veterans without access to their mental health medications are at risk for decompensation, hospitalization, and withdrawal symptoms that could lead to medical emergencies. Many Veterans went without medications while some were forced to utilize Psychiatric Emergency Services (PES) for medication renewals. The corresponding increase in volume of non-emergent visits was unsustainable, placing excessive amounts of stress on mental health clinicians and increasing wait times for the ED, PES, and outpatient pharmacy.

The solution was a pharmacist-run, outpatient clinic for patients who may need short-term medication management by a psychiatric clinical pharmacist until they were reassigned and seen by a new mental health prescriber. This proactive model allowed Veterans to continue receiving their mental health medication without placing an undue burden on the Veteran, mental health prescribers, and outpatient pharmacy. It also provided proof of concept for pharmacist-run mental health clinics, which was a new concept for our Mental Health Service. The success of this clinic has led to the creation of pharmacist-run benzodiazepine taper, stimulant, and medication management clinics. Recently, when our executive leadership reached out to the Mental Health Service to ask what they needed to improve access, their response was, "we want more clinical pharmacists."

Data from this clinic was collected from October 1, 2015, through February 29, 2016. This practice reached 81 unique Veterans and resulted in 152 medication interventions. A majority of the interventions involved medication renewal at 80 percent while 15 percent involved medication adjustments. Another outcome indicated a 21 percent reduction in PES visits during this period.

Key Information

The Pharmacist-Run Reassignment Clinic was implemented on October 1, 2015, at the Denver VAMC. Clinical pharmacists, in collaboration with the mental health outpatient director, led the clinic. The clinic pharmacist ensured that Veterans did not have an interruption in their mental health medications while they awaited reassignment to a new mental health prescriber. This proactive clinic also addressed medication management issues, such as completing a titration/taper, switching medications, managing side effects, and confirming that appropriate labs are monitored. The clinical pharmacist also aided in scheduling Veterans for reassignment to a new mental health prescriber.

Context

VA Eastern Colorado Health Care System (ECHCS) is a Joint Commission-accredited, complexity Level 1A facility, covering more than 44,000 square miles and serving Veterans in Eastern Colorado and surrounding states. The main facility in Denver serves 87,023 unique patients. The clinical pharmacist-run reassignment clinic addressed an access to care issue for Veterans who had lost their mental health prescriber. It also lessened the workload on PES staff to allow them to focus on Veterans with acute conditions (suicidal, homicidal, disability, etc.).

Practice Description

The clinical pharmacist identified Veterans who had lost their mental health prescriber and were almost out of medications. Using a data warehouse, "Medication Exhaustion Report," the clinical pharmacist would outreach to the Veteran to assess their mental health needs. Mental health medications were entered by the clinical pharmacist, along with laboratory orders and return to clinic orders, for scheduling telephone follow-ups. The clinical pharmacist assessed Suicidal Ideation (SI) at each encounter. Referral to a higher level of care was available when the Veteran's needs exceeded the pharmacist scope of practice.

Replicability

This practice can be easily replicated at other facilities with clinical psychiatric pharmacists with a scope of practice. Veterans who are without mental health prescribers can be identified using the data warehouse. This practice could be expanded to areas caring for high-risk or vulnerable Veteran populations, where gaps in medication therapy could lead to patient morbidity or place a high burden on health system resources.

Recognition

Anthony Pepe, Matt Gibu, Rebecca Barnhart, Lisa Smith

Bone Health Team to Improve Access to Osteoporosis Screening and Treatment

Karla Miller, MD, Grant Cannon, MD, Staff Physician
VA Salt Lake City Health Care System, Salt Lake City, UT
karla.miller@va.gov

This virtual bone health clinic improves osteoporosis screening, diagnosis, and treatment, while providing a convenient service to patients without adding copays and additional physician appointments.

Introduction

Mr. X is an 83-year-old Veteran who received a letter regarding bone health from the remote Cheyenne VAMC bone health team based in Salt Lake City, UT. He returned the letter and the attached questionnaire relating to risk factors for fracture. Noting a fracture of his left hip after a ground level fall, he was identified by the bone health team as a high-risk patient for future fractures and met the criteria for osteoporosis. We were able to discuss the importance of treating osteoporosis, and he chose to begin therapy. He was unaware that he had osteoporosis and was a candidate for treatment based on his prior hip fracture, until his encounter with the bone health team.

Osteoporosis is a silent, treatable, chronic, and under-diagnosed medical condition characterized by compromised bone strength, which results in an increase in low-trauma fractures. These fractures, with their associated morbidity and mortality, are of significant medical and economic impact. Key facts about osteoporosis include:

- Osteoporosis is a serious, disabling disease that affects both men and women.

- It is a common misconception that osteoporosis only affects women. In reality, osteoporosis is a disease of aging that affects both genders.

- Osteoporosis screening is recommended for all patients over the age of 50 with risk factors, all men over age 70, and all women over the age of 65.

- Only 40 percent of patients with a hip fracture ever regain pre-fracture level of independence.

- Men represent 30 to 40 percent of all osteoporotic fractures, and men who suffer a hip fracture are two to three times more likely to die than women are.

Key Information

The Salt Lake City (SLC) Bone Health Team was created as part of the Specialty Care (SC) PACT program and has been successful at increasing rates of osteoporosis screening in the SLC area. The team functions in coordination with PCPs. After establishment of a care coordination agreement, the SLC Bone Health Team contacts patients, invites them to enroll, performs risk assessments using the Fracture Risk Assessment Tool (FRAX), orders screening tests, and implements osteoporosis therapies when indicated. Throughout this process, the PCP is informed of actions through notes in the electronic medical record. The initial Bone Health Team in SLC screened 7,644 patients with 975 consultations. In comparing patients screened by the bone health team to patients not screened, there was a substantial increase in all measures of osteoporosis care. The measures include Dual-energy X-ray Absorptiometry (DXA) completion with a 77-fold increase, diagnosis of osteopenia with a 27-fold increase, diagnosis of osteoporosis with a seven-fold increase, and initiation of fracture reducing medication with a nine-fold increase.

Context

Having demonstrated that the SLC Bone Health Team can successfully deliver bone health services to urban and rural Veterans in the SLC system, we evaluated the potential to extend these services to all rural Veterans in VISN 19. We then examined the rural Veterans at risk for osteoporosis by facility. The populations considered at risk for osteoporosis should include all adults over 50. The National Osteoporosis Foundation recommends that all women over 65 and men over 70 undergo a DXA scanning. Developing a more efficient method of screening patients is critical. Our team is developing a system to apply risk assessment measures to this population and to extend the benefits of the bone health team for osteoporosis screening to all rural Veterans in VISN 19.

Practice Description

The current practice allowed us to establish a care coordination agreement with the PC team in the Fort Collins, CO, CBOC. Using this care coordination agreement, at-risk patients are screened using the FRAX tool, and then offered the potential for DXA screening and osteoporosis treatment. Information to the providers is given through notes in the EHR.

Replicability

It is possible to replicate this practice using electronic and telephone communication methods to contact patients and their provider. This allowed the dissemination of the bone health team outside of SLC and created a service enrolling patients at the Fort Collins CBOC using a care management program.

Recognition

Marissa Grotzke, Yanina Rosenblum, Phillip Lawrence, Karla Miller, Phillip Lawrence, Anna Atkinson, Donna Richards

Expanding Stroke Telerehabilitation to Rural Veterans

Andrew Butler, PhD, PT, MBA, FAHA, Professor and Senior Research Scientist

Atlanta VA Health Care System, Decatur, GA
andrewbutler@gsu.edu

This practice seeks to serve rural Veterans who are recovering from stroke using home-based, telerobotic-assisted devices to improve functional ability and quality of life, while improving access and cost savings.

Introduction

As the second leading cause of death worldwide and the leading cause of long-term disability, stroke creates an enormous financial and emotional burden on survivors, their families, and the health care system. Accounting for an estimated $1 billion in total annual VA costs, an estimated 15,000 Veterans are hospitalized annually for strokes, with half of survivors experiencing moderate to severe physical impairment and loss of quality of life.

Due to the need for frequent and long-term care, stroke has an even more pronounced burden in rural areas due to a lack of access. The VHA ORH will be responsible for an estimated annual 4,400 new stroke cases, requiring an estimated $25.6 million in outpatient care in the first six months after a stroke incident, in addition to the care of an estimated 22,600 existing rural stroke survivors. In an effort to expand care for rural Veterans with limited access to rehabilitation services, the Mentor Pro robotic therapy device actively engages Veterans in neurorehabilitation through task-specific goal-oriented skilled therapeutic exercises masked as video games. By eliminating transportation barriers, the ORH-funded project, "Expanding Stroke Telerehabilitation to Rural Veterans," investigated operational feasibility of delivering the Mentor Pro in-home telemedicine solution to people in rural Georgia and Alabama, resulting in increased functional independence, highly-satisfied Veterans motivated to complete prescribed exercises, improved access to care, and reduced per-capita health care costs. Use of the robotic rehabilitation telemedicine device has shown to increase the number of Veterans receiving physical rehabilitation by 116 percent, while reducing costs by 61 percent, with potential annual savings of $8 million in a national deployment.

In our recent practice, Veterans articulated an overall increase in functional ability and mobility from the use of the robotic devices. One Veteran remarked, "I noticed a difference almost immediately," while another mentioned, "It loosened up my leg a lot ...you see I can move my leg now." In some cases, Veterans ascribed significant gains in functional ability and improvement in quality of life because of the telerehabilitation robotic device; in some, functional mobility improved so much that they were able to walk considerable distances. One user recounted, "I couldn't move anything but now I can do all of this...I can go up and down the ramp out there now four times by myself...I couldn't do anything before."

Key Information

Between 2013–2015, Dr. Andrew Butler, research scientist at the Center for Visual and Neurocognitive Rehabilitation at the Atlanta VAMC and professor of physical therapy at Georgia State University, along with clinicians at the Trinka Davis Veteran Village, Blairsville, GA, CBOC, and Birmingham, AL, VAMC investigated a new way to rehabilitate the limbs of stroke patients using a specially designed robotic exoskeleton. This therapeutic device consisted of an actively assisted exoskeleton to strengthen the arm or foot paired with the visual feedback from a responsive, intelligent display, enabling enhancement of brain connections as part of the rehabilitation. The portability and connectivity of the device allowed for an in-home deployment. The Mentor Pro telerehabilitation robotic device has been shown to improve access to Veterans residing in rural areas who may otherwise have limited access to rehabilitation services after sustaining a stroke. The promising practice aimed to create a National Rural Stroke Telerobotic Rehabilitation Initiative Headquarters in Atlanta, GA, to establish, coordinate, train, sustain, and promote stroke telerobotic rehabilitation services at nationwide expansion and sustainment sites in Birmingham, AL, Carrolton, GA, and Blairsville, GA.

Context

This practice is headquartered at the Atlanta VAMC. Through partnerships with rural CBOCs in Carrolton, GA (Trinka Davis Veteran Village), Blairsville, GA, and Birmingham, AL, and with the assistance of additional clinician referral sources, this project has gained exposure across the southeastern US. The devices improved access to rehabilitative activities for rural Veterans with limited access to services, increasing the number of Veterans receiving physical rehabilitation by 116 percent. By providing an engaging and interactive therapeutic interface while eliminating the transit burden to centralized therapy services, the practice attained high Veteran satisfaction, improved clinical outcomes, increased access, and reduced costs. By providing remote therapy, the hand or foot peripheral component (HM/FM) devices alleviate time a Veteran spends without care due to therapist or appointment shortages.

Practice Description

Veterans participating in this practice were given use of a home-based robotic rehabilitation device for a maximum of three months and instructed to perform two hours of daily Robotic Assisted Therapy (RAT). RAT was delivered in the home telerehabilitation program using either a hand or a foot peripheral component (HM and FM, respectively) that connected to a computer to play video games onscreen. Veterans were instructed to start at low activity levels performed for one-hour daily and to increase to two hours per day within the first week. Veterans were able to take advantage of RAT flexibility by completing the daily prescription in a single two-hour session or in multiple sessions if their schedules prohibited the full dosage of therapy in a single session. The device recorded information, such as the range of motion achieved while playing the games, time spent using the device, and game scores.

A therapist trained in robotic therapy received referrals from collaborating physicians or NPs who pre-screened Veterans in their clinics. The therapist then arranged an in-home set-up and trained the Veteran and his or her caregiver on how to use the device and access the games. Veteran's device use and progress toward achieving greater wrist or ankle range of motion angles were remotely monitored through telemedicine by a therapist who called the Veteran weekly to discuss use and progress, provide encouragement, and address any issues or questions. The therapist was also able to assign and modify daily exercises to focus on specific areas or to motivate the Veteran as was clinically appropriate. Through a computer dashboard, the therapist was able to visualize Veteran progress and through weekly progress updates, the referring clinician was updated on each Veteran's progress.

Replicability

Leveraging staff and knowledge from existing local expansions and strong local administrative relationships, the Atlanta VAMC is an ideal headquarters for the National Stroke Telerehabilitation Initiative. No additional hires are necessary to incorporate this promising practice, as key project personnel can be reallocated from trained existing staff. Regional collaborations with researchers from the University of Georgia structured participant and clinician interviews. The project has also fostered a strong relationship within industry; the Mentor Pro robotic therapeutic device manufacturer has pledged technical support for all sustainment and expansion sites. Future projects looking to replicate and develop the success of the practice should focus on fostering strong relationships with referral sources in regional CBOCs and developing collaborations with industry and educational supporters who can provide technical and knowledge-based insights to adapt the project's aims to region specific needs. The promising practice has been a success due to improved outcomes, patient and therapist satisfaction, and local physician and therapist champions.

Improved clinical outcomes, high Veteran and therapist satisfaction, and the practice's ability to increase access and reduce costs should aid in replication at other facilities, both from a clinical and financial standpoint. From an operational standpoint, due to the nature of telerehabilitation and its mostly remote workflow, this practice has the unique position to extend centralized support services to new facilities. That is to say, existing Atlanta staff can provide both technical and patient support to expansion sites, thus dramatically decreasing the barrier to participation by integrating into existing workflows and eliminating the need to hire new staff. The Atlanta therapist remotely monitoring and managing Veteran care in Georgia and Alabama can easily extend those services to a Veteran in Montana or Oklahoma. Overall, we believe that this practice is highly replicable at future facilities from the perspective of reducing financial burden, improving clinical outcomes, and receiving operational support from Atlanta and existing sites.

Recognition
VACI, ORH

Training Community Clergy Partners to Increase Access to Care for Rural Veterans (Rural Clergy Training Program)

Keith Ethridge, Associate Director
National Chaplain Center, Hampton, VA
keith.ethridge@va.gov

The goal of the Community Clergy Training Program (CCTP) is to train community clergy partners to increase support for mental health and access to care for rural Veterans.

Introduction

Every community across the country has a house of worship, but many do not have health care facilities. On March 2, 2016, the National VA Chaplain Center and the US Army Reserve hosted chaplains and chaplain assistants from across the US representing all three divisions of the US Army. They met for a two-day Rural Clergy Training Program (RCTP) train-the-trainer seminar, which focused on reducing the risk of Veteran suicide and supporting Veteran mental health. The training educates community and military chaplains about the unique needs of Veterans, who often approach their religious leaders when coping with difficult issues, rather than seeking mental health support. The training provides coaching for religious leaders on methods for making appropriate referrals to military or VA health care services. Follow-up surveys suggest the training has a measurable effect of getting more Veterans the mental health care support they need. Trained clergy increased their VA referrals by 64 percent and their community health care referrals by 41 percent, according to preliminary data.

Participants have praised the training, saying it helped them understand how to better support Veterans in their community. "This is what we need to be able to reach our community, to help our Veterans, our soldiers and family members walk through difficult situations," said one participant. Another agreed, "It helped me to understand what was available to Vets through VA. It opened my eyes for things to look for especially with family members of Vets with PTSD. It helped me to better understand one of our parishioners who has PTSD from his service in the Korean War."

Participants have returned to their communities and active duty units to train other clergy. Using the knowledge and materials provided, they are leading small groups, where they discuss the unique local experiences of Veterans they encounter. This represents a significant expansion of the program, which also includes online trainings, a regular newsletter, and relevant webinars with expert speakers.

Key Information

In 2012, the National VA Chaplain Center and ORH collaborated to create the RCTP, through which more than 200 civilian clergy conducted training workshops at rural VAMCs. In its first two years, the training program delivered in-person workshops to clergy in 23 rural communities across the US. The program grew in recent years, reaching more than 1,000 participants with recurring online trainings. It also expanded to include train-the-trainer sessions, which create regional ambassadors who bring their knowledge to other clergy in their communities. This promising practice established a toolkit and web-based training model to educate clergy about the role they can play increasing rural Veterans and their families' access to care, and the signs that a Veteran may be in need of medical support. Through the initial training, supplemental webinars, and newsletter updates, program participants learn about the issues that the Veteran community faces. This program does not try to transform clergy into diagnosticians; rather, it educates rural clergy about VA and the community resources available and helps clergy understand the problems Veterans may develop due to military service. Clergy are being trained to recognize common symptoms of crisis and struggles with transition, including PTSD, military sexual trauma, and moral injury.

Context

More than 5.2 million Veterans live in rural areas. While rural life provides benefits, such as a tight-knit community and less crowding, research shows that rural Veterans experience a higher risk of suicide. Because they face greater geographic barriers to accessing health care, many search for assistance closer to home at local houses of worship. "Clergy are a trusted source for counsel and often the first-line contact in small, rural communities. The confidentiality they provide is important to Veterans, especially when discussing mental health issues," stated program lead Chaplain Keith Ethridge. However, clergy are often not aware of how to discuss common issues that Veterans face and often lack the knowledge about how to connect Veterans to mental health resources. This practice helps clergy in meeting that need.

Practice Description

In its first two years, the National Chaplain Center in Hampton, VA, and the Veterans Rural Health Resource Center in Gainesville, FL, collaborated to develop a training curriculum and reusable communications materials, organize and conduct in-person workshops, analyze data, conduct outreach, and do post-training evaluations. Webinars were also created. Training topics included re-adjustment and health care needs of combat Veterans, PTSD, the impact of stigma in seeking mental health care in rural communities, and how to refer Veterans to VA health care. Local outreach, by direct mail and relationship building, attracted the first classes of clergy to the trainings.

Based on the popularity of the webinars, increasing demand for training, and limitations of travel in rural areas, the program has focused on broader distribution of the training. Program organizers adapted the curriculum to an online format and created four recorded classroom-style modules, each covering a specific topic. In partnership with the VA Office of Informatics and Analytics, more than 800 participants inside and outside VA joined session broadcasts. Program organizers continue to provide support and guidance, while local champions recruit participants for group viewing sessions of the recorded online trainings. Increasingly, community organizations with established grassroots networks (the Church of God, the National Guard, etc.) and these local champions volunteer for train-the-trainer sessions to learn how to talk to other clergy about Veteran and military health issues.

Replicability

To earn the designation of Rural Promising Practice from the ORH, this program demonstrated 1) improvement in access to care; 2) evidence of improved direct program impact or clinical results for Veterans; 3) patient, provider, and/or caregiver satisfaction; 4) return on investment via reduced costs of care, but not at the expense of quality; 5) operational feasibility and replicability at other facilities or service sites; and 6) strong partnerships or working relationships that maximize efficiency or effectiveness.

The training program successfully created a tested and proven curriculum with support materials and used those resources to evolve from local in-person workshops to moderated viewing events of pre-recorded My VHA eHealth University (VeHU) sessions as well as train-the-trainer workshops. Results of work in FY 2015 indicate that facilitated My VeHU viewing events are an effective method to deliver training to rural clergy, and that community partners can organize and lead successful events when provided with program guidance, tools, and materials. Due to the success of the initial viewing, and with continued partnership support, program organizers have also helped organize a dozen additional viewing events, further making the program's services accessible to those who lack the ability or means to travel to live gatherings. Organizers are also creating more ways for participants to stay involved and continue sharing what they have learned. National partners will also receive a toolkit of educational and process materials to lead their own community "viewing events" using the My VeHU videos. These reusable resources and evergreen online trainings ensure that the program is replicable to any clergy members who want to learn more about Veteran and military-specific health, and how to connect those in need to the appropriate resources.

In 2016, program staff will supplement the My VeHU "Rural Chaplains and Clergy Caring for Veterans" training series with additional sessions from the My VeHU catalog. They also plan to collaborate with VA Health Services Research and Development Charleston Health Equity and Rural Outreach Innovation Center (HEROIC) to conduct research designed to evaluate the clinical impact of the training program.

Recognition

The administrators, practitioners, and partners who serve Veterans using this rural promising practice. For more information, visit www.ruralhealth.va.gov

VISN 12 Centralized Rural Telepharmacy Program

Sandra Calenda, PharmD, CACP, CPS; Dana Frank, PharmD, CGP, CPS; Helen Kasimatis, PharmD, CPS

Edward Hines Jr. VA Hospital, Hines, IL
sandra.calenda@va.gov

All Veterans deserve uniform access to care, including clinical pharmacy services. The use of centralized telepharmacy (i.e., Clinical Video Telehealth (CVT), telephone, e-consults, secure messaging, etc.) enables equal access to pharmacist Comprehensive Medication Management (CMM).

Introduction

A 65-year-old Veteran presents to his PC clinic for routine follow-up. At that time, his A1C is noted to be 11.9 percent. This patient has a long-standing history of poorly-controlled diabetes as indicated by A1C greater than 9 percent. The patient is referred to the CPS for diabetes management, as he needs his A1C to be under 8.5 percent to proceed with a much-needed rotator cuff repair surgery. Within three months of working with the CPS, the patient's A1C drops to 7.9 percent, the lowest A1C this patient has had in six years. The patient is able to have his surgery. This is just one of many patients who have seen improvement in their chronic disease state management after working with a CPS.

The benefits of utilizing a CPS in Medication Therapy Management (MTM) are well documented in literature. Due to the smaller patient panels and rural locations, many CBOCs within VISN 12 did not offer clinical pharmacy services until this program was initiated. With this program, patients at these CBOCs now have the same access to pharmacist provided MTM, as do their counterparts at the main facility.

Of the 86 patients actively being managed for diabetes in FY 2015, the average A1C went from 8.9 to 7.8 percent after the patients began follow-up with a CPS. Of the patients with A1C greater than 9 percent, and at highest risk of diabetes complications, the average A1C went from 10.5 to 8.2 percent, before and after CPS services. Positive blood pressure and lipid outcomes have been noted as well. Furthermore, many patients have had medication reviews, which is critical among the aging and medically-complex patient population.

Key Information

The Centralized Rural Telepharmacy program was initiated within VISN 12 in 2013. Initially, the CPS piloting the program provided virtual modality care for a CBOC at Hines VA, at Tomah VA, and at Iron Mountain VA. The implementation was a joint effort between the VISN 12 pharmacy executive and pharmacy leadership at each participating site. Due to the success of the initial pilot, the program has expanded to include two additional CPSs and now provides care to seven rural CBOCs.

Context

This program serves rural Veterans assigned to CBOCs within VISN 12. In total, approximately 17,400 enrolled patients at the sites are impacted by this project, with approximately 9,500 Veterans being enrolled at CBOCs that previously had no CPS services. The use of Clinical Video Telehealth, telephone clinics, e-consults, and secure messaging allows for the matching of panel size to the appropriate allocation of CPS with a scope of practice. The use of technology enables coverage of multiple CBOCs by CPSs, thus improving access and operational efficiency. The CPS is well positioned to undertake complex medication management cases, which aid to increase access to the PCP for more acute issues.

Practice Description

In March 2013, a centrally-based CPS began to provide care to rural CBOCs within VISN 12. The stakeholders included the VISN 12 Network Director, VISN 12 Pharmacy Executive, facility Chiefs of Staff, facility PC leads, and facility pharmacy leadership at each of the participating sites (Tomah, Hines, and Iron Mountain). Patient encounters were completed via CVT and telephone; e-consults and secure messaging options were initiated during this pilot. Due to smaller patient panels at the participating CBOCs, one FTE CPS was able to initiate and provide all the clinical pharmacy services for two CBOCs and further expand services for an additional CBOC utilizing existing infrastructure and resources.

Due to the success of the initial pilot, two additional CPSs began to support the program in December 2014, which allowed for expanded coverage to additional rural CBOCs. The individual CPSs were able to create rapport with their providers via teleconference, face-to-face meetings, and electronic communication. The existing positive culture within VISN 12 between CPSs and PCPs, the positive working relationship, and the available technology has allowed the CPS to provide MTM services to rural areas, successfully narrowing the gap for PC by using telepharmacy.

Replicability

Within VISN 12, the program has been successful for a number of years and the utility of this program is well known. The collaboration of many different parties was needed to implement this program. Guidance created by this program in the form of a checklist has been previously published and can be used to assist in the logistical setup. The CPSs involved in the program had been in a direct patient care role within VA for some time prior to implementation, which likely added to the success of the program due to prior experience in starting and managing clinics. With supportive leadership and telehealth infrastructure, this telepharmacy program can be expanded to any VA facility in need of services.

Recognition

Donna Leslie, Lea Morgan, James Rice, Julie Stein

Home Interdisciplinary Telerehabilitation Team

Don Hayes, Physical Therapist

VA Central Iowa Health Care System, Des Moines, IA
donald.hayes2@va.gov

Using video technology, Veterans are provided rehabilitation through a comprehensive team, including physical, occupational, and speech therapies. Providing these services in the Veteran's home for those living in rural areas improves their access to care.

Introduction

VA Central Iowa is located in a rural area. Rural health populations have traditionally been medically underserved. Research shows that rural Veterans have a higher incidence of physical illness and co-morbidities and lower scores on health-related quality of life measures than their urban counterparts. Despite greater health care needs, rural Veterans are less likely to access health services through VA or the private sector. Key barriers are lack of transportation, the distance to VA facilities, lack of telehealth services, lack of specialty services, inadequate knowledge of VA eligibility and services, difficulties in recruitment and retention of health care providers, and an increasing need for outpatient services.

This project supports an experienced Interdisciplinary Rehabilitation Team, including a physical therapist, occupational therapist, and speech pathologist embedded within a Hospital Based PC (HBPC) PACT. The vision is that the team will complete the environmental and physical assessment required for the External Peer Review Program (EPRP) with subsequent rehabilitation visits utilizing virtual care technologies. The project includes a model for improved identification and selection of prosthetics for patient safety and function in the home by rehabilitation professionals. Protocols, procedures, guidelines, and handbooks for home evaluation and treatment will be disseminated to the field to assist other sites in establishing similar programs.

Veteran and spouse feedback shows increased customer satisfaction:

"I can't believe that I just saw my doctor yesterday and you are already here the next day to take a look at what I need for my bathroom. Last time this took five months and I almost gave up on the whole thing. I need this stuff to get in and out of my shower."

"It is so great that you can come into my home to take care of my husband because it is so hard to get him in and out of the car."

Key Information

The Interdisciplinary Rehabilitation Team works under the overall programming of VA Central Iowa's Home Base PC Specialty PACT. The team includes physical therapists, occupational therapists, telehealth coordinators, and speech pathologists embedded within our Home Base PC Specialty PACT. Additional technical advice came from VACO leads in physical, occupational, and speech therapy. The providers then collaborated with the telehealth Medical Support Assistant (MSA) for optimal scheduling to include the Veteran's availability as well as travel time to and from the Veteran's home to ensure minimal to no overtime costs for the facility. The Rural Health Telehealth Clinical Technicians (TCTs) worked in collaboration with the Facility Telehealth Coordinator (FTC) and Nurse Manager (NM) to arrange travel and home visits. Under the direction of the FTC and NM, the TCTs were trained on the use of essential telehealth equipment needed to complete the visits. The FTC issued the tablets while providing training to the TCTs.

Context

This new and current process allows for use of technologies, such as Transportable Exam Station (TES) units, tablets, and Clinical Video Telehealth (CVT). This process has allowed for savings of drive time yet ensuring the right care at the right time. This process allows for programs, such as Hospice/Palliative, Geriatric Patient Aligned Care Team (GeriPACT), Spinal Cord Injury (SCI), and others to utilize a similar program.

Practice Description

Scheduling occupational therapy home safety evaluations now happens within two to three weeks. Veterans are seen within two weeks and photographic images are obtained by the Rural Health TCTs under the direct and live guidance of the trained therapist. Real-time communication via video maximizes the opportunities with every visit. Education is provided to the Veteran in their home.

PT is now able to see Veterans in their homes for postsurgical therapy sessions, home exercise instruction, and follow-up across our service area. Speech therapy is now able to provide voice therapy with the expansion of two methods provided by telehealth. The therapy may take place with the Rural Health TCT or with tablet capability.

Replicability

In the third and fourth quarters of FY 2015, 238 rural Veterans were served. The number of rural encounters equaled 1,143, of which 521 were via telehealth. This is a 30 percent increase in total visits and a 55 percent increase in telehealth visits from first and second quarters to the third and fourth quarters of FY 2015.

The telehealth encounters saved an average of 57 miles per visit. This translates into 29,697 miles saved for our clinicians as well as a cost savings of $17,075 in travel reimbursement. The team has presented on national training calls and the recorded sessions are available at http://www.rstce.pitt. edu/varha/.

In addition, the information was shared with the British National Health Service in collaboration with VISN 23.

Recognition

Mark Havran, Roberta Patterson, Pamela South, Kirsten Johnson, Donald Hayes, Kristen Ganfield, Joel Kennedy, Amy Ballou, Whitney Welp, Jamie Flatness, Roxanne McGee, Bobbi Karr, Ann Touney, Jennifer Hagerty, Jeremy Putzier, Nan Musson, Deb Voydetich

National Electronic-Consults Implementation

Susan Kirsh, MD, MPH, National Director Clinic Practice Management and Access; Katherine Williams, MPH, Health Science Specialist; P. Michael Ho MD, PhD

VHA Office of Specialty Care, Washington, DC
susan.kirsh@va.gov

Electronic-consults (E-consults) may improve the overall patient experience of care by reducing inconvenience and wait times for specialist consultation. E-consults provide an opportunity to improve care coordination for patients because of better PCP-specialist communication.

Introduction

The Office of Specialty Care supported the implementation of electronic-consults through pilot grants and weekly calls to increase the use of E-consults nationally. An E-consult is a request for specialty input on a patient regarding medications, tests, or a specific management question. This program was initiated in 2011 with an intent to replace face-to-face consults, as clinically appropriate, and with the goal of increasing patient convenience. The Specialty Care Evaluation Center (funded by the Office of Specialty Care and Health Services Research and Development) worked to identify the impact of the E-consult program. Providers, including both specialists and PCPs were surveyed to gain their perceptions of the impact of the E-consult program on patients and their own engagement.

What was revealed is the E-consult program has affected many aspects of care delivery. Almost two-thirds of clinicians (doctors, NPs, and physician assistants) agreed that the program increased their efficiency and allowed more time for patients that needed face-to-face visits. This was corroborated by data on patients who received an E-consult, where 43.2 percent were less likely to have subsequent face-to-face visits with the same specialty within three months following the E-consult. "It was the simplest and best thing to do for my patients; we welcomed it as a way to formally document work and make visits efficient." "I like E-consults, they're very detailed, the information they give you is educational." Nearly 63 percent of PCPs surveyed reported that the program had improved quality of care and care coordination for Veterans, and a similar proportion, 62 percent, agreed that E-consults improved access to specialty consultation for Veterans. Both PCPs and specialists shared they preferred fewer face-to-face visits and the Veterans appreciated less travel to get specialist input in their care. "It's another way of getting care to the patient when the patient needs it, without them having to wait for another appointment." For CBOCs during the time period of 2011 to 2014, approximately 6,875,631 total travel miles were saved and $2,853,387 in potential travel reimbursement costs were avoided as a result of E-consults.

Key Information

E-consults were developed to provide PCPs with a mechanism to ask advice and input from medical and surgical specialists through the EHR without the need for direct face-to-face visits. The goal of E-consults was to provide specialty care more efficiently, timely, and locally through enhanced coordination with PC. Weekly calls were held with the initial 12 sites implementing E-consults and the program office to support E-consult implementation by sharing progress and lessons learned. E-consult implementation required robust negotiation between local PCPs and specialty care clinicians at sites upon initiation.

Context

The delivery of patient-centered specialty care is challenging, particularly in a large geographically dispersed integrated health care system, such as VA. Of the 8.3 million Veterans receiving services annually, nearly 50 percent see one or more specialists. With specialists located predominantly in urban medical centers, Veterans often need to travel to receive specialist care or see a community provider, which may lead to challenges in coordination of care. The use of E-consults specifically targets the 41 percent of Veterans who live in rural areas. Patients in rural areas often have difficulty accessing specialty care and encounter problems with care coordination.

Practice Description

The E-consult program was initially implemented in May 2011 at 12 VAMCs in seven VISNs for specialties, including oncology, diabetes, endocrinology, dementia, neurosurgery, cardiology, hematology, liver transplant, pain medicine, and rheumatology. Later, the program became a national priority as a component of VA goals for Patient-Centered Care and Specialty Care Transformation worked with VISN leadership to expand the program nationally. Currently, there are 150 medical centers and 121 of these are utilizing E-consults for 58 specialties.

In most E-consult cases, the PCP will talk to the patient about the specialist's suggestions. This is a program benefit because the provider has a treatment relationship with the patient and can integrate the recommendations from the specialist into the Patient-Centered Care (PCC) plan. In the beginning, the Office of Specialty Care sat down with individuals from primary and specialty care to understand the most effective way to develop and implement the E-consult program. Additionally, the sites that were the most successful in utilizing the program also had specialists at the beginning of the program implementation sit down with PC and discuss the process of an E-consult and identified collaboratively who would be responsible for components, and whether using an electronic note template would be helpful.

E-consults may improve the overall patient experience by reducing inconvenience and waiting times for specialist consultation. E-consults promote the use of a standardized referral process with iterative communication that can lead to increased effectiveness of care delivered. E-consults provide an opportunity to improve care coordination for patients because of better PCP-specialist communication. In addition, when combined with the capabilities of an EHR, it is possible to identify populations who would benefit from additional specialty care expertise. "Consultation" may be pre-emptive, thereby avoiding preventable morbidity. This population management approach will need to be evaluated prospectively.

E-consults may reduce the per-capita cost of health care from the health care system perspective. Reductions may be accomplished by improved efficiency when using high-cost specialists. On the other hand, increased access to specialists may result in increased testing and consequent expense; health care value may improve, albeit without reducing costs. Additionally, efficiency may be improved by better coordination of care and less fragmentation of care.

Replicability

Since the initial pilot site implementation, the E-consult program has been replicated at most medical centers across VA. Given feedback from pilot sites that different amounts of time necessitated different workload credit options, the Office of Specialty Care supported enhanced workload credit. This change was very important in helping to make this program spread across VA.

The implementation of E-consults is a potential mechanism for VA to achieve the "triple aim" for optimizing health care delivery to improve patient health care experience and the health of the patient population while balancing per capita cost.

Recognition

Mike Doukas, Len Pogach, the Specialty Care Evaluation Center

Telehealth Patient Aligned Care Team Clinical Pharmacy Specialists

Jessie Litke, PharmD, BCPS, TelePACT CPS; Katie Erickson, PharmD, BCPS, TelePACT CPS, Telehealth Pharmacy Program Manager

VISN 20: Northwest Network, Boise, ID

jessica.litke@va.gov

Utilizing telehealth modalities, incorporation of CPSs on a Telehealth Patient Aligned Care Team (TelePACT) improves Veteran access to care and continuity of care.

Introduction

"You guys have given me more appointments and care than I have ever received before, and I've been at VA for a while. You guys are the top of the pinnacle." This direct quote is not an uncommon statement to hear from Veterans seen by Telehealth Patient Aligned Care Team CPSs within the Telehealth Hub. Unfortunately, multiple sites in VISN 20 struggle to retain PCPs, leaving Veterans with no designated PC team and disjointed follow-up.

One such example is Mr. X. The last contact he had with VA was an Emergency Room (ER) visit in August 2015, where his blood sugars and subsequent A1C revealed he had diabetes. The results were forwarded to his provider, but his provider was a locum that had recently left. He fell into the gap and the message was lost. As a patient now assigned to a Telehealth Hub panel with a TelePACT CPS, the CPS team caught his lab result during a regular review of the team's diabetes registry. He is now on medications; has had multiple Clinical Video Telehealth (CVT) and phone meetings with the TelePACT CPS, team nurse, and dietician; and is scheduled to see his PCP. These interventions are the product of a functioning telehealth CPS on a PACT. Through increased access, and a shared workload, the Veteran receives comprehensive care.

Key Information

VISN 20 is the most remote region in the country and struggles to maintain PCPs. The Telehealth Hub started as a pilot in FY 2014 through a grant from the Office of Connected Care. Based in Boise, ID, the Telehealth Hub provides PC teams to VA sites in VISN 20, providing rural Veterans improved access to PC services. Functioning under the PACT model, the Hub includes the following team members: MD/DO/NP/PA, PCPs, CPSs, psychologists, LCSWs, and Medical Support Assistants (MSAs). During FY 2015, the TelePACT CPS component grew to six pharmacists. This entailed collaboration among the Boise VA Telehealth Pharmacy Program Manager, Telehealth Operations Manager, Associate Chief of Pharmacy for Clinical Services, and Chief of Telehealth Services. The primary function of the TelePACT CPS on the team is to conduct direct patient care focusing on chronic disease management. In addition, the TelePACT CPS is an integrated member of the PC team who attends team meetings, collaborates with the team for panel management, and acts as a real-time drug information specialist. The Hub overall has demonstrated improved access through the empanelment of over 15,000 Veterans and more than 3,200 PC visits in the first quarter of FY 2016 alone.

Context

While the Telehealth Hub is located on the Boise VA campus, we are a VISN 20 resource. Currently, the TelePACT CPS team provides service to 14 different VA clinics composed significantly of rural and highly rural Veterans. The TelePACT CPS addresses the difficulty Veterans have accessing PC services in VISN 20 by providing stable, longitudinal, chronic disease management at these sites through telehealth and serving as a team provider with prescribing privileges within a scope of practice. This facilitates continuity of care and increases access while the site recruits permanent staff or secures telehealth providers on a permanent basis.

Practice Description

PACT team members may refer patients with chronic disease states, such as diabetes, hypertension, hyperlipidemia, and tobacco cessation, to the TelePACT CPS via warm handoff or consult. Patients may also be referred to the TelePACT CPS via patient population management review. The TelePACT CPS will determine appropriateness of the consult, work with MSAs to schedule patients, and meet with patients via real-time, secure, CVT or telephone depending on patient preference and proximity to VA clinic. Scheduling a CVT appointment requires that space be ensured, that there is clinic staff to room patients, and that technology is available.

Prior to working with a facility, a Memorandum of Understanding (MOU) and a Telehealth Service Agreement (TSA) need to be drafted to outline the terms of agreement. A VISN-wide MOU has been created and each facility has a TSA in place.

Replicability

This program has been successful due to the ability to recruit highly qualified CPSs, and a willingness to adopt.

Recognition

Toni O'Day, Paul Black, Matthew Rogers, Brenda LaDue, Danielle Ahlstrom, William Llamas, Cassie Perdew, Laura Schultz, Pharmacy leadership and telehealth staff at the following VA facilities: Anchorage, Mann-Grandstaff, Roseburg, Walla Walla, White City

Improving Access to Foot and Ankle Care Through Telepodiatry Initiatives

Jeffrey Robbins, DPM, Director Podiatry Service
VACO, Washington, DC
jeffrey.robbins@va.gov

The purpose of the Telehealth Podiatry program is to increase foot and ankle services to the Veteran in remote locations, especially those at risk for limb loss. It utilizes Store and Forward Telehealth (SFT) and Clinical Video Telehealth (CVT) to supervise care remotely using synchronous and asynchronous methods.

Introduction

Basic foot care is essential for patients with diabetes and other serious conditions that place them at risk for amputation. For Veterans living in remote areas, this becomes a challenge, as the availability of basic foot care is severely limited. Populations in remote areas are not large enough to justify the deployment of a full-time podiatrist. In addition, travel distances from main medical facilities prevent providers from traveling to remote CBOCs to provide this kind of care. That is why telepodiatry and telesupervision serve as effective methods to increase access for those remote CBOCs.

Key Information

Telesupervision of basic preventive foot care involves the provision of care by a non-podiatrist who is remotely supervised. This is accomplished in remote CBOCs using either Store and Forward Telehealth or Clinical Video Telehealth technologies. The Office of the Director of Podiatry Service in collaboration with the Employee Education System (EES) administers an ongoing basic foot care training course for health techs, RNs, LPNs, and Physician Assistants (PAs).

Context

Currently, there are 1.8 million patients in our VA system at risk for amputation, of which 690,000 are designated as high risk. The average age of these patients is approximately 70-years-old. With telesupervision, we have increased the numbers of telepodiatry visits in ten VISNs from 2,132 visits in 2013 to 4,972 visits in 13 VISNs in 2015.

Practice Description

The purpose of the Telehealth Podiatry program is to deliver podiatry services to the Veteran in a more convenient manner, so that more Veterans may be served and diabetic foot complications may be identified earlier in an effort to prevent limb loss. The program entails a video examination by the remote podiatrist who directs care as well as the onsite basic foot care provider. After completion, the basic foot care provider contacts the remote provider for inspection of results and discharge. The note is written by the onsite provider documenting the involvement of the remote supervisor and identifies the appropriate signatories.

Replicability

Since first established in VISN 5, the program has been successfully duplicated in 12 other VISNs. The hope is to further expand this program and increase capacity, especially in remote areas.

Recognition

Kathleen Cronin

Veterans Without Borders

Matthew Rogers, PA-C Telehealth Clinical Operations Manager

Boise VAMC, Boise, ID

matthew.rogers5@va.gov

A TelePACT Hub brings high-quality, team-based PC services to Veterans in areas facing a significant professional clinical staffing shortage.

Introduction

A rural Veteran in Alaska travels more than 70 miles via snowmobile to a road, where he hitches a ride to a CBOC for his annual medical visit. The CBOC he typically travels to has been unable to recruit providers, and has never been staffed to include CPS or psychologists on team. A Telehealth Patient Aligned Care Team (TelePACT) currently leverages technology to achieve economies of scale and provides CPS, psychology, and PC services in a true PACT model to the Veteran. The virtual TelePACT Team is spread between Boise, ID; San Francisco, CA; and Mat-Su, AK.

A large medical center in VISN 20 experienced unprecedented PCP attrition and had an on-average recruitment time of 24 months for PCPs. The medical center considered outsourcing the PC services to the community or contracting with a locum tenens agency, neither of which support Veteran-centric care. The TelePACT Hub offered a more viable solution; it included leveraging existing nursing staff and bringing on the PACT provider team virtually to ensure that an entire Veteran panel was managed with VA-trained staff. In addition, this solution provided continuity with the medical center, and the PACT teamlet was maintained. In this instance, the TelePACT Team functioned as virtual locums (with VA expertise) providing service to the Veteran panel for 20 months while securing a permanent replacement.

A small CBOC in rural Washington had an unexpected medical issue with one of their PCPs, which left the CBOC without a PCP for six months. Using the clinical staff within the Boise TelePACT Hub, the CBOC was able to maintain panel coverage and no patients were forced to seek care outside the VA system.

Key Information

The Boise TelePACT Hub was implemented in 2014 as a proof of concept and expanded to a broader pilot in 2015. Currently it is providing coverage to over seven PC panels across VISN 20. Today, the TelePACT Hub is able to navigate in and out of CBOCs and medical centers across VISN 20 to support and stabilize staffing, as needed. In addition, the TelePACT Team has developed a core set of expertise in PACT and, as they provide services from site to site across the VISN, they are able to assist sites in further development of their PACT model of care.

Context

VISN 20 is the most rural VISN in the nation and has, on average, more than 50 PC clinician vacancies per year. Most medical centers in VISN 20 incorporate PC Mental Health Integration (PCMHI) and CPS within their PC staffing model, but CBOCs are unable to provide this staffing level due to a lack of patient numbers. Piloted in 2014, the Boise TelePACT Hub created a core TelePACT Team inclusive of medical providers, PCMHI, and CPS to provide team-based TelePACT services via telehealth to CBOCs and medical centers across VISN 20. This provides sites across VISN 20 with more stable PC coverage and allows CBOCs and smaller clinics to provide CPS and PCMHI support where it would not be available.

Practice Description

The Boise TelePACT Hub consists of the following staff:

- Seven FTE PTPs (MD, DO, PA-C, NP)

- Six FTE CPS (PGY-2, board certified with prescriptive authority)

- Three FTE psychologists (post-doc or fellowship trained in ambulatory PC mental health)

- Two FTE LCSW (focused on medical social work and also provide therapy)

- 1.25 FTE PC psychiatrists

- One FTE neuropsychologist

- Two FTE Telehealth Clinical Technicians (TCTs) (to provide technical support and training to staff, orphans)

- Two FTE administrators (one FTE clinical oversight and one FTE admin, essentially a co-directorship)

- Three FTE administrative support (one FTE program specialist, one FTE data analyst, and one FTE secretary)

- Two FTE MSAs (two FTE required to manage schedules across systems, open encounters, consults)

To manage the needs of Veterans, the providers function in a transdisciplinary team, bringing the best skill set to the Veteran based on need. To facilitate this, the virtual provider team performs "warm hand-offs" across disciplines, as needed, and on demand. In an instant, patients can be working with a PCP, psychologist, pharmacist, social worker, or all of them at the same time, depending on the Veteran's needs.

As it has grown and evolved, the Telehealth Hub now has three primary reaches: 1) provide team-based transdisciplinary primary telehealth care to sites throughout VISN 20 with chronic short staffing challenges, 2) partner with the Centers of Excellence (COE) Graduate Medical Education (GME) program and begin teaching the next generation of providers about transdisciplinary telehealth care, 3) develop a research arm that evaluates the qualitative impact of telehealth services in PC.

Replicability

Expansion of this model to each VISN is possible. One or two hub sites could be located in each VISN to serve CBOCs that have a difficult time with the recruitment and retention of PC teams. The ideal situation is establishing a hub with provider staffing that can function in a true PACT model. Not only can this model support larger centers, it can bring additional resources to smaller CBOCs, where staffing a CPS or PCMHI team is not viable. A relatively small capital investment with ongoing operational funding would be sufficient to build and sustain a core TelePACT team.

Recognition

Sarai Ambert-Pompey, Sarah Curtright, Danielle Ahlstrom, Ami Student, Autumn Keefer, Jeff Sordahl, Jessica Litke, Cassie Perdew, Katie Erickson, Kay Burnett, Rory O'Connor, Ruth Campbell, Ashley Vanderdasson, Stephanie Bremser, Maisha Correia, James Weiss, Laura Schultz, Lawrence Brown, William Llamas, Shannan Brimmer, Oreana Harless, Victoria Richard, Terry Hardin, Teresa Boyd, Larry Hobson, Toni O'Day, Henry Elzinga, William Weppner, Jill Hedt, Paul Black, ORH

Clinical Video Telehealth Hub

Holly Stapley, RNMN, CVT Hub Manager

VA Pittsburgh Healthcare System, Pittsburgh, PA
holly.stapley@va.gov

The Clinical Video Telehealth (CVT) Hub provides Veteran-centric, evidence-based, general and specialized mental health services, in geographically remote areas where quality mental health care providers are in short supply.

Introduction

To be truly patient-centered, we have to be able to bring quality care to the Veteran. Many Veterans live in remote areas, where recruitment and retention of mental health providers is difficult. These are often areas without available behavioral health specialty care. In these cases, Clinical Video Telehealth services can provide access to quality care without inconveniencing the Veteran. In 2012, a Telehealth Hub was established in VISN 4 to meet the needs of underserved areas by providing mental health care to Veterans in need.

For this to be a success, Veterans needed to accept this modality of care. As we started this program, we discussed situations that demonstrated where we would have an impact. Key to our practice was the collaboration with other specialists who helped us treat patients with significant other medical conditions. As we progressed, we were able to work with PC to look at medication reduction in patients with polypharmacy. We also encountered patients who moved and we were able to see them at a new CBOC. We were able to see patients who went to Florida for the winter. We were able to include the family in counseling sessions. In all instances, we achieved a virtual environment and sought to provide seamless care.

Key Information

VA Pittsburgh initiated their CVT Hub in October of 2012. VISN leadership brought forth the action to plan, create, and implement a CVT Hub. Psychiatrists and psychologists, who would provide mental health services to VISN 4 and other sites experiencing mental health access issues, would staff this hub. The goal was to significantly expand access to general and specialty behavioral health care for Veterans at outlying facilities. The program would reduce wait times for behavioral health services, improve the timeliness of VA care, and reduce costly and lengthy travel for Veterans. The program would improve the effectiveness, geographic equity, efficiency, timeliness, and patient-centeredness of VA mental health care.

Prior to 2012, VA Pittsburgh had been providing CVT services to five CBOCs as well as limited group telehealth services to two local Vet Centers. By the time this program was implemented, VA Pittsburgh behavioral health providers had developed valuable experience and demonstrated commitment with services. VA Pittsburgh was receptive to participating in the initiative to create a CVT Hub. Existing staff initiated the project in 2012 to serve patients from two VAMCs within VISN 4.

Context

The initial goal was to recruit eight full-time licensed Behavioral Health (BH) providers: five psychiatrists and three psychologists. Administrative support would initially be provided by the Behavioral Health Service Line (BHSL) business office. Two clerical staff were assigned to this endeavor. Space was allocated at the Greentree Annex and outfitted with EX-90 telehealth technology.

As sites expanded, it became necessary to review the structure of the hub initiative. A business plan was put forward in June 2014 to request designated leadership and administrative support to the Telehealth Hub to further the mission of behavioral health access within VISN 4 and beyond.

Practice Description

The program's vision is that VA Pittsburgh Healthcare System Behavioral Health Hub will augment outpatient behavioral health capacities to meet VA's commitment to providing timely, high-quality behavioral health care to Veterans within and beyond VISN 4. The program mission is to:

- Fill identified gaps in BH mental health services.
- Increase access in geographically remote or challenging areas.
- Provide services in areas where it is difficult to recruit VA Mental Health Professionals.
- Increase efficiency in places where travel time to nearest VA clinic is excessive.
- Provide specialized services not available or in high demand at outlying sites.

The CVT Hub staff provides a comprehensive initial assessment, diagnostics, treatment recommendations, and treatment planning through psychiatry and psychology. Psychiatrists provide medication management, including monitoring of adherence, response, and side effects. Psychological services include numerous empirically supported and evidence-based practices, including:

- Cognitive behavioral therapy for depression, anxiety disorders, adjustment, anger management, and couples counseling.
- Interpersonally informed therapy for unipolar and bipolar depression.
- Acceptance and Commitment Therapy for anxiety and depression.
- Prolonged Exposure and Cognitive Processing Therapy for PTSD.
- Motivational Interviewing to promote and support behavior change and treatment adherence.
- Additional services for psychological problems, such as complicated grief, stress management, and coping skills.

Staff schedules are reviewed weekly to determine if sites are utilizing the slots that they negotiated. Block provider scheduling is utilized at each site, which allows them to have staffing consistency. It also allows the Veteran to utilize a consistent time block for recurring appointments. Staff does not leave their offices to locate patients; they are notified by the remote site when the patient is available.

A monthly call is set up for each site that allows the staff to touch base, determine if there are any concerns, and creates a collaborative relationship with each site. In addition, the monthly calls help each site work with the hub; helping to create an effective and responsive team at each location. The synergistic effect has led to greater collaboration to ensure broad access to mental health services for Veterans with unmet needs.

The CVT Hub has the ability to implement empirically supported therapies and best practices in ways that adhere as closely as possible to established treatment protocols. Charts are reviewed by the provider to review treatment outcomes.

These patients are treated and followed as part of the mental health caseload for either telepsychiatry or telepsychology. At present, the following sites are receiving service from the CVT Hub:

- Altoona VAMC (James E Van Zandt) and the following CBOCs: Dubois, Indiana, Huntingdon, Johnstown and State College
- Butler VAMC and the following CBOCs: Armstrong, Clarion, Cranberry, Mercer, and Lawrence
- Clarksburg VAMC (Louis A Johnson) and the Tucker CBOC
- Erie VAMC
- Wilkes-Barre VAMC and the following CBOCs: Sayre, Tobyhanna, Northampton and soon to be added Berwick (pending)
- Philadelphia VAMC and the following CBOCs: Fort Dix and soon to be added Saracini (pending)
- North Florida/South Georgia Healthcare system (seven CBOCs), VISN 8

We have received queries from other out-of-region sites but have reached our capacity and are unable to take on more sites.

To date, we have doubled the encounters in FY 2014 (from 824 to 1,726 in FY 2015), further meeting the needs of even more Veterans.

Replicability

This is a Veteran-centered program. We can safely and efficiently provide mental health care to a Veteran at a distant site, working collaboratively as part of the facility team where the Veteran receives care. We meet mental health needs through comprehensive evaluations, providing of evidence-based psychotherapy, medication management, and follow-up assessments for treatment adherence.

The overarching concerns are replicability, affordability, and sustainability. During this process, we have reviewed mapping, workload, and Veterans Equitable Resource Allocation (VERA) reimbursement. We have found that the program is still growing and may take several years to reach steady state—at which time we will be able to determine the financial profitability. In addition, we would like to document best practice outcomes and publish the results.

Recognition

Marcella Horvitz-Lennon, Morgen Kelly, VA Pittsburgh leadership

Telemedicine for Anesthesia Pre-Operative Assessment

John Sum-Ping, MB, ChB, FRCA, National Director, Anesthesia Service

VA North Texas Health Care System, Dallas, TX
john.sum-ping@va.gov

Patients living more than 50 miles from the main hospital can now have their pre-operative anesthesia evaluation performed at their local CBOC via telemedicine.

Introduction

Texas is large and many Veterans choose to live in rural locations. At VA North Texas Health Care System, Dallas Medical Center, we have quite a large catchment area. Traveling to the big city for care can be inconvenient, requiring hours of travel for the Veteran.

All patients who are scheduled for surgery or procedures requiring anesthesia need a pre-operative anesthesia evaluation. Patients who live more than 50 miles from the main hospital are able to schedule their pre-op evaluation at the local CBOC, and closer to where they live instead of coming to the main hospital. This is accomplished through the use of telemedicine. Because of this practice, we have seen patient satisfaction increase and savings to VA for travel expenses.

Key Information

Telemedicine has been implemented at several VA health care systems; however, use of telemedicine specifically for the Anesthesia Pre-Operative Assessment is relatively new. At VA North Texas, we implemented Telemedicine for the Anesthesia Pre-Operative Assessment in 2014. Successful implementation required collaboration between our Medical Administration Service (MAS) and Health Information Management (HIM) staff at the central and satellite locations to establish and maintain a scheduling profile.

Context

VA North Texas Health Care System is a progressive health care provider in the heart of Texas. Poised as VA's second largest health care system, it serves more than 117,000 Veterans and delivers 1.4 million outpatient episodes of care each year to Veterans in 38 Texas counties, and two counties in southern Oklahoma. The system has about 5,000 employees and 1,700 community volunteers, driven by the passion to serve Veterans.

Practice Description

The new practice involves scheduling patients, who live a significant distance (greater than 50 miles) from the main hospital, to be seen at the nearest CBOC and in the first two to three hours of the day. Typically, this time is not as busy at the main hospital because patients scheduled for surgery are either being interviewed by the surgical mid-level providers or getting their tests completed. Patients are satisfied because they do not need to travel far for their anesthesia pre-operative evaluation.

Replicability

Telemedicine for Anesthesia Pre-Operative Assessment was adopted to improve both Veteran access and satisfaction. Having appropriate telemedicine equipment at the CBOCs was crucial to the success of this practice. In addition, motivated anesthesia providers willing to provide care without the security of a face-to-face, hands-on interaction is required. The success of this effort should be easy to reproduce. The challenge will be getting appropriate equipment in the remote locations.

Recognition

VA North Texas Health Care System, Dallas, TX, and CBOCs

VISN 2 Behavioral Telehealth Center

Katharine VanTreese, LCSW Program Supervisor

VISN 2: Health Care Upstate New York, Albany, NY

katharine.vantreese@va.gov

By combining prevention-based programming and offering services using the telephone or home telehealth delivery, the Behavioral Telehealth Center (BTC) reaches Veterans throughout upstate New York to offer evidence-based care.

Introduction

Veterans are increasingly looking for individually tailored virtual care options that reduce travel time and cost, fit into their work schedules, and offer flexibility and convenience. The VISN 2 Behavioral Telehealth Center offers programming in several areas focused on preventive care and self-management of common problems, including dementia, depression, anxiety, adjustment disorders, tobacco use disorder, alcohol misuse, and obesity. Care is available at no cost (no copays or telehealth fees), from a patient's home, using telephone or home telehealth modalities.

- RAPID (Recognizing and Assessing Progressive cognitive Impairment and Dementia): Studies have shown that dementia patients are high health care utilizers (twice the outpatient encounters, hospitalizations, and length of stay of counterparts without dementia). Dementia is under-recognized in VA, and the RAPID program increases the rate at which we identify patients with dementia. Patients and their caregivers engaged in RAPID showed an average $2,700 reduction per patient in health care costs over six months.

- Primary Care Mental Health Integration (PCMHI) Care Management: In the first few years of implementing our virtual program, our penetration rate increased by 63 percent. Our penetration rate has been ranked in the top three or four in the nation for the past two years, and VISN 2 was the first VISN to "go green" on the national PCMHI implementation map with all sites meeting Uniform Mental Health Service Package requirements of the blended model. Additionally, we noticed that Veterans receiving appropriate levels of care had significant improvement in antidepressant medication adherence. We also implemented a Perinatal Screening program for all pregnant women in the VISN.

- TeleMOVE! saw a 57 percent increase in clinically significant weight loss (greater than 5 percent of body weight) between FY 2010 and FY 2011 which has been sustained over the past three years. We also noted a 65 percent increase in intense and sustained treatment (mov7 performance measure) from FY 2010 to FY 2012, which has also been sustained for the past three years. In addition, there was a 66 percent increase in MOVE! visits within the first three years of the implementation of TeleMOVE! from FY 2010 through FY 2013.

- TeleQuit Home Telehealth Tobacco Cessation: To date, 81 percent of Veterans who complete at least one cycle either completely quit tobacco (59 percent) or decrease their use (22 percent).

Key Information

When implementing a PCMHI Care Management program, our comparatively small, rural VISN decided that the best way to offer this service to the most people was to adapt the Behavioral Health Lab (BHL) telephone-based model to fit a call center "hub" covering the entire catchment area. Leaders in several positions collaborated to add other, related programs to the BTC, capitalizing on seed funds available for pilots (for example, Office of Telehealth Services (OTS) funding was used for Home Telehealth-Weight Management and Office of Mental Health (OMH) Request for Proposal (RFP) for PCMHI) as well as grants from the ORH. All services are offered virtually and focus on integrating PC with behavioral health and/or Geriatrics and Extended Care (GEC). It was implemented in a phased approach, beginning in 2007 and evolving into its current design in FY 2010. Four health technicians provide administrative support to all programs and one supervisor oversees the site; whenever possible, clinical staff (nurses, social workers, and mental health counselors), are cross-trained to offer workload flexibility. By combining support staff, space, program supervision, and having a wider coverage area, the VISN was able to reach a large number of Veterans with a minimal amount of staff.

Context

The BTC covers all of VISN 2 (now VISN 2 North) and is available to all Veterans enrolled in PC services. Services available span four major areas: 1) TeleMOVE! Weight Management (Home Telehealth, Telephone Lifestyle Coaching, and Monthly Support Calls; 2) PCMHI Care Management, which includes a baseline assessment of many psychological metrics, triage, and evidence-based protocols, such as antidepressant medication monitoring, brief therapeutic interventions, disease management protocols for anxiety or depression, tobacco cessation or alcohol misuse, or referral management to specialty care; 3) TeleQuit Home Telehealth, which offers a daily response, virtual care modality for smoking cessation; and 4) Recognizing and Assessing Progressive Cognitive impairment and Dementia (RAPID) program, which focuses on targeted screening to detect undiagnosed dementia and offers a phone-based group or individual counseling and education program for caregivers. These services could be offered at the facility level, but staffing constraints would not allow them to be equally available in all areas. In this context, the evidence base that supported implementing the program can erode as sites struggle with fidelity to practice standards and models.

Practice Description

Our design involved considerable collaboration with stakeholders throughout the VISN to address several gaps in care. We arranged for one system of pooling resources, offering virtual care and maintaining evidence-based practice standards. Unused space was found in an existing VAMC and network staff was hired to fill positions. Labor mapping, building accurate clinics, and stop coding all helped determine utilization by each facility, and educational efforts are ongoing to ensure that all providers understand how to use the BTC programs.

Replicability

This practice was possible in VISN 2 because of the following factors:

- Belief in "One VA" and commitment to reducing care silos

- Strong partnership across disciplines/service lines to form an interdisciplinary team that works with PACT
- Willingness to prioritize evidence-based, health promotion/disease prevention-based care
- An integrated CPRS network made sharing information and developing consults easy; however, it is not a requirement. Access agreements and MOUs would also allow for treating a Veteran outside of one's VAMC
- Leadership vision and support for the "big picture" plan allowed this design to be implemented and to thrive. Another facility, group of facilities, VISN, or region would simply need to be willing to dedicate some staff time to have access to all the programs available through the Center

Recognition

Bruce Nelson, Margaret Dundon, Laura Wray, Mary Schohn, Eva Dickinson, facility and network partners and leaders

Drive-Thru Flu Shot Clinic

Cecilia Beauprie, Chief Nurse of Outpatient Nursing Service
Edward Hines Jr. VA Hospital, Hines, IL
cecilia.beauprie@va.gov

Imagine a Veteran in their car, SUV, or motorcycle cruising through a drive-thru, putting the vehicle in park, being greeted by a smiling nurse, then pulling up his/her sleeve and receiving the flu shot without getting out of the vehicle; all this in 15 minutes.

Introduction

A Drive-Thru Flu Shot Clinic (DTFSC) at Edward Hines Jr. VA Hospital facility in Hines, IL, was stood up at the beginning of the flu season to serve Veterans to be vaccinated without scheduled appointments. The drive-thru flu shot clinic has been in place for several years and has received nothing but praise from hundreds of Veterans.

Key Information

Flu shot champion, Cecilia Beauprie, Chief Nurse of Outpatient Nursing Service (ONS) led the design and implementation of the DTFSC at Edward Hines Jr. VAMC. Effectively collaborating with a multi-disciplinary flu immunization program team, the DTFSC has operated since 2008. The drive-thru's first location was a driveway beside a garage of one of the vacant residential buildings on campus. The location has moved to a parking lot in front of the hospital building, near the entrance gate and close to the main road for quick entry and exit. The program has a van containing supplies, and a room for the nurse to shelter on cold or rainy days.

Context

Edward Hines Jr. VAMC, located 12 miles from downtown Chicago, sits on a 147-acre campus and offers primary, extended, and specialty care as a tertiary care referral center for VISN 12. Specialized clinical programs include blind rehabilitation, spinal cord injury, neurosurgery, radiation therapy, and cardiovascular surgery. The hospital serves as the VISN 12 southern tier hub for pathology, radiology, radiation therapy, human resource management, and fiscal services. Hines VA operates 483 beds and six CBOCs in Elgin, Kankakee, Oak Lawn, Aurora, LaSalle, and Joliet. More than 800,000 patient visits occurred in FY 2015, providing care to more than 57,000 Veterans from Cook, Du Page, and Will counties.

The DTFSC was initially a strategic novelty to promote influenza immunization to Veterans with no clinic appointments during the flu season, younger Veterans who prefer not to spend time inside the building waiting areas, and elderly Veterans who decline to use valet parking but have difficulty walking to the VA building from the parking lot. The DTFSC receives inquiries about the program before the flu season begins each year. DTFSC has been achieving the objectives of the Influenza Immunization program, and in a 20-day period, immunizations are administered to an average of 800 Veterans. This allows approximately 2.5 percent of Veterans seeking flu vaccinations to be served with no hassle. Preventing influenza and/or minimizing the severity of influenza for 800 Veterans in a given year, exceeds the expectations of the DTFSC.

Practice Description

Notices and promotions about the DTFSC are sent out to all Veterans through letters, the facility website, Facebook, and a phone messaging system. A driver-friendly location in the parking lot of the campus is identified, providing easy access and quick egress so Veterans can remain in their vehicles. The vehicle serving as a nursing station holds a supply cart with vaccines and related supplies. Review of influenza immunization procedures, preparation of flu shot checklists, and other documentation are completed. Last but not least, the clinic secures and trains at least one nurse (RN or LPN) to administer the flu vaccine injections over a 20-day period in September to October, and during flu season. The practice is supported by protocol based on the national directives and approved by the Medical Executive Committee of the facility.

Replicability

Our practice has been duplicated in the CBOCs in the last three years and by another VA facility in VISN 12. A facility having an appropriate location in its parking lot and a well-established process are the elements of a successful DTFSC.

Recognition

Cecilia Beauprie, Flu Immunization Program Oversight Team, John Evans

CARE COORDINATION

eScreening Program

Niloofar Afari, PhD, Director of Clinical Research, VA Center of Excellence for Stress and Mental Health

VA San Diego Healthcare System, San Diego, CA

niloofar.afari@va.gov

eScreening is a mobile technology that improves care coordination and business processes. It offers Veteran-directed screening, real-time scoring, individualized patient feedback, instantaneous medical record clinical documentation, immediate alert to clinicians for evaluation and triage, and monitoring of treatment outcomes.

Introduction

The eScreening program is a promising practice that was developed to facilitate the screening process and improve care coordination and measurement-based care for Veterans. eScreening is a dynamic mobile technology that provides efficiencies in screening, treatment, and monitoring practices.

Veteran patients have benefitted from direct provider interventions when the results of their assessments indicated an emergent need for care. eScreening makes emergent care a reality for Veterans.

Key Information

VACI, VHA Innovation Program, and the Office of Mental Health (OMH) teamed up to develop and pilot the eScreening program. The program enables clinical reminders, health factors, Mental Health Assistant data, and clinical text notes to be synchronized into the VHA electronic medical record (CPRS) and shared instantaneously among providers. The program is adaptable to multiple settings, including care coordination, mental health, and PC clinics, to rapidly and easily identify those who may be in need of mental health support or intervention and monitor progress in treatment.

Context

Results of a FY 2013 pilot study with over 1,300 Veterans seen at the VA San Diego Transition Care Management program indicate that eScreening can significantly improve care coordination and business process compared to paper screening, including:

- Faster documentation of completed clinical reminders, averaging 19 days less than paper screening
- Decreased need for additional clinical follow-up from 84 to 59 percent
- Increased completion of comprehensive suicide risk assessment of appropriate Veterans to nearly 90 percent
- Reduced redundancy yielding an estimated savings of 6.5 provider hours for every 100 patients and 4.4 patient hours for every 100 patients seen
- Increased operational efficiencies yielding an estimated savings of $100 for every 100 clinical reminders completed

Practice Description

eScreening is now an established clinical practice at the VA San Diego Healthcare System. From January to November 2015, our Transition Care Management team used eScreening to assess 884 Veterans, reducing the documentation burden by an estimated 17 minutes per Veteran.

Replicability

eScreening has been implemented at the Long Beach Medical Center and is slated to go live at the Las Vegas and San Francisco Medical Centers in 2016. Given the growing list of facilities that have requested eScreening, demand for its use across the VHA enterprise is high.

Regional Liver Cancer Tumor Board

David Kaplan, MD, MSc, FACP, Director of Hepatology

Corporal Michael J. Crescenz VAMC, Philadelphia, PA

david.kaplan2@va.gov

Combining a regional telehealth-supported Liver Cancer Tumor Board, a web-based submission process, and a consolidated database to manage and track communications has shortened time for Veterans to receive their evaluation and first treatment, and has reduced unnecessary biopsies.

Introduction

Hepatocellular Carcinoma (HCC) is the cancer with the most rapidly increasing incidence in the VA health care system and the US as a whole, due primarily to long-standing Hepatitis C infection, alcohol use disorders, and obesity. HCC most often can be diagnosed by a well-skilled radiologist and rarely requires biopsy confirmation. Furthermore, unlike most other cancers in which only medical, surgical, and radiation oncology expertise are generally sufficient for management, optimal care for HCC requires a wide variety of expertise, including input from hepatologists, hepatobiliary surgeons, interventional radiologists, medical oncologists, radiation oncologists, and palliatricians. Most VA centers do not have ready access to all these disciplines.

In eastern VISN 4, four VA stations are located within a one-to-four-hour drive from a tertiary, academically-affiliated VA. As a result of increasing referral rates from "spokes" VA clinicians to the "hub," several patterns of suboptimal patient management were observed. First, many patients with clear radiologically-confirmed HCC were not being diagnosed based on imaging and being referred for unnecessary liver biopsies, delaying care by months in some cases. Second, many of the imaging protocols employed at the spokes VAs were not optimized for liver cancer diagnosis. Third, diagnosis referrals to HCC specialists were often delayed until after patients saw local non-expert oncologists, often receiving inappropriate firstline therapy. Fourth, patients who were candidates for liver transplantation were not being referred in a timely fashion. Fifth, patients who were candidates for curative resection were not being referred in a timely fashion. Sixth, multiple patient travel episodes were required for all relevant hub specialists to evaluate some individuals. Lastly, follow-up imaging results on patients treated at the hub and sent back to referring spokes were not being communicated back to the hub for appropriate follow-up.

Context

The Philadelphia VA is a large tertiary, urban, academically-affiliated VA serving a population of over 2,000 Veterans with chronic Hepatitis C as well as patients with other chronic liver diseases.

Practice Description

To address these communications and practice issues, we instituted a Regional Liver Cancer Tumor Board, leveraging VA telehealth and intranet resources. First, we formalized the hub Liver Cancer Tumor Board to include all relevant specialties at a mutually convenient pre-clinic meeting time.

We identified an available room for long-term use and outfitted that room with necessary telehealth equipment to support live face-to-face case presentations with spokes providers. Telehealth Service Agreements (TSAs) and intrafacility consults were established to facilitate telehealth co-management of patients. A referral form was created using Microsoft Sharepoint software, accessible to all team providers via VA intranet. A local Microsoft Access-based Case Management database was created by Dr. Kaplan to automate: 1) receiving and processing case referrals; 2) generating a weekly agenda; 3) staging of cancers; 4) recording tumor board recommendations; 5) communicating via e-mail to referring providers and relevant specialists the tumor boards recommendations; 6) recording tumor board attendance; and 7) generating tumor board minutes. Telehealth visit slots were created in the Gastointestinal (GI) HCC clinic to facilitate video-consultation with patients living greater than a one-hour drive from Philadelphia. Dr. Jordan Booty developed a set of standard computerized tomography (Computerized Tomography) CT and Magnetic Resonance Imaging (MRI) protocols for HCC that were communicated back to the spokes sites' radiologists. The LIRADS reporting system was introduced via radiology teaching webcasts to radiologists interested in learning this new standard.

Participating sites include Philadelphia (hub), Coatesville, Wilmington, Wilkes-Barre, and Lebanon VAs. The effort was led by Dr. Kaplan with critical collaboration from MDs, PAs, NPs, and cancer care coordinators at the spokes VAs. Lynn Watson, Director of Telehealth services at the Philadelphia VA, was instrumental in facilitating the telehealth backbone. The Tumor Board began its weekly meetings July 22, 2014.

We presented the findings from the first year of the intervention at the Liver Meeting (AASLD) in San Francisco in November 2015 (abstract #521). Sixty-one (61) patients diagnosed prior to 7/22/14 and 63 patients in the ten months following the intervention were compared with regard to times from imaging abnormalities to receiving care. Time from abnormal imaging to specialist evaluation decreased from 44 to 21 days (p=0.0018), a change most profoundly seen at the spokes (from 55 down to 23 days, p=0.0004). Unnecessary biopsies were reduced (p=0.006) and the number of resections increased (p=0.025). Treatment occurred nearly one month earlier (p=0.025) after initial identification of an abnormality on surveillance or diagnostic imaging.

Replicability

This care coordination model is highly replicable in other regions with central specialty care and spokes with reduced access to these services. Application requires a hub team focused on patient care and patient satisfaction willing to break down silos to optimize outcomes. The coordination database reduces the administrative support needed to manage a large panel of patients.

Peer Support Groups in Chronic Disease Self-Management

Laura Mortensen MSN, RN, Veterans Health Education Coordinator
Veterans Health Care System of the Ozarks, Fayetteville, AR
laura.mortensen@va.gov

At the Veterans Health Care System of the Ozarks (VHSO), a collaboration and grant award in June of 2014 led to Veterans becoming AmeriCorps members and training in the Stanford University Chronic Disease Self-Management Program (CDSMP). These Veterans facilitated exceptional peer support groups that improved the partnerships between staff and Veterans.

Introduction

Eight Veterans and their caregivers, each diagnosed with a chronic condition, met for the first time at the Farmington, AR, library to start the six-week Strength to Serve (S2S) program. As a result of their positive experiences within the group, they decided to continue their monthly meetings at one another's homes and maintain the support they had established in class. The S2S program offered information, instruction, and most important peer support in dealing with the daily frustrations of managing a chronic disease. These CDSMP classes were facilitated by Veterans who were not medical professionals but trained as AmeriCorps members at the VHSO.

Key Information

An action item originated from the Office of Patient Care Services and presented an opportunity to explore the use of health coaches to help educate Veterans in self-care and disease management. S2S was an AmeriCorps/Partners in Care Foundation initiative that identified and trained individuals to serve as health coaches and used the nationally recognized CDSMP developed at Stanford University. Through collaboration with the Northwest Arkansas Area Agency on Aging, the Veterans Health Education Coordinator (VHEC) at VHSO was awarded the S2S program in June of 2014. Over the course of the next year, 285 referrals were made to the CDSMP groups. Of this number, 67 percent were Veterans and the rest were family members and caregivers. Health coaching was provided to 160 participants, of which 65 percent were Veterans. There was a 46 percent completion rate for Veterans, which means they completed at least four of the six classes.

Context

VHSO serves over 56,000 Veterans in 24 counties, with 22 of them considered rural or highly rural. Each PC team manages 1,200 individuals with an average of 24 percent diagnosed with one or more chronic conditions. Reaching Veterans is a challenge due to geographical barriers. Enabling them to manage their chronic conditions is one of the most important tasks Veteran education can assume. The establishment of an AmeriCorps team at VHSO resulted in outreach in communities where these rural Veterans received support and education necessary to manage their conditions.

Practice Description

The Stanford University CDSMP consists of peer-led groups of individuals diagnosed with a chronic disease meeting once a week for two hours for six weeks. They complete a prescribed lesson plan that originated from Stanford University. They explore self-management techniques and address daily issues of fatigue, stress, medications, sleep, coping, family dynamics, and exercise. The groups are led by lay facilitators who have a purpose to guide and provide the scripted lesson plan.

VHSO's S2S Team planned a kickoff event on October 1, 2015, and ran the CDSMP, later renamed Strength in Self, until September 1, 2015. The CDSMP classes were held at the main facility, our CBOCs, and community facilities. We partnered with senior centers, American Legions, Veterans of Foreign Wars of the United States (VFW) organizations, and churches to provide classes close to where our Veterans lived. The facilitators traveled to these locations to promote groups and increase participation.

Replicability

The S2S program at VHSO resulted in several outcomes that were positive for the facility, our Veterans, and the AmeriCorps members. First, VHSO was recognized as one of ten VAs awarded this program across the nation. Secondly, many Veterans who completed the classes requested more interactions and services. From those, requests for participation in our Tai Chi and Qigong programs grew. Other complementary activities became more visible. Finally, the AmeriCorps members themselves developed strong ties with VHSO and are now advocates for the facility. One has continued his designation as a Worker Without Compensation (WOC) and works tirelessly on Veteran councils and grants. Others return to the facility to volunteer for projects and events.

This type of program is easy to reproduce at other health care facilities. The CDSMP is available to anyone who is interested and able to locate a master trainer in the area. The only barrier to having a program like this is to identify enough volunteers interested in becoming lay facilitators. The outcomes are exceptional and lead to improved partnerships between staff and Veterans. The S2S program was a great success due to the fact that 50 percent of the team was composed of Veterans. Their experiences and integrity gave the program credibility and ensured its success.

Veteran-Community Partnerships

Kenneth Shay, DDS, MS, Director, Geriatric Programs

VACO, Washington, DC

kenneth.shay@va.gov

A Veteran-Community Partnership (VCP) is a VA-initiated, but VA and community-maintained, partnership whose sole focus is to enhance coordination of care and services (e.g., caregivers, end-of-life care, homelessness; etc.) for Veterans. The strength of VCPs lies in the camaraderie and commitment to Veteran causes that VA and community partners share and act upon in their local and regional networks.

Introduction

Mr. X is a non-service-connected, Gulf War-era Veteran living in an impromptu campground in a highly rural area of a northwestern state. His neighbors in the "tent city" where he lived became aware of problems with his health when his poorly-controlled diabetes led to serious infections in his feet and legs. He reluctantly agreed to seek treatment at the local county hospital. A social worker at the hospital had recently been contacted by a social worker at the VA CBOC and together the two of them, in collaboration with colleagues at both VA and in various community service agencies, had received training in establishing a Veteran-Community Partnership focusing on homeless and indigent Veterans. The hospital social worker, therefore, had an enhanced familiarity with Veteran benefits and knew personnel at the CBOC whom she could contact on his behalf. With her support and assistance, Mr. X enrolled for VA benefits. He started receiving his care at the CBOC, enrolled in a VA vocational rehab program, and was able to qualify for US Department of Housing and Urban Development-VA Supportive Housing (HUD-VASH) program housing. Due to several years of poorly-controlled diabetes, his eyesight began to fail and, through contacts established with the VCP, staff at the CBOC were able to put him in touch with a guide dog service that furnished him with a helper animal free of charge because of his Veteran status.

Key Information

VHA's 2009 Geriatrics and Extended Care (GEC) Strategic Plan noted that only a minority of Veterans turn to VA for their health needs, and of those who do, the majority also get some measure of their health services in the community. As Veterans over the age of 65 make up over half of the Veterans seeking VHA care in a year, and nearly all are Medicare-eligible, the prevalence of dual users in the elderly Veteran population is even greater. Yet as of 2009, there was no system-wide effort to support the coordination of care and services for Veterans between VA and non-VA providers and agencies. In 2010, GEC undertook development of VCP to address this need. Working with a contractor skilled in partnership-building and a national stakeholder council of subject matter experts in community cares, three sites (in Michigan, New York, and New Hampshire) piloted the concept of a VA-initiated, but VA and community-maintained, partnership with the sole focus of enhancing coordination of care and services for Veterans. The uptake was astonishing and was not limited to geriatric patients, which was the original model. The concept was then shared with a succession of VISNs and individual sites. The coalescing element for each new partnership is an agreed-upon, shared focus on the part of VA and the community partners: some VCPs focus on caregivers, some on end-of-life care, some on homelessness, some on returning Veterans, and some on Veterans with dementia. At present, there are over 50 VCPs operating in 14 VISNs, and new sites are scheduled for training and startup.

Context

As VCP was in its second year, GEC learned of the initiation of the Office of Community Engagement (OCE), led by Dr. Jennifer Lee. Dr. Lee and her deputy, Lelia Jackson, were instrumental in coordinating partnership development, with the result that VCP and OCE spring from many shared values and priorities concerning VA facilities' integration with communities. OCE and Ms. Jackson, its present director, continue to work closely with VCP, with Ms. Jackson serving as an active member of our Stakeholder Advisory Council and Dr. Kenneth Shay, the director of the VCP activity, contributing to a variety of OCE activities. More recently, the initiation of "MyVA Communities," a Secretary-level initiative for leveraging community interest in Veterans' issues, has introduced an invaluable set of potential collaborators for VCPs. MyVA Communities is a community-led effort on behalf of Veterans and encompasses ties not only to VHA, but to VBA and NCA entities as well. As such, cooperation between a local MyVA Community group and a co-located VCP can advance the agendas of both groups, with particular focus on identifying and addressing health-related challenges facing Veterans in the region.

Practice Description

The power of VCP is in its flexibility and ability to translate shared goals into actions by VA and community partners on behalf of the Veterans they serve. Experience has taught us that community-level interest is invariably favorable but that local VA ability to participate is variable. As such, VCP needs to begin at a VA where one or more staff who already work at the interface between VA and the community (e.g., social workers, outreach coordinators, voluntary services, etc.) identify the various individuals in the community with whom they interact on behalf of Veterans, and then set up a meeting with all VA and community people. Shared goals and additional VA and community partners are identified and the group coalesces over succeeding weeks and months as they work toward the goals they have identified, whether it has to do with a particular group of Veterans, caregivers, or addressing some other important concern. As new ideas are brought to the group, either the full group or a subgroup tackles the next challenge, reinforcing the group's ties and increasing their visibility and sense of community. What all VCPs accomplish is greater awareness on the part of the community partners of what VA offers, how resources can be made available to Veterans, and what an incredibly important part of the community VA can be. And VA partners expand their awareness of the community resources that can be brought to bear on Veterans' needs as well as to whom to reach out to make that happen. VCPs can play a singular role in addressing the Under Secretary's priority of "Restoring Public Trust" in VA by demystifying and humanizing VA to the public through interpersonal interactions and shared goals and accomplishments.

Replicability

The strength of VCPs lies in the camaraderie and commitment to Veteran causes that VA and community partners share and act upon in their local and regional networks. Dr. Shay is contacted on a regular basis by community agencies with interest in teaming up with a local VA to start a VCP, and by singularly ambitious VA personnel (e.g., Chiefs of Voluntary Services, Outreach Coordinators) who have heard about VCP at an educational session or the website (www.wehonorveterans.org/va-

Veteran-organizations/Veteran-community-partnerships) and have similar activities underway (and wonder if they can use some of the materials that have been developed to facilitate creation and maintenance of a VCP). As mentioned previously, there are presently over 50 VCPs in operation, with more coming online all the time. The program is successful and grows because it taps into a strong existing desire within the community to help those who have put their lives on the line for the country. In doing so, it enhances VA staff ability to do their jobs on behalf of Veterans.

Recognition

VA staff, Sarah Hyduke, Gwynn Sullivan, Jennifer Lee, Lelia Jackson

Simultaneously Improving Diabetes Care and Performance Metrics: An Interdisciplinary Approach with the Center of Innovation

Alyse Chandler, PharmD, BCPS, CDE, Endocrine CPS

Ralph H. Johnson Medical Center, Charleston, SC

olivia.chandler@va.gov

The A1C project is a multi-disciplinary initiative that uses a trained Endorcine Service Team to proactively enroll Veterans (many rural) with A1C greater than 9 percent in a telephone clinic aimed at lowering blood glucose levels and managing diabetes.

Introduction

The A1C project was a multi-disciplinary initiative that aimed at lowering the blood glucose of patients with A1C greater than 9 percent enrolled at the Ralph H. Johnson VAMC (RHJ VAMC). The mission was funded by the Office of Health Equity with the help of the Center of Innovation (COIN) research. The Endocrine Service Team, which consisted of an attending, CPS, dietitian, NP, and two RNs, was the primary player in this initiative. These individuals are trained diabetes educators and are recognized by the American Diabetes Association. Elevated A1C was a health issue at RHJ VAMC, as we were failing our External Peer Review Program (EPRP) measures for diabetes control. This intervention and project was direly needed for the health of our Veterans.

As the endocrine CPS, I was actively involved in enrolling patients into my telephone clinic. I was able to reach patients living in rural areas and manage their diabetes without the added burden of traveling to their nearest clinic. Between October 1, 2015, and March 1, 2016, 67 percent who had at least one visit with a CPS showed a reduction in A1C. Of those patients, more than 60 percent achieved the facility metric of an A1C less than 9 percent. During the two-year research initiative, almost 1,000 patients were referred to a CPS for diabetes management. Because the Endocrine team was consistently involved with these patients, we were able to lower their A1C and ultimately prevent complications associated with diabetes if left untreated. Patients were also provided with diabetes education (i.e., through group classes or one-on-one sessions) and follow-up appointments with the Endocrine team to foster personal coaching. This environment gave our Veterans ample opportunities to succeed in managing their diabetes. Patients and caregivers were very responsive to the multi-disciplinary approach with their care and because of this their burden of elevated blood glucose was manageable.

There have been numerous success cases with the A1C project. One example is a 63-year-old male with an A1C of 9.6 percent referred to endocrine pharmacotherapy services. At his initial visit, he was only on one oral medication and basal insulin. He was also referred to receive Care Coordination Home Telehealth (CCHT) services for diabetes because he was unable to come for live visits. The endocrine pharmacist used the blood glucose data submitted by CCHT to adjust his medications. He was started on prandial insulin to help control blood glucose around mealtimes. After titrating insulin, his A1C has decreased from 9.6 to 5.9 percent without having any hypoglycemic episodes. His A1C decreased to goal within a seven-month period. Although he utilized only the endocrine telephone clinic, the patient's blood glucose was decreased by close follow-up by the endocrine pharmacist using CCHT data. This example shows how beneficial a team-based approach can be to help improve the health of our Veterans.

Key Information

The A1C project was started at the RHJ VAMC in 2014. COIN had seen the necessity for reaching our Veterans with A1C greater than 9 percent. The COIN team is responsible for rural health and diversity health care, and many of our patients in outlying clinics have uncontrolled diabetes. This project expanded from our main VA to the other CBOCs (i.e., Myrtle Beach, Beaufort, Savannah, Hinesville, Goose Creek, and Trident). Dr. Kathie Hermayer, MD, was the lead who collaborated with the Endocrine team to facilitate this project. It began in 2014 and initially started with the Endocrine team (NP, registered nurses, dietitian, and clinical pharmacist) but eventually included other clinical pharmacists at the CBOCs as well as telehealth services. This team-based approach allowed greater possibilities and resources for our Veterans to utilize. They would no longer feel they had to deal with diabetes alone but now they were encouraged by a team of health care professionals and given a chance to take control of their health.

Context

The Veteran population at RHJ VAMC is primarily middle-aged African American men who served in the Vietnam War (including Agent Orange exposure). There are six CBOCs that are affiliated with VA. As part of the A1C project, this included patients in the rural communities and the main VA. Patients living in the rural communities have difficulty obtaining VA services due to distance/travel to the clinics. This challenge was addressed by managing patients' diabetes by telephone visits. Patients could also be enrolled into CCHT services to allow them to transmit their blood glucose readings to an RN. The readings were a great tool for pharmacists and physicians to help manage patients' diabetes.

Practice Description

The endocrine team had a RN who used the portal (PC list of patients with uncontrolled disease states, such as diabetes) to research which patients needed endocrine intervention. If they had an A1C greater than 9 percent, they were referred to receive diabetes education (given by Certified Diabetes Educator (CDE), endocrine pharmacist, RN, and dietitian), pharmacotherapy services (either live or telephone visits), endocrine NP appointments, and CCHT services. The endocrine RN would review the patients' charts for medication adherence and if labs were needed. After the patients were referred to the endocrine pharmacist, the pharmacist would contact patients and set up visits to establish care. Appointments were made based upon patients' needs. Face-to-face and telephone visits were offered to all Veterans. Most of the appointments were followed up within one to two weeks to ensure patient adherence and continue coaching patients to better health. After patients were confident in their ability to manage their diabetes and blood glucose was better controlled, the telephone visits were spread out to three-to-four week intervals.

Replicability

This model is similar to PACT models used in PC; however, the main difference is the endocrine team focused on A1C greater than 9 percent. The endocrine RN was able to specifically focus her attention to enroll patients into pharmacotherapy services or the endocrine NP clinic. While the PACT model does address A1C greater than 9 percent, it also focuses on other disease states that may take the nurses' attention/time away from addressing each patient. With the A1C project, however, hyperlipidemia and hypertension were also addressed during the visits.

Recognition

Kathie Hermayer, Lisa Oliver

ED Nurse Navigator

Danielle Marks, MSN, RN, Assistant Nurse Manager, Emergency Department

Salem VA Medical Center, Salem, VA

danielle.marks@va.gov

The priority of the ED Nurse Navigator is to ensure that unresolved care needs are met after Veterans are discharged from the ED and to provide opportunity to identify obstacles in care transitions and work interdepartmentally to overcome them.

Introduction

"Nurse Navigators steer patients through the health care labyrinth."—K. Rothwell

The priority of the ED Nurse Navigator is to ensure that unresolved care needs are met after Veterans are discharged from the ED. Additionally, the role gives ED personnel a direct, consistent person they can rely on to ensure follow-up. Lastly, the role provides an opportunity to identify obstacles in care transitions along with the ability to work interdepartmentally to overcome them.

In 2015, the program was named a Best Practice by Booz Allen Hamilton and the Office of Inspector General. Cumulative data from March 2015 to February 2016 indicates that 19 percent (3,002) of the Salem VAMC ED's discharges were flagged by nursing staff as having unresolved care issues at discharge. The ED Nurse Navigator reviewed 100 percent of those discharges, intervened in 33 percent (995), and provided direct care coordination in 30 percent (303). Furthermore, since program implementation, VA's Emergency Medicine Management Tool (EMMT) reflects a drop in 72-hour return for admit data from 1.8 percent (last in the nation) to 0.6 percent (compliant).

Key Information

Nurse Navigation began in 1990 to address disparities and improve access to care, and was traditionally used for oncology patients. In 2012, the Salem VAMC ED submitted a request for a funding proposal intended for an ED Nurse Navigator pilot program. The request was funded and initially followed female Veterans who were discharged from the ED to ensure resolution of symptoms and seamless transition to supportive services, such as Women's Health Clinic and PC. That pilot program showed a 20 percent improvement to follow-up of female Veterans discharged from the ED and a 12 percent increase in enrollment in Women's Health Clinic. In March of 2015, the decision was made to expand the program to all "high-risk" ED discharges, regardless of gender.

Context

The Salem VAMC opened in 1934 and currently serves approximately 112,500 Veterans living in a 26-county area of Southwest Virginia. In addition to the main facility in Salem, services are offered at CBOCs. We recognized that ED staff typically work under extreme time pressure, and patient discharge and follow-up responsibilities were spread out informally among staff. Our prior efforts to improve ED operations focused on patient-staff interactions during the ED visit. Little attention was given to patients' experiences in the days and weeks afterwards. Subsequently, Veterans were returning to the ED with the same or even worsening complaints over and over again. This program began as a safety net to ensure continuity during outpatient transitions of care.

Practice Description

ED Nursing Management led program implementation by collaborating with IT to change the discharge template to a dialogue note and embed a mandated flag prompting the ED Nurse to indicate if the Veteran was leaving the department with an unresolved care issue. The flags generate an ad hoc report that can be pulled in VistA by discharge date. The ED Nurse Navigator prints this report within seven days of ED discharge and reviews the EHR to ensure that the Veteran is scheduled for or has received appropriate follow-up. If no follow-up is documented, the ED Nurse Navigator calls the Veteran to ensure resolution of symptoms and, if needed, works with other departments to coordinate unresolved follow-up needs.

Replicability

Most, if not all, VAMCs have "high-risk" patients who are more likely to return seeking urgent/emergent care if their unresolved needs are not met. The capability for this program is likely present in all facilities with an operating ED. The VA runs the largest integrated health care system in the country. The interconnectedness between the ED, PC, and Specialty services forms a unique collaborative which removes traditional barriers to cohesive care.

Recognition

Robin Krupin, Mary Wright

Veterans Health Information Exchange

Margaret Donahue, MD, Director for VLER Health Program Office, Co-director for Interoperability Office, Health Informatics, Office of Informatics and Analytics, VHA

VACO, Washington, DC

vlerhealthexchangeteam@va.gov

The Veteran Health Information Exchange program gives VA and participating community care providers secure access to certain parts of the Veteran electronic health record.

Introduction

Many Veterans are concerned that their community HCPs do not have access to their medical history. The Veterans track, maintain, and often provide hard copies that they physically carry from one clinician to another. The Virtual Lifetime Electronic Health Record (VLER) Health program enables sharing health information between VA and community health partners, so Veterans do not have to manually transfer their health records nor worry about unnecessary or duplicate procedures. Further, the program provides both VA and community health partners with the necessary health data to ensure efficient, timely care to their Veteran patients.

Veteran access to care is paramount and VA is committed to making health care between VA and community health care providers as seamless as possible for the majority of VA patients who also receive care outside VA. VLER Health is Veteran-centered and holistically focused across the care continuum. It has improved Veteran satisfaction and care quality. Ultimately, the Veterans Health Information Exchange (VHIE) allows Veterans to more readily identify with the interoperability and functionality of the program. Moreover, the VLER Health program promotes a clear call to action for Veterans to be a partner in managing their individual health care.

Key Information

VLER Health is host of the VHIE, a multi-faceted business and technology initiative. VLER contains a portfolio of health information-sharing capabilities between VA and community health care providers and is designed to share Veterans' health information electronically, safely, and privately between VA, other federal agencies, including the DoD, and community health care facilities that are members of the secure eHealth Exchange. Its goal is to better inform care providers, improve continuity and timeliness of care, enhance awareness among all involved parties, and help to eliminate gaps in a patient's health record.

Practice Description

VA Direct Secure Messaging is a secure mail "push" initiative that provides electronic transmission of outpatient referral information from the DoD to external providers, with the return of clear and legible consult reports to support clinical decision making and continuity of care. The VA Direct allows VA users to send and receive specific information to community health care providers via secure email-like messaging through a trusted network of 45 community health care providers. Examples of use case opportunities consist of Non-VA Care Coordination (NVCC) Referral

Management, Long-Term Care Admissions, Mental Health, Alert Notification, and My Health*e*Vet Blue Button.

VLER Health Exchange is the "query-retrieve" technology that allows clinicians to securely and seamlessly discover and exchange health data between VHA and community health providers. The VA Exchange capability is currently available at all VAMC locations nationwide and over 70 community health systems. VA continues to partner with other federal agencies including Indian Health Services and Social Security Administration to enable secure, trusted exchange of health care information. Currently, health data that is available for exchange are allergies, problems, advance directives, medications, vital signs, immunizations, smoking status, chemistry and hematology results, radiology results, pathology results, surgical procedures, clinical procedures, discharge summaries, history and physicals, consult notes, future appointments, and outpatient encounters.

VLER Community Engagement is responsible for securing Veteran Consent and for providing on site and remote training for Veterans and VAMC clinicians on the benefits of using VLER Health Exchange, Direct Secure Messaging, and Blue Button Download. VLER has 56 Rural Health Community Coordinators (RHCC) onsite at VAMCs deemed rural by the ORH. Twelve remote Community Coordinators (RCCs) work in VAMCs and are responsible at VISN level locations across the US VA will continue expanding by adding community health care providers and health information exchanges (HIEs) nationwide.

Replicability

VLER Health is defined as a portfolio of secure solutions for exchanging health data with community care providers that are based on national standards over trusted networks. The performance goals set for FY 2015 were accomplished through integrated efforts in four specific areas of concentration: 1) Partner Engagement and Onboarding for Direct and Exchange; 2) Improving Veterans Authorizations; 3) Enhancing Clinical Adoption through Technological Improvements; and 4) Expanding our Reach with Community Engagement.

Recognition

Jamie Bennett

Empowering Patients and Improving Care Coordination by Providing Access to Their VA Health Record

Carolyn Turvey, PhD, Research Health Scientist; Dawn Klein, MSW, Research Coordinator
Iowa City VA Health Care System, Iowa City, IA
carolyn.turvey@va.gov

Our program trains Veterans to use My HealtheVet, the VA patient portal/personal health record, to generate a printable summary of their VA health record. They can use this to share with their community providers to improve the continuity of care.

Introduction

With more and more Veterans receiving care outside VA, efficient ways to inform non-VA providers about Veterans' VA health history is critical to quality care. Our program trained a Veteran and his spouse to use My HealtheVet, the VA patient portal/personal health record, to generate from his home computer a printable summary of his VA health record. Sometime after this training, the Veteran suffered marked chest pain. He and his wife went to the local non-VA Emergency Room (ER), where the providers asked the Veteran about his current medications. Though his wife had a handwritten list, it was incomplete and did not have doses for many of the medications. As her spouse was transferred from their local critical access hospital to a higher level of care, the wife returned home briefly and remembered she could access her husband's VA Health Summary using My HealtheVet. She used My HealtheVet to generate his summary and shared it with the ER doctors. They stated that it had critical information because it indicated her husband was on a blood thinner of which they were not aware. In light of this information, they delayed a procedure until they had tapered the blood thinner adequately. Had they gone ahead with the procedure as planned, the Veteran may have suffered serious consequences. While reflecting on this event, the spouse said:

"Everything happened so suddenly. I had all these things to worry about and did not know how I would keep everything straight. I remembered the VA Health Summary and printed it. I would not have been able to remember [my husband's] allergies and medications without the summary. Having it there helped me talk through his medications and conditions with the doctors. The doctors found it very useful."

Key Information

Our training program aims to engage Veterans in their health care by providing them access to their VA health record. One way Veterans can engage in their care is to share their information between VA and non-VA providers to improve coordination of care. This is important for Veterans receiving benefits through VA purchased care programs, such as the Veterans Choice Act, as well as other Veterans who seek community care using their other insurance, such as Medicare. In 2010, My HealtheVet launched the Blue Button feature to provide Veterans access to their VA medical record information. VA was one of the first health care systems to provide patients electronic access to portions of their medical record and the ability to download and print their VA Health Summary.

Our prior research found that Veterans valued the Blue Button, but were not certain how to use it. We developed a training program that taught Veterans how to download their VA medical record and how they could improve their health care by sharing this VA Health Summary with their non-VA providers. We have been training Veterans to do this since 2013. To date, our outreach programs have tended to focus on rural Veterans because they are more likely to be dual users (that is, Veterans who receive care from VA and non-VA providers).

Context

This training was developed and designed by Carolyn Turvey, PhD, and Dawn Klein, MSW. It has been distributed nationwide through several collaborations with VA operational partners and community provider organizations. One collaboration between the Iowa City VA Health Care System, My HealtheVet Program Office, ORH, and Department of Health and Human Services Office of the National Coordinator implemented this outreach and training in nine sites nationwide—Maine, Iowa, Kansas, Nebraska, Montana, Florida, Minnesota, New York, and Utah.

Practice Description

The training includes an online video and accompanying paper-based training. The training first presents why it is important for community providers to have VA health information so they can make better treatment decisions (for example, about medications) and help to save time and money by avoiding repeat tests or procedures. Then, the training provides step-by-step instructions on how to generate a VA Health Summary, including a recommendation that Veterans bring a copy of this summary to their next community provider medical visit. The multi-agency multi-site collaboration described previously trained 620 Veterans. Of these, 77 percent said that using the VA Health Summary will help them be more involved in their health care. We also surveyed their non-VA providers, of whom 90 percent endorsed that information from the VA Health Summary improved their ability to have an accurate medication list and make treatment decisions about medications. In addition, 50 percent of these community providers reported they did not order some laboratory tests or other procedures because of information available. This training has since been disseminated nationwide.

Replicability

To broaden the reach and impact of this training, we made both the video and paper-based training materials available to all Veterans nationwide by including a Spotlight Article on the My HealtheVet home page. This article included a link to an online video available on VA YouTube, "Your VA Health Summary—Share for Better Care" and "VA Health Summary Quick Guide." The Your VA Health Summary video was featured for a month with more than 600 views, and there were over 1,100 downloads of the Quick Guide. In addition, during this time, the number of unique Veterans accessing their information increased.

These educational resources are easily available online for patient education wherever and whenever they are needed. My HealtheVet coordinators, VA clinicians/staff, and community non-VA providers can encourage and engage patients to review and share their information available in My HealtheVet.

Recognition

Veteran participants, Health IT Partners, community health care organizations, VA site coordinators, My Health*e*Vet coordinators, Health Information management, ORH, My Health*e*Vet program office, Theresa Hancock, Chip Harman, Kim Nazi

Improving Delirium Assessment Among the Older Veterans Population

Evelyn Metz, APRN, DNP, FNP-C, AGANP-BC, VHA-CM, Clinical Nurse, ECHo Level III Faculty, CAM-S Delirium QI Project Coordinator
Durham VAMC, Durham, NC
evelyn.metz@va.gov

The Confusion Assessment Method (CAM-S) is an evidence-based clinical practice that helps diagnose delirium to ensure proper and prompt care.

Introduction

Improving delirium assessment among the older Veterans population through the implementation of the short form Confusion Assessment Method is an evidence-based clinical practice that stemmed from the improving the Care of Elder in Hospital (ECHo) Durham VAMC (DVAMC) initiative. CAM-S is a copyrighted assessment that DVAMC was given permission to use by its author. Beginning from the ED, nurses' skills in diagnosing delirium have increased since CAM-S was incorporated in the Evaluation and Management (E&M) note in the ED and the Review of System (ROS) note in Medical/Surgical and Patient Acute Rehabilitation Care (PARC) units.

The impact of CAM-S delirium assessment on Veterans and their families has been significant. Veterans and family members are being educated in an interactive way by providing them with the approved ECHo Delirium, Dementia, and Depression Patient Education Brochure. Families and Veterans have expressed their appreciation of how delirium is being addressed by nurses and medical teams, as demonstrated by the following examples:

5. Ms. X., a Veteran's wife shared, "The education brochure had clearly explained what my husband showed tonight; he was in pain, and became agitated and not acting like himself. Thank you." (January 2016). Mr. X's pain was addressed immediately; his pain is a precursor to agitation and delirium, which were averted. Mr. X was discharged the following day.

6. Mr. Y is a 65-year-old Veteran who presented in the ED related to a surgical complication. Utilizing the CAM-S, the nurse noted that he scored positive with delirium. The provider was notified immediately, which steered Mr. Y to a prompt delirium management beginning from the ED. Upon transfer to the surgical intensive care unit, the ED nurse communicated to the admitting nurse that Mr. Y scored positive with delirium. Proper care was afforded to Mr. Y, which led to appropriate measures dealing with his delirium and within 24 hours his delirium was resolved (April 2015).

The employee impact of the CAM-S initiative has been demonstrated. Clinical nurses' confidence in recognizing delirium increased after they received delirium/dementia training. Although it varies from unit to unit, with regards to delirium management, collaboration between nurses, mid-level providers, residents, and physicians have dramatically increased. For instance, when nurses communicate that a patient might benefit from pharmacological intervention because of lack of sleep at night even when pain/comfort is not an issue, providers are proactive in exploring apposite pharmacological agents to promote sleep. Likewise, when pain management is insufficient, providers listen to individual nurse's suggestions of providing patient relief.

Key Information

Delirium is a condition of a sudden alteration in an individual's mental status accompanied by easily distracted behavior, manifested by a fluctuating course of symptoms. According to experts, delirium is often unrecognized by ED providers due to lack of proper and routine screening. Being the point of entry for hospital admissions, the ED plays a vital role in the evaluation and management of older patients presenting with altered mental status; therefore, CAM-S was implemented in the ED for three months (March to June 2015). As a member of ECHo Committee, a clinical nurse who was engaged in her doctorate study led the collaborative effort and was instrumental for forming a team. The ED Medical Director, Educator, Quality Improvement (QI) liaison, few nurses, acting manager, computer programmer specialist, ECHo Committee, and nursing leadership collaborated with the effort. Implementing CAM-S matters because as experts indicate, when delirium is missed, individuals were likely to die within six months of onset; therefore, preventing delirium has a direct implication in the older Veterans mortality and morbidity and overall Quality of Life (QOL).

Context

As a designated tertiary health care facility, DVAMC has a 248-bed capacity and is fully accredited to provide emergent, psychiatric, inpatient, extended, and rehabilitation care. As a part of the Veteran Services Integrated Network (VISN 6), DVAMC provides innovative and comprehensive health care to more than 200,000 unique Veterans in 26 counties in central North Carolina. Consequently, DVAMC functions as the referral center for Veterans within VISN 6. Annually, our facility treats at least 63,248 Veterans in various clinical settings. Of this figure, at least 44 percent were aged 65 years or older; accordingly, 35,000 were seen in the ED. Individuals who are 65 years or older are susceptible to develop delirium; without deliberately assessing older patients' mental status, delirium presence is overlooked. Due to the fact that over half of Veterans seeking health care at DVAMC present through the ED, the ED plays an important role in providing the baseline delirium assessment of the older Veterans population.

Practice Description

The Rosswurm-Larrabee Evidence-Based Practice Model served as the framework for the CAM-S implementation. This model guided the Strengths, Weaknesses, Opportunities, and Threats (SWOT) analysis to demonstrate the role of the ED toward improving the older Veterans care. Articles relating to delirium and appropriate assessment tool were synthesized; thereafter, evidence gathered was presented to the ED Medical Director, ED Quality Improvement Project Liaison, ED Educator, nurses, and Associate Chief of Nursing Services (ED, ICUs, and Surgical Services). Geriatric experts were consulted and CAM-S was thoroughly reviewed. Accordingly, a Delirium QI Project Protocol was prepared and submitted to the Institutional Review Board (IRB), which was approved.

Following the CAM-S training guidelines, the ED nurses were provided with two weeks hands-on training. The training involved patient case scenarios, group discussion on CAM-S utilization and interpretation of delirium score, interventions, etc. Pre and post delirium and dementia knowledge survey questionnaires were utilized to assess the effectiveness of the training method. A few nurses came on board and served as ED nurses CAM-S support. The ECHo Team supported the ED project and has been instrumental in its dissemination to the other clinical areas: medical/surgical and PARC units. Accordingly, nurses in the medical/surgical and PARC units were trained in the same manner.

Replicability

Because of the growing population of older Veterans and our facility's continuous focus on improving Veterans care across the spectrum, CAM-S was successfully implemented and disseminated at DVAMC. Being an evidence-based and research-driven institution, we all have a common goal: improving Veterans' QOL and increasing patients' satisfaction through the utilization of cost-effective and efficient health care innovation. Addressing geriatric care, such as routinely assessing their cognitive status through CAM-S, has been proven effective. Therefore, this initiative can be easily replicated to the following clinical settings: CBOCs, short/long-term care, ambulatory care, hospice, and wherever patient care is provided. Currently, CAM-S delirium assessment is on its way to our hospice unit.

Recognition

John Villani, Luna Ragsdale, Ellie McConnell, Maria Orsini, Michelle Simpkins, Amy Howard, ED Nursing and Medical Staff, Carol Howard, ECHo Committee Members, ICU, 6A&B, 7A&B, PARC Nursing Educators, Nursing Leadership, Gigi Smith, Marcia Engle, Vivien Collins, Tamatha Cales, Natalie Kean, Linda Rown, Sheeba Chacko, Monalesia Chapman, Cristina Hendrix, Sharon Gorden, Greg Eagerton, Sharon Inouye

The Delirium Toolbox

James Rudolph, MD, Director, Center of Innovation in Long Term Services and Supports
Providence VAMC, Providence, RI
james.rudolph@va.gov

The Delirium Toolbox identifies Veterans who are at risk for delirium and empowers frontline staff to mitigate that risk. Delirium occurs in 25 percent of older hospitalized Veterans and prevention can be effective.

Introduction

Mr. X is an 86-year-old Veteran who was admitted to the hospital with a urinary tract infection. On his admission, a nurse performed a delirium risk assessment. The Veteran stated that he was tired due to poor sleep in the hospital and that he was quite bored, because he had forgotten his reading glasses at home. He had difficulty stating the months of the year backwards. Mr. X was found to be at high risk for delirium due to his sensory deficit, his cognitive deficit, and his infection.

From the Delirium Toolbox, the nurse provided Mr. X with a pair of reading glasses to correct his sensory deficit, a puzzle book to address his boredom and keep him cognitively stimulated, and a pair of ear plugs to improve his sleep. His delirium risk level was included in the nursing assessment in his medical record to alert his care team. As a result of these interventions, Mr. X was able to read his patient education materials, remain cognitively active, and sleep better. After treatment for his infection was completed, he was able to return home.

Key Information

The Delirium Toolbox is a risk modification program that empowers nurses to improve the care of older Veterans who are admitted to the hospital. The Delirium Toolbox focuses on identifying high-risk patients, empowering nurses to employ risk modification strategies, and monitoring for changes in cognition. The Delirium Toolbox has been implemented in the VA Boston (2011–2013), VISN 1 (Togus, Providence, and White River Junction (2012–2013)), and five VISN 9 facilities (2015). The Delirium Toolbox utilizes a train-the-trainer system to build champions in expansion facilities and a coaching system to provide consultation and empowerment. These champions, nurses, and other hospital staff are the drivers of the Delirium Toolbox program at each site. The Delirium Toolbox findings were published in 2014. Veterans who received an item from the Delirium Toolbox had a shorter length of stay (-0.7 day), reduced restraint use (-4 percent), and a trend toward lower variable direct costs (-$1,390 per patient). After start-up, the Delirium Toolbox costs about $5,000 annually, resulting in a return on investment measured in days.

Those with delirium are at a higher risk of being placed in a nursing home, which can be reduced by implementing the use of the Delirium Toolbox. This quality improvement practice is designed to identify and modify delirium risk proactively to improve patient outcomes and lower hospital costs.

Context

Delirium is an acute change in cognitive function (acute brain failure) that preferentially affects older, cognitively impaired, and medically ill patients. Delirium occurs in up to 25 percent of medical inpatients, 50 percent of surgical patients, and 75 percent of older intensive care patients. Delirium is associated with increased morbidity, mortality, costs, and a decline in function. There is no approved treatment for delirium. As a result, delirium prevention programs are paramount in mitigating related morbidity and mortality and preserving independent function, particularly in integrated health systems which care for a population of patients (such as VHA). The Delirium Toolbox was developed at the VA Boston Healthcare System (VABHS) with funds from a T-21 initiative to Prevent Institutional Long-Term Care.

Practice Description

The components of the Delirium Toolbox are: 1) identify patients at high risk for delirium; 2) empower frontline caregivers to reduce delirium risk with low-cost items to improve sensory input, promote sleep, and enhance cognitive stimulation; and 3) monitor longitudinally for changes in arousal indicative of delirium.

1. Identify high-risk patients: Nursing assesses many of the core risk factors for delirium in the process of admitting and caring for patients. We compiled these factors into one location in the medical record. We utilized the Delirium Toolbox to improve knowledge of delirium, its risk factors, and prevention strategies. Additionally, we recently developed and validated an electronic prediction rule for delirium risk.

2. Modify risk with items from the Delirium Toolbox: The Delirium Toolbox contains items to increase cognitive stimulation (cards, puzzles, stress balls), improve sensory input (hearing amplifiers, reading glasses), and promote sleep (earplugs, eye masks, headphones). Most importantly, the items in the Delirium Toolbox empower nurses to modify delirium risk with low-cost items. This empowerment is unique, because most assessments do not allow nurses to take tangible actions.

3. Monitor for changes in arousal: Cognizant of nursing workload, we developed and validated a scale for delirium, the modified Richmond Agitation and Sedation Scale (mRASS). The mRASS simply asks patients to describe how they are feeling and the nurse scores it. If the mRASS fluctuates, the patient should be assessed for delirium. Use of the mRASS encourages a common language among nurses and physicians with respect to changes in mental status. Our subsequent work has identified that abnormal mRASS is associated with negative hospital events including restraint use, in-hospital mortality, length of stay, discharge to a rehabilitation facility, and hospital variable direct costs.

Replicability

With the age and co-morbidity of Veterans projected to increase over the next 20 years, the clinical challenges of delirium will not subside. The mounting evidence that delirium is associated with other negative hospital events strengthens the imperative that delirium be addressed systematically. In this spirit, we recently developed and validated an electronic prediction rule for delirium risk identification. Increased delirium awareness and demand for identification and management protocols will continue to grow.

A collaboration of the Office of Patient Safety, the New England Veterans Engineering Resource Center (VERC), the Office of Geriatrics and Extended Care, and the Delirium Toolbox team developed and administered a Rapid Process Improvement Workshop for the Delirium Toolbox in FY 2015. We targeted five VA facilities in VISN 9. Nurses were the prime recipients of the educational initiative. Information about epidemiology, recognition, prevention, and management of delirium was disseminated through a multi-modal educational initiative and nurse "champions" were trained to advocate for recognition of delirium risk and reinforce early intervention on their wards. Not only did the Delirium Toolbox educational program increase knowledge of delirium, the number of patients screened for delirium risk increased over the course of the program.

Like most clinical demonstration projects, success of propagation is dependent on the commitment and captivation of champions disseminating the program at their facility. Creating delirium champions will develop a sustainable and expandable model at each medical center. The Delirium Toolbox is accessible to nurses on each ward so they are able to offer appropriate supplies to patients. In addition to this tangible component, education is provided to nursing staff regarding how to identify and intervene to manage delirium risk.

Recognition

Office of Geriatrics and Extended Care, VA Providence Center of Innovation in Long Term Services and Supports, Office of Patient Safety, New England Veterans Engineering Resource Center, Elizabeth Archambault, Kelly Doherty, Brittany Kelly, Ken Shay, Karen Massey, Orna Intrator, Peter Mills, Julia Neily, Lisa Zubkoff, Kristine DeSotto, Elizabeth May, Matt Rutherford

Geriatric Resources for Assessment & Care of Elders

Cathy Schubert, MD, Section Chief of Geriatrics

Richard L. Roudebush VAMC, Indianapolis, IN

cathy.schubert@va.gov

The Geriatric Resources for Assessment and Care of Elders (GRACE) home-based geriatric care management team collaborates with PACT and Veterans to help Veterans "age in place" and maintain function and quality of life. GRACE is associated with reduced acute care utilization and thus cost savings to VAMC.

Introduction

Mr. X was an older Veteran experiencing frequent falls and hospitalizations, who was frustrated and suspicious of physicians and health care personnel. He was thought by providers to have cognitive impairment and to be taking his medications improperly. The GRACE NP and social worker conducted an in-home geriatric assessment and discovered that Mr. X had profound hearing loss that was previously unrecognized. The GRACE protocols for hearing impairment and medication management were triggered and included several interventions for better care and outcomes. Specifically, the GRACE team typed out questions and always used written communication during visits. According to his daughter, Mr. X grew to really enjoy the GRACE team visits because he felt like they were listening to him. Extensive medication management using written communication led to Mr. X's using a pill box, discontinuation of dangerous over-the-counter medications, and better understanding and adherence to his medication regimen. Mr. X was not found to have cognitive impairment after all but only profound hearing loss which made him seem confused at times. Mr. X has had no further falls or hospitalizations since the GRACE team became involved with his care.

Quotes about GRACE:

- Veteran: "I am amazed at how you guys keep track of me! GRACE is amazing! I surely do appreciate you guys. You are a great team to have caring for me."

- Caregiver: "The GRACE team saved my husband's life and my sanity. I had hit rock bottom when the team came to our home and didn't know how we were going to continue like this. The entire team is warm and sensitive to our needs. I would like to thank GRACE from the bottom of my heart for giving me my old husband back!"

- Primary Care Physician: "Thank goodness GRACE is involved on this patient!"

In its first two years, GRACE enrollment was associated with a 7.1 percent reduction in ED visits, 14.8 percent fewer 30-day readmissions, 37.9 percent reduction in hospital admissions, and 28.5 percent decrease in total bed-days-of-care, saving VAMC an estimated $200,000/year over and above program costs for the 179 Veterans enrolled in GRACE at that time. A full description of GRACE implementation and outcomes in its first two years at the R. L. Roudebush VAMC has been accepted for publication (Schubert CC, Myers LJ, Allen K, Counsell SC. Implementing GRACE Team Care in a VAMC: Lessons Learned and Impacts Observed. Journal of the American Geriatrics Society, in press.).

Key Information

GRACE was implemented at the R. L. Roudebush VAMC in Indianapolis, IN, in April 2010. Because of its interdisciplinary nature, several service lines worked together to implement GRACE. The GRACE program is a part of the Geriatrics and Extended Care (GEC) Service Line and reports to the GEC Chief under Patient Care Services. The GRACE Medical Director/Geriatrician is the Geriatrics Section Chief within the Medicine Service. Because GRACE works closely with Primary Care/PACT in the care of older adults, collaboration with the Chiefs of Ambulatory Care and PC was also vital to implementation and sustainment.

Context

In 2010, there were over 15,000 Veterans aged 65 or older who were receiving PC services at Roudebush VAMC. These patients accounted for approximately 4,500 ED visits and 2,700 hospital admissions, having an average length of hospital stay of 5.1 days, and a 30-day readmission rate of 14 percent. Nearly 300 carried a formal diagnosis of dementia or Alzheimer's disease (which was likely a gross underestimate of disease burden as dementia is often undetected in PC until advanced stages), and over 2,000 required assistance from family/caregivers in one or more activities of daily living, thus meeting the definition for frailty. This population, typically burdened by multiple chronic illnesses, is at high risk for needing institutional extended care in a nursing home. GRACE seeks to mitigate this risk by improving care quality and by enhancing the experiences of older Veterans facing the challenges of aging, disability, and serious illness by providing optimal care coordination and management across the care continuum.

Practice Description

The GRACE model includes home-based geriatric assessment and care management by a NP and social worker who collaborate with the PCP and a geriatrics interdisciplinary team and are guided by 12 care protocols for common geriatric conditions.

Veterans aged 65 an older who are provided PC at the Roudebush VAMC and admitted to the inpatient medicine service are identified by the GRACE Medical Director/Geriatrician to receive GRACE Team Care. The Medical Director/Geriatrician visits eligible patients during the hospital stay and provides geriatric medicine consultation as appropriate, working in collaboration with the hospital attending physician. She also assists with transitional care planning to ensure consideration of alternatives to institutional extended care and help avert hospital readmissions. Eligible patients who are discharged and agree to participate in the GRACE program are provided a transitional home visit within five days of hospital discharge by their assigned GRACE NP and social worker. GRACE staff then provide longitudinal care management using the GRACE model and in accordance with each Veteran's needs and health care goals.

Replicability

Factors that contributed to the success of GRACE included the following: early engagement of an invested, supportive leadership who were provided with regular updates on the program's progress and positive impact, especially on acute care utilization; recruitment of energetic GRACE team staff with experience in geriatrics and interdisciplinary team care; and the natural alignment of the concepts behind GRACE with VA's implementation of the medical home in PC (PACT).

Aspects of the GRACE model have been also implemented in the Atlanta and Cleveland VAMCs and could be successful in any VA setting that cares for high volumes of older, medically complicated Veterans.

Recognition

Steven Counsell, Rebecca Parks, Carrie Ortwein, Julia Dolejs, Cheril White, Deborah Pruitt, Erica Gallmeyer, Justine May, Lauren Diekhoff, Jennifer McIntosh, Deborah Wilson, Brad Mossbarger

Implementing Innovations in Rehabilitation to Promote More Rapid Goal Attainment

Dennis Sullivan, MD, Director of the VISN 16/CAVHS Geriatric Research Education and Clinical Center

Eugene J. Towbin Healthcare Center, Little Rock, AR
dennis.sullivan3@va.gov

By changing the culture of care in a hospital rehabilitation unit, getting patients out of bed to ambulate as much as possible, and using innovative techniques to accurately document each patient's level of activity, the D.A.S.H. (Daily Ambulation Strengthens Heroes) project is improving both the care Veterans receive and the clinical outcomes they experience.

Introduction

Mr. X is an 82-year-old white male who was admitted to the Geriatric Evaluation and Management (GEM) unit after a serious episode of pneumonia that resulted in a prolonged hospitalization and the development of profound weakness. Although he was going to Kinesiotherapy (KT) for 30 minutes per day, on average, four times per week, he was otherwise spending most of his time in bed. Upon meeting the Veteran and explaining the initiative to increase ambulation during hospitalization and how it would benefit him, he was eager to participate. He stated, "I want to walk and get better. I know I need to get out of this bed." A walker was provided for his use and staff worked with him to set ambulation goals and to walk with him at least once a day until he was able to do so safely by himself. His total time out of bed and distance walked each day were monitored and this information was used by the staff to guide their care ensuring that Mr. X received the help that he needed. By the end of the first week, he was ambulating twice a day with a staff member and he had doubled the distance he could walk before needing to rest. His overall disposition/mood also improved as he enjoyed getting out of his room and interacting with the staff while ambulating in the halls. After each walking session, he always requested to remain in the program. At the time of his discharge, it was obvious how proud he was of his accomplishments.

Key Information

The project utilizes Quality Improvement (QI) principles to implement an innovative evidence-based program that promotes early and progressive ambulation for older Veterans admitted to GEM units for recuperative care and rehabilitation. The D.A.S.H. program addresses a critical need. Older Veterans often spend most of their time in bed while hospitalized, even though it is well established that the more time they spend out of bed ambulating, the better their clinical outcomes. Contributing to the problem, the clinical staff is often not aware of the amount of time each Veteran is out of bed. The project goal is to improve processes of care and eliminate barriers to ambulation to ensure that the Veterans in the GEM Unit reach their rehabilitation potential. Specific ambulation goals are set for each Veteran based on input from the Veteran and key professional staff. Utilizing newer technologies, the staff is then provided an ongoing objective record of how much time each Veteran is out of bed and walking each day. This feedback informs the staff of the Veteran's progress in meeting his/her ambulation goals and provides an indication as to when more assistance may be required.

Context

The target population for this project consists of older Veterans admitted to a GEM unit at the Central Arkansas Veterans Healthcare System. These patients are in the recuperative phase of a serious illness. At admission to the unit, they are generally too weak and deconditioned to return home, even with family members. As a majority live in a rural setting, few homecare resources are available to them. It is only the care provided on the GEM units that helps these Veterans to regain a level of function that allows them to return home. Walking for strength is a key component of the rehabilitation efforts.

Practice Description

This project consists of an innovative evidence-based program that helps older hospitalized Veterans get out of bed and walk more each day. A component of the project is the use of new technologies that inform the GEM unit staff of each Veteran's progress in meeting his/her walking goal. The new technologies have two parts that form an innovative "Patient Monitoring System'" a high resolution Real-Time Locating System (RTLS) and special nanoelectronic mattress overlays. The RTLS system tracks each Veteran's progress when in the unit, giving an accurate account of time out of bed, distance walked, and gait speed. Mattress overlays tell the amount of time in bed and in the future could be used as a source of information to assess risk for pressure sores or other problems.

Replicability

Locally, the D.A.S.H. project was initiated as a collaboration between the Geriatric Research, Education, and Clinical Center (GRECC), Nursing, Geriatrics and Extended Care, Physical Medicine and Rehabilitation, and Engineering Services at the VISN 16/Central Arkansas Veterans Healthcare System (CAVHS). Nationally, the project represents collaboration between the VISN 16 and VISN 8 GRECCs and the VISN 8 Center of Innovation on Disability and Rehabilitation Research. The program is evidenced-based and nurse-driven, modeled after successful clinical trials that demonstrate the benefits of early and progressive patient ambulation. Although the Patient Monitoring System (PMS) utilizes advanced technologies and is being developed by the GRECC through a contract with a private corporation, the main focus of the project is improving processes of care. These care processes are being improved utilizing existing FTE through a cooperative effort of the collaborating services. The goal is to eventually disseminate the program to all hospital wards throughout the entire VHA. As the newer technologies are further refined, the cost of the PMS will decrease eliminating the only major barrier to dissemination.

Recognition

Office of Geriatrics and Extended Care, the Offices of Rural Health and Health Equity, VISN 16, CAVHS, VISN 8 Center of Innovation on Disability and Rehabilitation Research

Multi-Disciplinary Heart Failure Disease Management Program

Siddique Abbasi, MD, Staff Cardiologist
Providence VAMC, Providence, RI
siddique.abbasi@va.gov

The Heart Failure program is a multi-disciplinary model of heart failure management that leverages the expertise of multiple disciplines (including pharmacy, nutrition, nursing, social work, cardiology, and psychology) to provide optimal guideline-directed medical care.

Introduction

Heart failure is the leading cause for inpatient admission among Veterans. In addition to carrying a five-year prognosis similar to many high-grade cancers, the diagnosis of heart failure leads to frequent clinic visits, rehospitalizations, and a radical change in the quality of a Veteran's life. Moreover, the diagnosis of heart failure places a tremendous demand on family and caregivers. Veterans must make radical alterations to their diet, constantly monitor their fluid weight, and take a variety of new medications. These changes can overwhelm a Veteran and their family. A common difficulty that arises when a Veteran receives a heart failure diagnosis is that they feel inundated with new information.

Recently, a Veteran and his daughter came to the Heart Failure clinic after an inpatient stay for decompensated heart failure. He had been very independent and functional prior to this new diagnosis, so the news came as a shock to him and his daughter. They both wept as I explained to them what changes would occur in the coming months. However, I explained to them that the Heart Failure program at the Providence VAMC would provide them with an integrated, multi-disciplinary approach to managing heart failure and making this transition as seamless as possible. Specifically, I told the Veteran that the Heart Failure program had a pharmacist to oversee his new medication regimen, a nutritionist to oversee the changes in dietary restrictions, and a psychologist to help him to cope with the anxieties of his new illness. I told him that he would also have access to shared medical visits, in which he could discuss his new illness with other Veterans to better understand that he could still live a meaningful life. We also discussed that in the event he was hospitalized, our Heart Failure team would see him, he would receive education, and he would be given close follow-up (within two weeks) after discharge. In reviewing our own facility's data, we found that Veterans who were seen in our ambulatory Heart Failure clinic had a rate of death/30-day rehospitalization of 6.4 percent compared to 11.8 percent in those who did not attend Heart Failure clinic.

When the Veteran visited the clinic six months later, he had completed the four-week shared group visits, he experienced monthly monitoring in Heart Failure Clinic, and he had not had any further hospitalizations. Most importantly, he was able to process his new diagnosis, accept it, adjust aspects of his life, and live a rich and rewarding life.

Key Information

The Heart Failure program originated from a Health Services Research and Development Service (HSR&D) research grant executed by Dr. Hank Wu, which was supported by partnerships with various departments, including the Hospitalist service, Pharmacy, Telehealth, Nutrition, and Psychology. Prior to the initiation of these programs in 2009, the 30-day readmission rate for heart failure in the Providence VAMC was at 34 percent, far worse than the national average. However, by 2014 and forward, the 30-day heart failure readmission rate had improved to approximately 20 percent, far exceeding the national average.

The promising practice used at the Providence VAMC is to employ a chronic care model of heart failure management that leverages the expertise of multiple disciplines (including pharmacy, nutrition, nursing, social work, cardiology, and psychology) to provide optimal guideline-directed medical care. Important elements of this model include:

- Transition of Care consultation to provide seamless transition between the hospitals to home.
- IV Diuretic Outpatient Clinic to provide volume assessment and aggressive diuresis to Veterans with New York Heart Association (NYHA) Class IIIB or Class IV symptoms.
- Shared Medical Visits to provide four educational modules in which Veterans can learn from a pharmacist, nurse, nutritionist, and psychologist about the multi-faceted treatment of heart failure.
- Inpatient Cardiology Consultation to provide assessment and recommendations to admitted heart failure patients.
- Heart Failure Clinics to provide close (within two weeks) follow-up to patients at risk for rehospitalization.

Context

The Providence VAMC is a primary and secondary health care facility serving Veterans in Rhode Island, southeastern Massachusetts, and eastern Connecticut. The medical center has 238 beds, 250,000 outpatient visits per year, and adds 400 to 500 new patients each month. The Providence VAMC discharges approximately 150 unique heart failure patients annually. Heart failure is the most common reason a Veteran is admitted as an inpatient. Readmission rates were above national averages in the late 2000s, giving rise to programmatic initiatives to treat heart failure in a chronic care model. The Providence VAMC has been a pioneer in incorporating nurses, NPs, and pharmacists into the care delivery for heart failure patients.

Practice Description

The implementation of the Heart Failure program occurred in several stages. In 2009, a multi-disciplinary heart failure outpatient clinic was implemented to improve access to care and to provide close follow-up to patients recently admitted for heart failure. Within one year, 30-day readmission rates had fallen from 34 to 24 percent. A major challenge that remained was helping to transition patients from the hospital back to their homes. Inadequacy of discharge planning, lack of timely follow-up, lack of patient/caregiver education, and poor continuity of care remained problematic. As such, a Heart Failure Transition of Care Team was developed in 2011, incorporating pharmacists (spearheaded by Dr. Tracey Taveira), nurses, and NPs. As a result, inpatient readmission rates continued to improve. In 2012, the Providence VAMC added an Ambulatory IV Diuretic Clinic for patients with advanced heart failure, and added the shared medical groups for heart failure. In so doing, we were able to keep at-risk Veterans from admission to the hospital (where they would be susceptible to deconditioning and infections/iatrogenic problems). By attending the Shared Medical Group visits with a focus on heart failure, Veterans were able to educate themselves and establish ties to other Veterans experiencing heart failure.

Replicability

The practice was successful at the Providence VAMC, because we had institutional support from our local leadership (Drs. Satish Sharma, Susan MacKenzie, and Sharon Rounds), vision by leadership in Cardiology (Dr. Hank Wu), and a robust partnership with pharmacy (Dr. Tracey Taveira) and research (Dr. Lisa Cohen), mental health (Karen Oliver), and nutrition (Dr. Amy Barrett). A significant factor that contributed to the success of the program was the collaboration with our pharmacists, NPs, and nurses, who were able to oversee the IV diuretic clinics, ambulatory Congestive Heart Failure (CHF) clinics, and transition of care consultations. Our VA has piloted pharmacist-led interventions successfully, and these successes led to trust between cardiology providers and pharmacists.

Recognition

Hank Wu, Satish Sharma, Tracey Taveira, Jennifer Jantz, Linda Coulter, Harsha Ganga, Stephen Bessette, Lisa Cohen, Jen Robitaille, Amy Barrett, Deborah McAuliffe, Karen Oliver

Readmission Prevention of Heart Failure

John Mills, BSN, RN, Care Manager
Sioux Falls Vet Center, Sioux Falls, SD
john.mills2@va.gov

Education interventions delivered by a multi-disciplinary team can lead to improvements in quality of care for patients with Heart Failure (HF) disease that reduce 30-day readmission rates and improve patient perceptions of care.

Introduction

Heart Failure patients have a high propensity for frequent readmission within 30 days from discharge. In analyzing the Sioux Falls VA Health Care System's historical Strategic Analytics for Improvement and Learning (SAIL) data, a review of past HF readmission percentages revealed four-quarters of ranking in the lower 50th percentile for HF readmissions within 30 days of discharge in comparison to other VHA facilities across the country. The 2014 Q4 SAIL data Congestive Heart Failure (CHF) readmission rate was 19.337 percent at the Sioux Falls VA Health Care System at the start of our project.

The Readmission Prevention of HF project charter was to assemble a multi-disciplinary team to address the high propensity of frequent readmission of HF patients within 30 days from an inpatient discharge. The team membership included the following disciplines: cardiology, nursing, pharmacy, physical therapy, occupational therapy, and nutrition. The main goal of this HF multidisciplinary team was to identify and implement needed interventions to reduce HF readmissions.

Deficiencies in discharge planning and education resulted in an approximate 20 percent rate of HF patient readmission within 30 days. A significant number of those readmissions were reduced through development of a structured HF discharge plan, which addressed the fragmentation of care that occurred when patients transitioned from inpatient to outpatient care. After six months of implementation of the Readmission Prevention of HF project, we collected quantitative data. Sixteen patients agreed to participate in the program. Out of this group, only one patient was admitted within 30 days of discharge for the same condition of HF. This gave us a 6.25 percent readmission rate for patients attending the HF group. The success of the HF project also impacted the overall SAIL data, decreasing the readmission rate to 18.927 percent and placing our facility in the upper 50th percentile of performance. Qualitative data collected also showed evidence of improved perceptions of care delivered to HF patients.

Key Information

The multi-disciplinary team identified the following four key challenges in HF discharge management: 1) lack of communication and coordination resulted in HF patients not receiving adequate follow-up due to fragmented inpatient to outpatient transition, 2) patients lacked HF education and knowledge about HF physiology and self-management skills upon discharge as evidenced by poor compliance with self-management of their condition, 3) there was poor patient compliance to medication regimes, and 4) providers were not titrating patients' medications effectively after discharge to optimize treatment. Therefore, a specialized cardiology HF clinic was needed for improved medical management of this patient population. Failure to address discharge planning and a lack of follow-up have significant financial effects on a health care system. A substantial reduction in frequent HF hospital readmissions can lead to significant reductions in the cost of care.

Context

The HF project was initiated at the Sioux Falls VAMC in Sioux Falls, SD, with the following inpatient bed count: six intensive care unit beds, 19 medical/surgical telemetry beds, 58 long-term rehabilitation beds, and six mental health beds, totaling 89 beds. Approximately 980 people are employed at this facility. The population served was comprised of recently admitted HF exacerbation patients who agreed to participate in a group education class and a specialized HF clinic. Patients had to be living independently and cognitively capable of participating in a class.

Practice Description

To have a successful transition from inpatient to outpatient care, we implemented the following four evidence-based components: 1) improved admission and discharge assessments, 2) effective teaching and patient learning, 3) patient-centered handoff that included family support, and 4) scheduled outpatient follow-up appointments after discharge.

Patients were scheduled for follow-up visits two to three weeks after discharge because most readmissions of patients with HF often occur within this timeframe. Patients attended a one-time multi-disciplinary-taught group class that educated HF patients and their caregivers about self-assessment skills to recognize the onset of an HF exacerbation and patient-driven interventions to prevent hospitalization. Each patient also had a medical appointment in a specialized HF clinic run by a cardiologist to ensure optimization and proper titration of all cardiac medications.

Replicability

Other network organizations can implement successful system-wide replications of this project to reduce HF readmission with a multi-disciplinary team approach. With no necessary extra cost or staff, this HF project was easily sustained. By using a multi-disciplinary team approach, we achieved improvements in HF quality of care patient outcomes. Changes in the quantitative and qualitative data measurement for discharge planning with HF patients showed improvements in 30-day readmission rates and patients' perceptions of care. National and network benchmark SAIL data measures reflected improved practices. Improvements in resource management from the new HF discharge process improved effectiveness of outpatient care that resulted in reduction of potential patient care cost associated with high readmission rates of this population.

Recognition

Robert Talley, Sarah Dekramer, Kristen Gerdes, Carla Goetsch, Kendra Scheidt, Jaclynn Chin, Kelley Oehlke, Erin Christensen, Steffanie Danley, Randi Sayles, Tarryn Jansen, Kathryn Schartz

Home Management of Patients on Home Intravenous Therapy

Amalia Garcia, RN BSN CCM, RN Care Coordinator
San Francisco VA Health Care System, San Francisco, CA
amalia.garcia@va.gov

This project implemented a systematic process to oversee Veterans receiving home Intravenous (IV) therapy, ensuring safe completion of the therapy.

Introduction

The aim of the project that began in July 2014 was to establish safe and high-quality monitoring and response systems for patients receiving IV antibiotics in the outpatient setting. The project was developed to reduce complications of IV therapy related to adverse events (drug-related side effects and toxicity, inappropriate removal of access device, and unplanned ER and admission visits during the therapy).

A multi-disciplinary improvement process committee, including Infectious Disease (ID) physicians and pharmacists, nursing leadership, social work, medicine, outpatient medicine, purchased skilled RNs, and Project RED (now known as RN Care Coordinators [RNCCs]) found that there were no defined roles and a lack of communication at hand-offs. There was no systematic process to ensure that providers reviewed labs, acted on them, and scanned them into the medical record. There was also a lack of standardized process for follow-up at the end of therapy, and limited monitoring to ensure efficacy of treatment.

Key Information

Assessment of appropriateness for home IV therapy was developed for each patient who wanted to go home while on IV antibiotic therapy. Medical/surgery teams, RNCCs, and the pharmaceutical company (private home infusion agency) assess patients for appropriateness for home IV before discharge.

When a Veteran is found to be an appropriate candidate for home IV, arrangements are made through a pharmaceutical company (provides IV meds and IV supplies) and a Home Health agency (for home IV/teaching, monitoring, PICC line care, blood draws). This frequently was associated with the patient's appreciation of being able to go home, decreased hospital length of stay, feeling of accomplishment in participating with one's care, being with family, and avoiding complications related to hospitalization.

The promising practice was implemented at the San Francisco VAMC and involved treatment of patients throughout Northern California and as far away as Reno, NV, and Fresno, CA. The implementation was with the coordination of the RN Coordinator, ID service, and ID pharmacist. The coordinated care project started in July 2014 with 42 home IV patients and 34 patients who completed their therapy at a Skilled Nursing Facility. In 2015, there were 60 patients on home IV, and an additional 30 patients completed their treatment at an SNF.

Context

The San Francisco VA Health Care System is a comprehensive network that provides services through the San Francisco VAMC (SFVAMC) and six community-based outpatient clinics in Santa Rosa, Eureka, Ukiah, Clearlake, San Bruno, and downtown San Francisco. It has a long history of conducting cutting-edge research, establishing innovative medical programs, and providing compassionate care to Veterans. The SFVAMC has 124 operating beds and a 120-bed Community Living Center (CLC). It provides care for more than 310,000 living in an eight-county area of Northern California.

Practice Description

If we determine that a Veteran is going to be discharged on home or Skilled Nursing Facility (SNF) parenteral antibiotic therapy, a series of safety measures follow.

The Parenteral Therapy team includes the ID team, who provides recommendations regarding the necessity of the antimicrobial antibiotic therapy, medication selection, dosing, and duration of therapy. To ensure that a Veteran does not get a Peripherally Inserted Central Catheter (PICC) placed unnecessarily, the ID and PICC teams communicate early on about the possibility of antibiotic therapy. The PICC RN evaluates the appropriateness of the long-term PICC placement initiated for the purpose of the antimicrobial therapy at home. We identify an outpatient medical provider to follow the patient at home before he is discharged. The RNCC evaluates the patient for appropriateness for home IV therapy, coordinates home health referrals, monitors the patient weekly to ensure that surveillance labs are done; results are reported, scanned in the medical record, and acted upon in real time.

The medical center:

- Selects a home infusion specialty service that will provide consultation, infusion equipment, medication, patient education, and monitoring to deliver safe and individualized care.

- Monitors the appropriate delivery of the parenteral antibiotic by calling the patient the first business day after discharge.

- Ensures that the patient has appropriate follow-up care at the medical center and confirms that the intravenous catheter has been removed at the end of therapy.

- Monitors quality of care and patient satisfaction by tracking a variety of metrics.

Replicability

We implemented this practice to establish safe, high-quality monitoring and response systems for patients receiving IV antibiotics in the outpatient setting, including at home or at an SNF.

Other facilities need to identify issues relevant to the development of a complex interdisciplinary team. We recommend the organization of a multi-disciplinary committee to identify problems, identify aims and measures to improve, and confirm a process to measure outcomes.

Recognition

Harry Lampiris, Daniel Maddix, Steve Collinson, Greg Burrell, Estela Dau, Dolores Swanson, Lourdes Hampton, Bermesola Dyer, Cindy Villegas

Improving Immunosuppression Monitoring and Care Coordination in Veteran Transplant Recipients

David Taber, PharmD, BCPS, CPS - Transplantation

Ralph H. Johnson Medical Center, Charleston, SC

david.taber2@va.gov

This clinic improves immunosuppression therapy monitoring and management in Veterans with organ transplants. Key initiatives include optimizing documentation and care coordination with outside facilities and reengaging Veterans to obtain appropriate laboratory monitoring and follow-up care within our VA facility.

Introduction

Solid organ transplant is the gold standard treatment for patients with end organ diseases of the kidney, liver, heart, and lungs, as it substantially improves survival and quality of life. Current immunosuppressants used to prevent rejection in transplantation are highly effective but carry the burdens of considerable toxicities, multiple drug interactions, and highly complex regimens. These attributes place Veteran transplant recipients at very high risk for developing drug-related problems, including adverse drug events, non-adherence, and medication errors. Our preliminary research demonstrates that medication errors occur in nearly two-thirds of transplant recipients, leading to hospitalization in one in eight recipients. Those who experience significant medication errors are at considerably higher risk of graft loss and death.

Most Veteran transplant recipients are dual users, receiving their health care across multiple systems. This can lead to discordant care and increase the risk of drug-related problems. We conducted a single-center study demonstrating substantial issues in care coordination for our Veteran organ transplant population, including 91 percent of patients having discrepancies in their documented medication regimens between VA and non-VA systems, 40 percent having inadequate immunosuppression drug levels measured to monitor therapy, and more than 80 percent having duplicative laboratory assessments. Based on this, we set out to implement a technology-enabled, pharmacist-led initiative to improve care coordination and immunosuppression therapy monitoring and management in our Veteran organ transplant population. Over the past 18 months, we have made substantial improvements in the monitoring of immunosuppression therapies and care coordination of these Veterans, including a substantial improvement in immunosuppression monitoring, increasing from approximately 58 percent at baseline to over 90 percent with the most current data. In addition, our initiative has increased the number of Veterans with an accurate transplant diagnosis from 88 to 100 percent and increased Veteran transplant recipients seen within a year from 88 to 96 percent.

There is one particular patient story that comes to mind that I think epitomizes this program and its potential impact on Veteran care. There is a Veteran kidney transplant recipient at our VAMC that received his transplant nearly 40 years ago (1977). He was receiving his immunosuppression through our VAMC, but was not having laboratory monitoring done for these agents through the VA system. It was assumed that this was being done at his transplant center, and vice-versa, with no communication between the parties. Through this initiative, we identified that he was lacking appropriate laboratory monitoring, reached out to this Veteran, and brought him in for testing. The results revealed a significant issue with his white blood cell counts. He was referred to hematology, which performed a bone marrow biopsy and discovered early stages of myelodysplastic syndrome, which can be caused by one of the immunosuppressants he was receiving. After coordination with his transplant center, his immunosuppression regimen was modified to remove the offending agent and replace it with one not likely to induce this issue. Subsequently, his blood counts returned to normal and the myelodysplasia appeared to have stabilized, if not reversed. We were happy to have identified this issue in the early stages of development, something that likely would not have occurred without engaging this Veteran and working with him to implement appropriate laboratory monitoring.

Key Information

We developed this initiative to improve care coordination and immunosuppression monitoring and management for our Veterans with organ transplants. Although not a large population of patients, organ transplant recipients are known to be at very high risk for drug-related problems and discordant care. The initiative uses technology to identify Veterans at our VAMC who had organ transplants, are receiving immunosuppression therapy, and require follow-up laboratory monitoring. This is a pharmacist-led program, whereby the CPS uses the data generated from the dashboard to identify potential issues, reach out to the individual Veterans to determine where he or she is receiving care, and coordinate appropriate follow-up monitoring and care. At times, this may include reengaging the Veteran to seek care within the VA system and/or appropriately documented monitoring of care that provided outside the VA system. We hope that the substantial improvements we have demonstrated in improving immunosuppression monitoring and care coordination will eventually lead to improved outcomes within this high-risk Veteran population. We plan to expand this program to include technology-enabled surveillance, including monitoring for medication non-adherence, drug-drug interactions, and worrisome trends in laboratory values. We also hope to lead in rolling out this program to other centers that care for Veteran organ transplant recipients.

Context

The Ralph H. Johnson VAMC and six surrounding CBOCs serve Veterans residing in the low country of South Carolina. This ongoing initiative has focused on providing improved immunosuppression monitoring, management, and care coordination for those Veterans who received organ transplants, totaling approximately 105 to date within our catchment area. We have also provided leadership to help improve care for the VISN 7 Veteran organ transplant recipients, totaling over 750 patients. A major challenge that this initiative addressed was improved communication and care coordination for high-risk Veterans who clearly receive their care across multiple health care systems, both within and outside the VA system. Reengaging Veterans who do not utilize the VA system for care and follow-up was another challenge that we have sought to improve. The results are promising, and we are working to expand this initiative to optimize care for this population across our VISN and beyond.

Practice Description

The practice involved adapting a dashboard that VISN 12 developed, which identified Veteran organ transplant recipients who were receiving immunosuppression medications through the VA system without appropriate laboratory monitoring. After the dashboard was functional and validated within VISN 7, the CPS utilized this information to engage identified Veterans and determine mechanisms to improve therapy monitoring and management. This included optimizing documentation and care coordination with outside facilities, as well as reengaging Veterans to obtain appropriate laboratory monitoring and follow-up care within our VAMC. The initiative was truly multi-disciplinary, and involved VA leadership, VA informaticists, VA pharmacy department personnel, PCPs and professionals involved in these Veterans' care outside the VA system. Without a coordinated effort from all these disciplines, the initiative would not have been successful.

Replicability

This practice was successful because it was thoughtfully planned, based on a similar initiative from VISN 12, had strong leadership and VA support, included a multi-disciplinary team, and worked to be Veteran-centered by engaging Veterans to determine the method they most preferred for follow-up care. Support from leadership at VA and full engagement and buy-in from the Veteran population were key to success. This practice is clearly reproducible, as evidenced by the fact it was adopted from a program from VISN 12. Keys for reproducibility include the same factors that made the program a success at our facility: strong leadership, Veteran-centered care and engagement, multi-disciplinary team involvement, and a CPS that has the knowledge, expertise, and motivation to make this a successful endeavor.

Recognition

Sharon Castle, Cory Fominaya, Beth Bryant, Shree Patel, Samantha Wright

Integrated Dual Diagnosis Treatment

Alisa Sprague, MHICM, CRC, MFH, CAP, Program Manager
Louis Stokes Cleveland VAMC, Cleveland, OH
alisa.sprague@va.gov

Integrated Dual Diagnosis Treatment (IDDT) is an evidence-based practice for more effective management of those with co-occurring severe mental illness and substance use disorders.

Introduction

For a long time, Mr. X struggled with his addiction and mental illness. He attempted to live independently and work but routinely failed due to his addiction, mental health symptoms, and repeated psychiatric hospitalizations. In 2009, Mr. X's case manager helped him move into yet another apartment where he sat on his bed for days on end drinking and using crack cocaine. It was at this point that his Mental Health Intensive Case Management (MHICM) case manager started to talk with him about attending IDDT groups. After some deliberation, he began attending groups at the Psychosocial Recovery Resource Center (PRRC) and slowly started to consider the possibility of making a change. He was surprised about being allowed to make his own choices rather than being told he needed to quit using and be compliant with treatment. While meeting with his mental health provider at the PRRC he said, "I think I need inpatient treatment."

While Mr. X was in residential treatment, providers worked together to find him a group home where he could continue to work on mental health and addictions recovery, and to attend groups at the PRRC. The peer support specialist shared how helpful Alcoholics Anonymous (AA) had been in his recovery, and at that point, Mr. X thought, "If he can do it, maybe I can too." He started going to AA, and while attending VA IDDT groups, asked his providers what he would need to do to obtain his own apartment, because his goal was to become independent. His case manager assisted him in finding an apartment that was located on a bus line. The IDDT team consisted of an intensive case manager, peer support specialist, recovery coach, and others who helped Mr. X learn skills necessary for independent living.

Mr. X has now been substance free for three years and has lived in his own apartment for over two years. He no longer needs intensive case management and outreach, and volunteers at a local health care center. Support systems have helped him to find meaning in his life and will help him continue his recovery journey. Mr. X's story is just one example of how the Louis Stokes Cleveland VAMC (Cleveland VAMC) IDDT team impacts Veterans.

Key Information

The MHICM team and PRRC have partnered together at the Cleveland VAMC to offer IDDT services. In 2013, training in IDDT was made possible for both teams, as well as providers from other programs, through a contract with the Case Western Reserve University Center for Evidenced-Based Practices (CWRU-CEBP). Alisa Sprague, MHICM Program Manager, coordinated these efforts. One of the most promising aspects of IDDT is its evidence-based foundation. Research shows that individuals with dual diagnosis (i.e., severe and persistent mental illness plus a serious substance use disorder) who receive IDDT treatment have fewer psychiatric hospitalizations and relapses, lower rates of incarceration, and fewer instances of homelessness than those who do not participate in integrated treatment services. The PRRC and MHICM programs were chosen as ideal programs because of the high numbers of Veterans with dual disorders participating.

Context

The Cleveland VAMC is the third largest VA facility in the country. With the introduction of the VA Uniform Mental Health Services Handbook (VHA Handbook 1160.01) in 2008, we have seen an increase in evidence-based services available for Veterans with various complex conditions. Despite all the resources within our VAMC, one of the most difficult groups of individuals to serve in an outpatient setting is Veterans who struggle with dual diagnoses. Cleveland and several other VA facilities have spent a considerable amount of time and effort providing programs and resources to address each of the various health, mental health, and psychosocial needs facing our nation's Veterans. However, there are many challenges associated with treating individuals with dual disorders in an integrated manner. Many Veterans continue to move from program to program or are involved in multiple, separate services, but research supports that integrated treatment is much more successful and effective for the dually disordered population. IDDT attempts to integrate treatment for individuals so one team of professionals can deliver mental health and substance abuse services. IDDT implementation has improved the Cleveland VAMC's ability to engage and support each Veteran in his or her recovery while simultaneously addressing complex needs, with the goal of each Veteran having the tools to pursue personally meaningful life goals and roles.

Practice Description

IDDT uses a stage-based approach to treatment. We tailor interventions each individual's internal motivation and unique life circumstances. IDDT provides a flexible approach to "meet the individual where they are" in their willingness to make personal change. We utilize the stage-based approach in assessment, care planning, and treatment. During the Engagement stage, staff works to develop a relationship with individuals who usually do not feel they have a mental health or substance abuse problem. Assertive outreach and patience are key variables to success at this stage. The Persuasion stage is when Veterans are beginning to contemplate making a change. During this stage, staff uses individual and group interventions to reduce any ambivalence the Veteran has about addressing their mental health and/or substance use disorder. During the Active Treatment stage, Veterans learn skills and actively use those skills to cope with mental health symptoms and substance abuse triggers. In the final stage of Relapse Prevention, Veterans are involved in more meaningful life activities as they actively manage their recovery and have reduced reliance on staff supports. It is important to note that each treatment stage has a specific clinical focus with clear, motivational, psychosocial, and pharmacological interventions.

To begin implementation of this model, our staff completed more than 20 hours of classroom training on the IDDT model with team-based consultation from CWRU-CEBP. Three fidelity reviews were conducted to ensure proper implementation of the model. PRRC and MHICM have regular meetings and developed referral criteria and a consult system that allows both programs to review, track, and monitor new referrals, as well as determine what levels of services are needed to address Veterans' individual needs. Staff identifies each Veteran's stage of treatment after the initial assessment and incorporates that information into the treatment plan and progress notes. Veterans are staged throughout their participation in the program and interventions are adjusted accordingly.

Ultimately, the goal is for individuals to move through all the stages, graduate from the program, and have improved treatment and recovery outcomes.

Outcomes show increased acknowledgment that substance use is problematic, willingness from the Veteran to begin discussing and addressing substance abuse, longer periods of abstinence between relapse, increased use of self-help groups, and an increased interest in working or meaningful activity. For many of these individuals the process results in more stable housing over time. The Veterans also report a reduction in symptoms, Suicidal Ideation (SI) and attempts, violence, and victimization. They also talk about improvements in their physical health and success at maintaining community living.

Replicability

It is imperative for other facilities interested in using the IDDT model to have the support of their leadership and the resources to work with the consultants over a period of time (at least two years). The model is easily adapted into programs currently working with patients with a dual diagnosis, but coordination among the programs is vital. Peer Support Specialists are crucial members of the team, as we saw in the story of Mr. X. When feasible, it is also helpful to have one dedicated medication provider for the team, so there is familiarity with the model and consistency for the Veteran served by the IDDT team.

Recognition

Susan Fuehrer, Paul Konicki, David DiTullio, Michael Biscaro, MHICM and PRRC teams, CWRU Center for Evidence-Based Practices

Pre-Operative Surgical Patient Navigation and Care Coordination: The RN Surgery Navigator

Shari Kym, MSN, RN-BC, Nurse Manager Surgery Clinics
VA Southern Nevada Healthcare System, North Las Vegas, NV
shari.kym@va.gov

The RN Surgery Nurse Navigator role uses a patient-centered care approach in providing comprehensive pre-operative patient education and care coordination to prevent surgery cancellations.

Introduction

An orthopedic patient and surgeon agree for knee replacement surgery in 45 days. The patient signs the consent and staff books the Operating Room (OR) time. Staff gives this patient a 25-page booklet to read and remember within the next 45 days. In addition to that, the Veteran must be cleared for surgery and have key tests done by medicine, cardiology, laboratory, radiology, and anticoagulation clinic. The patient must find a responsible adult and transportation. The Veteran is alone in dealing with his health issues and pain. He forgets key pre-operative appointments and instructions. His surgery date is November 11, but cardiology doesn't realize this and schedules his stress test on December 3. He loses his transportation and forgets to go to anticoagulation clinic. He reports to the OR on November 11 after drinking his coffee, despite learning 45 days ago he was not to eat or drink before surgery. The OR has no choice but to cancel his surgery.

Imagine this scenario with the addition of a RN navigating this patient through the complex health system, supporting his goals, and providing in-depth education and reinforcement while coordinating his pre-operative medical needs. This RN will prevent a surgery cancellation, and produce positive outcomes, including patient and staff satisfaction. The Veteran is often a complex patient with multiple medical problems and psychosocial issues. These patients require surgery from time to time. In the midst of having a health issue requiring surgery, these patients are faced with navigating their own path in a complex, inflexible health care environment. Many of these patients do not have the capacity or resilience to navigate the fragmented pathway to meet their surgery date, resulting in a surgery cancellation. The surgery clinic has grown rapidly with a new medical center opening in 2012, doubling its capacity, and OR cases also grew from 100 to over 200 patients per month. A rising surgery cancellation rate was observed in the last quarter for FY 2014 and beginning quarter FY 2015 with nearly one-quarter of the surgeries scheduled being canceled. These high rates led to frustration for the staff, family, and patients. This process was developing a perfect storm, requiring a new way of thinking about how we deliver care. In drilling down to why these cancellations were happening, we concluded that no one was taking ownership of these patients. We piloted the RN Surgery Navigator role in March 2015 and the surgery cancellation rate dropped from 23 to 14 percent with just one navigator. We added additional navigators and our latest surgery cancellation rate as of March 2016 is 6 percent. With fewer cancellations, we are seeing improved surgery efficiency, improved access for patients, and improved staff and patient satisfaction.

Key Information

The staff observed an increasing surgery cancellation rate. In drilling down as to why these cancellations were occurring, we observed two trends. First, the Veteran was not receiving timely patient education and reinforcement, resulting in unintended non-compliance in pre-operative instructions. Second, the patient was not getting their medical risk stratification and optimization within the time allotted before their preferred surgery date, and had social issues that led to cancellation. The process desperately needed patient navigation and care coordination.

We initiated the RN Surgery Navigator role in the Pre-Operative Clinic. It was a collaboration with Surgery Services and Nursing Services in achieving a "surgical home" for the Veteran. We also had supportive data from the National Surgery Office that sponsored a Pre-Operative Value Stream Analysis and Rapid Performance Improvement Workshop during the second quarter of FY 2015. The Nurse Manager led the change with recruiting a former pre-operative clinic nurse and leveraging her knowledge and experience in creating the unique role combining patient navigation and care coordination. We officially implemented this on March 2, 2015 in orthopedics and general surgery clinics, using monthly tracking of surgery cancellation rates as a metric for improvement.

Context

The VA Southern Nevada Healthcare System is a growing organization in both population and maturity as it recently moved to a standalone medical center in 2012. Previous OR operations occurred at Nellis Air Force Base with the US Air Force Joint Venture. The number of Veterans served is steadily rising with 57,383 in FY 2015, and an estimated user rate of 79 percent. Unique features of the Southern Nevada Veteran population include its draw from rural desert areas (Southern California to Southern Utah), a transient population as a tourist destination attracting seasonal visits, and Veterans' complete lack of social support systems and isolation. The surgery clinics have seen a steady rise of around 4,000 patient visits per month and slightly over 200 OR cases per month. An average OR case is approximately two hours with average costs at $1,000 per hour. Monthly surgery cancellation rates started climbing to an all-time high of 23 percent, which contributed to OR inefficiencies, patient and staff dissatisfaction, and elevated costs for non-productivity up to $100,000 per month.

Practice Description

We looked to best practices at other VA facilities to learn about their processes, successes, and lessons learned. We also looked at the private sector and reviewed the literature. We found that most areas did not combine the navigation and care coordination roles. We adopted a combined navigation and care coordination role with a patient goal-oriented strategy (the goal for the Veteran is to report to the OR for their scheduled surgery on the confirmed date, ready to go) and set metrics we wanted to meet (decreasing surgery cancellation rate to less than 9 percent). We developed a unique statement of role functionality and appropriate competencies to be achieved.

We presented the role to leadership, including the Nurse Executive and Associate Nurse Executive, and they approved it as a pilot. A nurse volunteered to assume the pilot role for three months. Together, we established a patient flow map and tracking tool. The Performance Improvement nursing team for tracking patient cancellations had already been established and continued their valuable reporting of our progress. We launched on March 2, 2015, focusing on two clinics: General Surgery and Orthopedics. Reports by the PI team in April revealed a significant drop in cancellation rates from 23 to 14 percent. We added additional navigators focusing on cancellation outliers in urology, plastics, and ophthalmology clinics, and our cancellation rate decreased to 7 percent. As General Surgery and Orthopedic Clinics grew, we added an additional navigator, and cancellation rates have leveled off at 6 to 8 percent, well below our goal. We have now looked beyond our OR program and are providing services for selected clinics for non-VA care navigation for patients going to other VA facilities via Integrated Family Community Services and into the community.

Replicability

Any outpatient area that requires complex care coordination and patient education like gastroenterology, oncology, and cardiology, could easily replicate this role. It could also be expanded to incorporate both in-network and out-of-network care. The use of CPRS across services lends to the success of the role, but also has limitations regarding alerts and conflicts in scheduling, and in this respect, a nurse is needed to implement the process. The Navigation and Care Coordination role reviews what services will be required for the Veteran, coordinates these services in order to prevent a surgery cancellation, introduces the Veteran to the services, and ensures the Veteran is proactively approached to establish their plan of care. The patient also receives face-to-face patient education and telephone follow-up reinforcement. Areas still to be resolved include appropriate labor mapping and true capture of productivity.

Recognition

Jennifer Strawn, Keesha Davis, Margarita Vistan, Rose Labarcon, Imelda Roque, Cathy Roma, Connie Hudson, Roma Polce, Julian Losanoff

Psychosocial Distress Monitoring and Navigation in Oncology

Donna Rasin-Waters, PhD, Psychologist

Brooklyn Campus of the VA NY Harbor Healthcare System, Brooklyn, NY
donna.rasin-waters@va.gov

The practice employs a systematic approach, involving psychological distress screening and personalized navigation plans, at oncology visits to help Veterans successfully complete their medical treatment.

Introduction

Mr. X, a Vietnam-era Veteran, was facing aggressive prostate cancer when he was triaged by the oncology nurse and given the National Comprehensive Cancer Network (NCCN) Distress Thermometer and Problem Checklist. When he rated himself as severely distressed, the nurse walked him across the hallway to the psychologist who was available two afternoons a week during the new patient clinic hours. The psychologist and oncology social worker could also be called upon for highly distressed Veterans receiving cancer treatments throughout the rest of the week. Mr. X was severely distressed about his cancer diagnosis and noted worry, depression, fear, and nervousness on his Problem Checklist. In addition, he checked off that he was homeless, had transportation issues, and had family problems. A Cancer Navigation Plan Note was completed in CPRS with the Veteran, encouraging regular contact with the psychologist during daily radiation therapy for the next eight weeks. The Navigation Plan, printed out in user-friendly format and given to Mr. X, also provided information about housing assistance and travel options. With Mr. X's consent, the psychologist also contacted family members to arrange a collateral visit with the goal of resolving a current dispute. Over the next two months, Mr. X was encountered 38 times for brief health and behavior interventions, collateral family meetings, and hands-on navigation. Mr. X needed the support of being walked over directly to VA Supportive Housing (VASH) for appointments and follow-up, as he was too distraught to go on his own. He was placed in the nearest shelter so he could access public transportation to his medical appointments. He needed frequent calls and a flexible appointment schedule to adhere to daily radiation therapy appointments. Following completion of radiation treatment, Mr. X met with the psychologist, as needed, when he came for less frequent hormone treatment. His distress level dropped below the threshold and he was able to continue to follow up with housing and family issues on his own with encouragement from the psychologist.

Mr. Y, another Vietnam-era Veteran, also diagnosed with prostate cancer, scored below the threshold for distress when triaged by the oncology nurse. He also saw the psychologist the same day, and a Cancer Navigation Plan Note in CPRS was completed and printed out for him. Mr. Y was provided with the resource information necessary to tackle current problems related to transportation. Having met the oncology psychologist, Mr. Y learned he could request an appointment at any time should his level of distress increase during medical treatment. He also stated he understood the navigation information and planned to go to the VA travel office to address transportation issues.

While both Veterans were seen the same day, their navigation plan outcomes were quite different. The Veteran with very low distress could navigate the complex VA system with necessary information provided. The severely distressed Veteran regularly encountered the psychologist for treatment adherence, crisis intervention, and hands-on navigation. Both Veterans successfully completed their medical treatment while addressing psychosocial issues. Prior to the psychosocial distress monitoring and navigation intervention, the oncology staff considered that Mr. X may have been lost to treatment due to non-adherence and problems that may not have even been evident to the medical staff.

Key Information

The VA New York Harbor Healthcare Systems Brooklyn Campus implemented the Commission on Cancer (CoC) standards requiring cancer programs to provide access to patient-centered services, such as psychosocial distress screening and navigation. Donna Rasin-Waters, PhD, Psychologist, led the implementation as part of a subcommittee of the VA NY Harbor Cancer Committee formed to address the CoC standards. The subcommittee wanted to develop a systematic way of providing navigation through a very complex system of services that differentiated Veterans who needed staff to assist them from those who could pull resources on their own if provided with information. The team did this by looking at the level of distress a Veteran reported at their first oncology visit.

Context

The VA New York Harbor Healthcare System (VA NYHHS) is an A1 facility serving Veterans in the New York City Metropolitan area, with facilities in Manhattan, Brooklyn, St. Albans, and various CBOCs.

Practice Description

Implementation of the NCCN Distress Thermometer and Patient Checklist by the triage nurse occurred from April 2011 to February 2014 on 396 Veterans using a Psychosocial Distress Screening Note, a CPRS template developed by the subcommittee to record the data. Metrics indicated six of the top 12 problems reported by Veterans in oncology were directly related to mental and behavioral health issues (worry, depression, nervousness, sadness, fears, loss of interest). This prompted the development of embedded mental and behavioral health services in the oncology clinic with the goal of immediate access to the oncology psychologist following triage by nursing through warm hand-offs. In 2015, we used these metrics to develop local resources for an individualized Cancer Navigation Plan Note, another template in CPRS developed by the team. Each Veteran received a personalized navigation plan printed out in user-friendly language. Veterans scoring the highest, as in the severe range of distress, received the most personalized, ongoing, and hands-on navigation. A Veteran satisfaction survey completed about the navigation plans on 58 Veterans found that all but two had kept their navigation plans, knew where they were at home, and would refer to them in the future.

This practice, meant to fulfill the CoC standards for distress monitoring and patient navigation, can be adapted through the following steps:

1. Form an interdisciplinary committee or team to discuss which service will regularly screen Veterans with the NCCN Distress Thermometer and Patient Checklist.

2. Discuss which mental and behavioral health providers will be readily available for warm hand-offs, to develop individualized navigation plans with Veterans from the Distress Thermometer and Problem Checklist data, and to provide follow-up, as needed.

3. The nurse manager, psychologist, and/or social worker trained nurses to triage Veterans using the screening tool to standardize the administration of the tool and reinforce the warm hand-offs, especially for severely distressed Veterans.

4. These templates (Psychosocial Distress Screening Note and Cancer Navigation Plan Note) can be utilized to collect metrics and create individualized navigation plans.

Replicability

This promising practice was successful due to the persistence of the psychologist, Chief of Hematology/Oncology, and program specialist who met regularly to refine the program, get input from the social worker and nurse manager, as needed, develop the CPRS templates, go over metrics, and ensure severely distressed Veterans were being followed. It is replicable once a system for same-day access to mental and behavioral health services is established for Veterans who are screened in the oncology service.

Recognition

Donna Rasin-Waters, Carol Luhrs, Maura Langdon, Louisa Daratsos, Johanna Maldonado

Cleveland VA ALS Center of Excellence

Frances McClellan, RN, MSN, ALS Coordinator; Stephen Selkirk, MD, PhD, Medical Director
Louis Stokes Cleveland VAMC, Cleveland, OH
frances.mcclellan@va.gov

The ALS Center of Excellence is an Interdisciplinary team that provides coordinated health care to Veterans with Amyotrophic Lateral Sclerosis (ALS). This approach has provided rapid access to care, improved delivery of Durable Medical Equipment (DME), and increased Veteran and family satisfaction.

Introduction

There is high-quality epidemiologic evidence supporting an association between the development of ALS and prior military service. These findings provoked VA to request that the Institute of Medicine (IOM) conduct an independent study of the potential relationship between military service and ALS. In 2006, the IOM found that military service increased the lifetime risk of ALS by 1.5 times. In 2008, ALS became a presumptively compensable illness, which means that Veterans diagnosed with ALS are entitled to 100 percent service-connected disability status and all benefits afforded to it. Currently there are over 2,000 Veterans nationwide with ALS receiving care in the VHA system.

ALS is a neurodegenerative disease of unknown etiology. The average life expectancy of an individual diagnosed with ALS today is two to five years, and 95 percent of patients will die within five years of their diagnosis. The diagnosis is life altering and devastating to Veterans and their families. Starting in 2008, the Cleveland VAMC Spinal Cord Injury (SCI) service began to receive referrals to care for severely ill patients with ALS. At that time the staff, paradigm, and protocols required to provide high-quality care for Veterans with ALS were not in place. Since then, the Cleveland VAMC has established a Certified Center of Excellence for ALS care.

Key Information

In 2008, the Cleveland VAMC SCI Center initiated a committee to improve the care of Veterans with ALS. The committee consisted of the Chief of Neurology, Robert Ruff, MD; the Chief of SCI, Chester Ho, MD; the SCI Service Rehabilitation Program Manager, Frances McClellan, RN, MSN; and the SCI Neurologist, Stephen Selkirk, MD, PhD. This committee examined the strengths, weaknesses, and opportunities facing ALS care at the Cleveland VAMC. They worked with a variety of services, including pulmonary/sleep, Prosthetics, Gastrointestinal (GI), anesthesiology, and speech to develop new and innovative processes that would ultimately improve care for Veterans with ALS. Starting in 2009, new processes were set into place that improved access to care, efficiency in the delivery of care, effectiveness of care, and patient satisfaction. In addition, we established an ALS Interdisciplinary team that included neurology, ALS coordinator, respiratory pulmonary/sleep, SCI therapy services, SCI nursing, SCI psychology, SCI social work, hospice, prosthetics, SCI telehealth, speech and language pathology, nutrition, the local ALS Association (ALSA), and the Paralyzed Veterans of America (PVA). With this in place, The ALS Center was founded in 2009 with the mission of providing coordinated care to Veterans with ALS and their families according to best practice standard of care guidelines put forth by ALSA and the

American Academy of Neurology (AAN). In 2014, the Cleveland VAMC ALS Center became the first VA facility in the country to receive the designation of a Certified Center of Excellence from the National ALSA. The Cleveland VAMC ALS Center of Excellence is only the second center in the state of Ohio and one of 32 centers in the US. This prestigious designation is perhaps most important to Veterans treated in Cleveland as several studies have demonstrated that patients cared for at ALSA-certified centers have a higher quality of life, longer survival times, greater access to disease-modifying medications, DME, hospice, Percutaneous Endoscopic Gastrostomy (PEG) tube insertion, and non-invasive positive pressure ventilation.

Context

The ALS Center of Excellence is embedded with the SCI System of Care at the Cleveland VAMC. We currently serve 105 Veterans with ALS from Ohio, southern Michigan, and western Pennsylvania. A team of professionals works together, led by the ALS Center director and coordinator, to provide high-quality multi-disciplinary care. The ALS coordinator is responsible for identifying new patients, making initial contacts, helping the Veteran get into the VA system, scheduling appointments, presenting new and follow-up patients at the team meetings, following up and ensuring implementation of all team recommendations, ensuring benefits are established for disability compensation, and being available to Veterans and families throughout their journey with ALS.

The processes that were developed as part of this interdisciplinary team included:

- A distinct prosthetic template and an identified prosthetic agent to prioritize DME purchasing and delivery. This decreased the delivery of DME from several weeks to one to three days enhancing our ability to provide emergent care.

- A Comfort Bi-level Positive Airway Pressure (BIPAP) protocol was established that allowed a day sleep study lasting three to four hours, instead of an overnight sleep study which was a significant barrier for the Veteran and family, reducing the time to study to one to two weeks.

- The DME equipment reuse program allows us to retrieve unwanted and undamaged high-end equipment; clean them, store them, and reissue them to other Veteran with ALS. This has enabled the ALS Center to provide necessary DME more rapidly, and at minimal cost.

- We initiated the ALS Telehealth program to provide specialty care to Veterans who live far from the ALS Center and cannot easily travel to us. The program allows us to do remote clinic-to-clinic visits (CVT) with our SCI and PCPs at other SCI facilities in Ohio, Michigan, and Pennsylvania when the patient is present with them. It has also allowed us to do video-to-home visits with patients who live rurally and are not close to any local VA facility. We arrange for procedures to be done in their local community and then have the ALS team see the patient via a secure video visit. We have also used this modality when Veterans are on hospice care. The use of telehealth in this setting has been shown to improve patient and family satisfaction, reduce caregiver burden, and reduce travel costs.

- The ALS Center has improved coordination of care for this complex patient population. The Veteran who comes to clinic has all necessary tests done on the same day, reducing the need for multiple trips.

Practice Description

A core group of ALS providers identified our Strengths, Weaknesses, Opportunities, and Threats (SWOT analysis). Strengths identified that the SCI program had an existing interdisciplinary team that understood patients with complex, high level disabilities, DME needs, and a hub and spoke system of care in which collaboration and referrals occurred seamlessly. Our weaknesses included standard processes for consulting specialists that took too long and were not consistent with the rapid progression disability this population of Veterans experienced. The opportunities included building processes that would work for this population and extending the team. Threats included a non-funded program, a disease associated with high costs, poor Veterans Equitable Resource Allocation (VERA) reimbursement, acceptance of care from Veterans with ALS who had never accessed VA, and the potential for other services to not allow an allocation of provider time. We developed processes to improve core issues, resulting in the development and implementation of a coordinated interdisciplinary care team and an ALS Center of Excellence at the Cleveland VAMC. The practice led to increased access to care, DME distribution, support services, reduced costs, and improved satisfaction of patients, families, and staff.

Replicability

This practice was adopted and successful because leadership realized the complexity of care required and the lack of processes in place to provide care to Veterans with ALS. There was an attitude that VA could provide high-quality care comparable to identified ALS Centers of Excellence across the country. In addition, the staff of the Cleveland VAMC collaborated with our team to develop solutions to each problem. The SCI neurologist and the ALS Coordinator work to continually address and improve processes as the program evolves. VAMCs of similar size should certainly be able to replicate a process and Center similar to ours. Smaller VAMCs could work with larger regional programs via telehealth.

Recognition

Robert Ruff, Chester Ho, Mary Ann Richmond, ALS Interdisciplinary Team from Cleveland

Development of a Multidisciplinary Transitions of Care Service for Chronic Obstructive Pulmonary Disease Management

Ed Portillo, PGY1/2 Health System Pharmacy Administration Resident

William S. Middleton Memorial Veterans Hospital, Madison, WI

edward.portillo@va.gov

A novel, interdisciplinary Chronic Obstructive Pulmonary Disease (COPD) Clinic was developed at the William S. Middleton Veterans Hospital to help service Veterans. The service has been developed in response to a growing need for population-health based initiatives centered around COPD care.

Introduction

Mr. X is a 65-year-old male who presented to the ED with a COPD exacerbation. It was the Veteran's second COPD exacerbation within a year and he drove three hours to the William S. Middleton VA ED for urgent care. The Veteran had experienced shortness of breath and coughing for over a week, and realized his condition required immediate attention. After waiting for evaluation in the ED, he was sent home with a prescription for prednisone and doxycycline for continued management at home.

This narrative describes what many consider to be the standard of care for COPD treatment throughout private sector and VA. When patients experience a COPD exacerbation, they often receive an antibiotic and steroid in urgent care. The fact is, COPD is the third leading cause of death worldwide and the mortality rate one year after a hospitalization from COPD ranges from 22 to 43 percent. After Mr. X's exacerbation, his lung function may have never returned to baseline and his quality of life may never have been the same. However, since his ED visit, our multi-disciplinary COPD service has kept him exacerbation-free and feeling great.

COPD hospital readmissions are tracked nationally on the Strategic Analytics for Improvement and Learning (SAIL) dashboard, and numerous ED visits are attributed to COPD exacerbations. This clinic service addresses the unique needs of our Veterans with COPD, and has significantly increased Veteran access to COPD care post-discharge.

Key Information

The William S. Middleton Veterans Affairs Hospital implemented this promising practice from November 11, 2015 to March 1, 2016. This service was offered to all Veterans who presented to the ED or Hospital with a COPD exacerbation. Participating Veterans had to receive PC at the VA West Annex Clinic for service participation. The project was led by the pharmacy department, with key collaborators in respiratory therapy, nursing, pulmonary, and PC. This service matters because the prevalence of COPD among the Veteran population is four times that of civilians. We owe it to our Veterans to be national leaders on COPD care.

Context

The William S. Middleton Veterans Affairs hospital is a 129-bed acute care facility with six community-based clinics. The COPD readmission rate at our VA based on recent SAIL data is 17.9 percent, which is much higher than the facility's overall readmission rate of 13.1 percent for all conditions. The average age of Veterans who enrolled in this service is 71-years-old, with 100 percent being male with previous tobacco use (38.9 percent remain tobacco users). The average number of COPD exacerbations in the past year for service participants was 1.8, with 57.8 percent leading to a hospitalization. The average Global Initiative for Chronic Obstructive Lung Disease (GOLD) stage of Veterans enrolled was GOLD 2. The challenge that this practice addressed was how to best provide timely, effective COPD care, which was successfully attained through leveraging our PACT in PC.

Practice Description

Veterans were referred post-discharge to be seen in clinic by a PACT pharmacist provider, where a 45-minute focused COPD visit was conducted. All pharmacists involved in this service followed GOLD guidelines and utilized their scope of practice to prescribe inhalers and steroids/antibiotics for use with the COPD Action Plan and order labs. Nurse care managers performed patient education on the COPD Action Plan. Veterans were also contacted during a telephone appointment two months post-exacerbation to reinforce adherence, with updated pulmonary function tests ordered three months post-exacerbation.

Replicability

This service was successful at our Madison VA facility given the facility-wide interest in improving COPD care. Four workstreams were developed for service completion with involvement from pharmacy, respiratory therapy, PCPs, and nursing. This service can easily be applied at other VA facilities.

Recognition

Berook Addisu, Prakash Balasubramanian, Jim Lewis, Jean Montgomery, Ellina Seckel, Andrew Wilcox

Mental Health Transition of Care Service

Sadie Roestenburg, Mental Health Clinical Pharmacist

VA Salt Lake City Health Care System, Salt Lake City, UT

sadie.roestenburg@va.gov

This pharmacist-led mental health Transition of Care (TOC) service provides medication reconciliation, as well as improved safety and access to care for Veterans as they transfer back from non-VA hospital settings.

Introduction

Transitions of care are key times when patients need extra assistance in understanding the changes that occurred during their hospitalization. Often times there are problems regarding medication access and understanding changes in treatment. These transitions of care are crucial times to help improve safety, improve access to medications, and reduce risk of destabilization or rehospitalization. There was one Veteran in particular who was discharged from a non-VA psychiatric hospital. He had severe dementia and multiple medical problems. He presented to the outpatient pharmacy to fill his discharge medications. The outpatient pharmacist contacted the Transition of Care pharmacist to facilitate medication fills. The Veteran had minimal paperwork and did not know what changes were being made by the non-VA facility. The TOC pharmacist met with the Veteran and contacted the discharging facility to clarify orders. It was discovered that the Veteran was being continued on an inappropriate insulin and anticoagulation regimen. These orders were clarified with the Veteran's PCP to not be continued. The additional medications were reviewed, reconciled, and filled for the Veteran, and an updated medication list was provided. Additional providers involved in the Veteran's care were notified of the transition. All the changes were reviewed with the Veteran's wife to ensure continuity of care. Had this TOC interaction not happened, the patient would have not known what to do with two injectable medications that were inappropriate to continue and may have led to serious potential side effects and safety issues.

A pharmacy resident research project reviewed 79 charts for Veterans who were transferred back to VA care from non-VA facilities (from March 1–30th, 2016). Sixty-one of these were related to mental health admissions. A total of 18 patients (29.5 percent) were evaluated by our TOC pharmacy service within this timeframe. Of them, 55.5 percent (10/18) presented to their seven-day follow-up. Of Veterans without pharmacy TOC involvement 27.9 percent (12/43) presented to their seven-day follow-up. Additional data on the overall impact of this service is needed.

Key Information

Two mental health pharmacy residents initiated this process in collaboration with the mental health pharmacists, mental health leadership, the Access Crisis Team (ACT), and pharmacy leadership. This has been an ongoing process and there are still many aspects that are currently under development. The initial development phase was Fall 2014 to Spring 2015, and this service has been in the pilot phase since Spring 2015. The goal of this service is to facilitate smooth medication transitions for Veterans with mental health concerns who are admitted and discharged from non-VA mental health facilities back to the Salt Lake City (SLC) VA care. Veterans may be admitted for mental health diagnoses to our ED, and then get transferred to another psychiatric facility outside of VA due to bed space, etc. Veterans are also often directly admitted to non-VA facilities. This process is difficult to capture each day and it can become a daunting task to find out which Veterans have been admitted to non-VA facilities. Medication changes are often made at these non-VA facilities without a medication reconciliation being done when the Veteran comes back to the SLC VA for their usual medical and mental health care. Veterans often present to the outpatient pharmacy with complicated discharge medication lists and confusion about what medications they should be taking, which can be a major medication safety and access concern.

Context

The George E. Wahlen VAMC in SLC, UT, is a 121-bed hospital with nine community-based outpatient clinics in the surrounding area. This facility serves more than 50,000 Veterans. With regard to mental health services, there is an inpatient psychiatric unit (21 acute beds), a 15-bed substance abuse residential unit, as well as extensive outpatient mental health and substance abuse services. Currently there are five mental health clinical pharmacists at this facility. This Mental Health TOC Service is meant to provide medication reconciliation for any Veteran who is discharged from a non-VA facility back to VA care. With 20+ non-VA facilities around the area, the challenges that are addressed with this service involve improving medication safety, access, and reconciliation for these transitions of care. These transitions are often complex medically and logistically, and may lead to destabilization of our Veterans.

Practice Description

Prior to initiating this service, there were multiple meetings with mental health and pharmacy leadership to help define what this pharmacy process would entail. This practice involves the mental health clinical pharmacists obtaining information through various ways (faxed paperwork, providers, ACT team, other pharmacists, social workers, etc.) regarding Veterans being discharged from non-VA facilities for mental health diagnoses. Discharge instructions and medication orders are faxed to a mental health administrative clerk when available, which is then sent to all mental health pharmacists. Each pharmacist has an "on-call" day for TOC duties, and any staff member can reach them. The mental health pharmacist then provides a medication reconciliation and helps to facilitate access to the correct medications, as well as to identify any medication issues that need to be resolved. The goal is to facilitate a smooth transition back to VA care, but also to help minimize medication errors, improve safety, and remind Veterans of their upcoming appointments. The mental health pharmacists involve the Veteran in this medication reconciliation process when able. The Veterans are educated about the changes made during hospitalization, which can help to improve adherence. We are still working on the best way of capturing more Veterans being discharged from outside facilities for mental health hospitalizations, as well as working to involve mental health providers and other members of the teams to help coordinate transitions of care.

Replicability

We adopted this practice due to the high-risk nature of Veterans who are discharged back into the community from a mental health hospitalization. Patients were presenting to the outpatient pharmacy and the pharmacists felt uncomfortable with reconciling the medication lists without review from a mental health CPS. The program was developed to minimize the gaps in TOC. The specific factors that have made this service possible are a combination of motivated, dedicated, mental health pharmacists, as well as support from mental health and pharmacy leadership. Due to the time requirement of this service, at this point we are unable to offer the complete, comprehensive TOC medication reconciliation service that would be optimal for these patients. We are in the process of requesting additional resources for the Mental Health or Pharmacy departments to better accommodate this necessary service.

The conditions that would be required for others to replicate this service are an adequate number of pharmacists with dedicated time allowed for this practice (being "on-call" and/or a dedicated pharmacist), a care coordinator for TOC if available, and a standardized way of identifying and capturing all Veterans discharged from non-VA facilities.

Recognition

Melissa Brewster, Christine Holman, David Denio, Chris Stock, Abril Atherton, Sadie Roestenburg, Traci Turner, Katelin Campbell, Allison Arterbury, Joel Grussendorf, Julia Boyle, William Marchand, Debra MacDonald, Bruce Bilodeau

Bringing Awareness of Amputation Prevention to the Inpatient Setting

Ashley Roach, Clinical Faculty

VA Portland Health Care System, Portland, OR
ashley.roach2@va.gov

By bringing awareness of amputation prevention to the inpatient setting, Veterans who are at risk can be identified and referred for follow-up care as well as engage in patient education to reduce their likelihood of future amputation.

Introduction

Amputations and disease processes, which can lead to amputation, can affect the quality of life of Veterans and represent a significant economic burden to health care systems. The rate of amputations at the VA Portland Medical Center has been one of the highest in the nation. Bringing awareness of amputation prevention to the inpatient setting provides an opportunity for staff to interface with Veterans in order to improve outcomes. Prior to conducting an amputation prevention education session to nurses on an inpatient floor, a majority of the nurses were unaware of the rate of amputations at their facility and the initiatives being taken to reduce them. After the education session, all the inpatient nurses agreed that this information was relevant to their practice and agreed on the need to increase awareness of this issue.

As a result of the identified need to increase amputation prevention awareness in the inpatient setting, nursing students became involved in conducting assessments for Veterans at risk for amputation. In eight days, students in the VA Nursing Academic Partnership (VANAP) VA Scholar cohort from Oregon Health & Science University (OHSU) School of Nursing assessed 33 patients and engaged them with motivational interviewing and teach-back education. Seven referrals were made for follow-up care. These Veterans might have fallen through the cracks had they not been assessed. Because of the success during this short trial period, there are plans to continue to implement this type of education in the future.

Key Information

The promising practice of increasing awareness of amputation prevention in the inpatient setting was implemented primarily on an inpatient ward at the VA Portland Health Care System. The project was led by Ashley Roach, OHSU VANAP clinical faculty, in partnership with other VA Portland Health Care System VANAP faculty. Other key participants included Dr. Foy White-Chu, Prevention of Amputations in Veterans Everywhere (PAVE) Committee Chair; Dr. Michele Goldschmidt, Health Promotion and Disease Prevention Program Manager; Audra Pfund, Clinical Nurse Leader; and Keith Keller, Nurse Manager. After questioning inpatient nurses, a need was identified: there was little or no understanding of the need to reduce amputation rates and the efforts being made to do so. This is significant because inpatient nurses have the opportunity to engage and support Veterans, especially if the Veteran has not been seen recently in the outpatient setting. By increasing awareness of an important and relevant issue, the problem can be addressed from multiple angles.

Context

The VA Portland Medical Center serves over 88,000 unique Veterans coming from a large geographical area. While many Veterans are seen in the outpatient setting on a regular basis, some Veterans who are hospitalized may not have been seen for a routine checkup in recent months. Identifying and assessing patients at risk for amputation on the inpatient side provides an additional opportunity to ensure that all patients who are at risk are getting the services and support that they need.

Practice Description

Over the course of six months, VANAP nursing faculty collaborated with health care system staff to implement several opportunities to increase awareness of amputation prevention measures. An evidence-based fact sheet was developed and disseminated to all VA health care system staff that outlined the current problem and areas for intervention including information on how to assess patients and provide patient education. Faculty provided nurse in-services and conducted a virtual journal club on an inpatient vascular surgery floor to increase awareness and facilitate discussion. Partnering with health care system staff, VANAP faculty held a "Peripheral Arterial Disease Awareness Day" event in the hospital lobby. This event drew staff and patients and included distribution of cookbooks and patient education materials. In addition, faculty delivered individualized patient education on an inpatient floor, and developed a learning activity for student nurses to use to assess and teach patients.

Replicability

We adopted this practice because of the recognized need in our facility to reduce the number of amputations. There was also an identified gap in the understanding of the problem, especially in the inpatient setting. Collaborating across care and academic settings and with multiple stakeholders was a key factor in ensuring the success of this project. Early support from the PAVE committee chair and buy-in from the inpatient ward manager were also essential elements to ensuring success. This project could be replicated in other facilities through collaboration with local PAVE committees. In addition, staff on inpatient units can work with unit councils to implement learning activities and educational sessions to increase awareness on their specific units.

Recognition

Foy White-Chu, Michele Goldschmidt, Audra Pfund, Keith Keller, Mary Lloyd-Pena, Pat McAndrew, Sharon Wallace, Michele Cooper, Paula Gubrud-Howe

VA Coordinated Transitional Care

Amy Kind, MD, PhD, Associate Professor, Assistant Director-Clinical; Laury Jensen, BSN, RN-BC, Program Manager

William S. Middleton Memorial Veterans Hospital, Madison, WI
laury.jensen@va.gov

The Coordinated Transitional Care (C-TraC) program is a low-cost transitional care program that uses hospital-based nurse case managers, inpatient team integration, and in-depth, standardized post-hospital telephone contacts to support high-risk patients and their caregivers as they transition from hospital to community.

Introduction

Mr. X was hospitalized with a gout flare and discharged to his Adult Family Home in the community with two new medications, an antibiotic, and a steroid. During the medication reconciliation completed during the initial transitional care call it was discovered that the caregiver was unaware of the new medications and the patient could not recall receiving them. They were unable to find the medications in his belongings. The C-TraC RN was able to obtain replacement prescriptions for him and have them delivered that same day. Without these medications his condition would have worsened and he likely would have been readmitted to the hospital within the next few days.

During the initial C-TraC call to an elderly man receiving his Primary Care through another VA facility, the RN found the patient was taking three different doses of the same medication from three different sources. The C-TraC RN intervened and potential harm to the patient due to medication toxicity was avoided.

Patients who participated in the C-TraC program experienced one-third fewer rehospitalizations than those in a baseline comparison group, producing an estimated savings of $1,225 per patient net of programmatic costs.

Key Information

The transition from hospital to home can be treacherous for vulnerable patients. Poor quality transitions can result in medication errors, discontinuity in care plans, and confusion or dissatisfaction for patients. Such transitions likely contribute to the rehospitalization of one in five patients within 30 days of hospital discharge. To address this need within the VA system, Dr. Amy Kind and RN Laury Jensen developed the C-TraC program. The program was developed and trialed at the William S. Middleton Memorial Veterans Hospital in Madison WI, in 2010–2012 utilizing funding through a VA T-21 Patient-Centric Alternatives to Institutional Extended Care Grant. C-TraC is a low-cost telephone-based transitional care program that utilizes hospital-based nurse case managers, inpatient team integration, and in-depth post-hospital telephone contacts to support high-risk patients and their caregivers as they transition from hospital to community.

Context

The William S. Middleton Memorial Veterans Hospital is an 85-bed acute care hospital providing tertiary medical, surgical, neurological, and psychiatric care, along with a full range of outpatient services. It serves 130,000 Veterans living in 15 counties in South Central Wisconsin and five counties in northwestern Illinois. Due to the large geographical area covered by the Madison VA traditional transitional care programs, in-home visits were not feasible. C-TraC was designed to address this geographical challenge by utilizing telephone-based interventions. The program targeted community-dwelling Veterans at high risk for poor post-hospital outcomes being discharged from medical-surgical hospital units. Veterans with cognitive impairment, or age 65 and older that either lived alone or had a previous hospitalization within a year were targeted.

Practice Description

Through chart review, the C-TraC nurse case managers identify Veterans eligible for participation in the program. They participate in inpatient discharge rounds establishing a relationship with the inpatient team and participate in the development of the plan for patient care post hospitalization. The C-TraC nurses offer geriatric and transitional care advice to inpatient providers and make recommendations for home health, therapy, geriatric evaluation, palliative care, and hospice consults as appropriate. Close to the time of patient discharge, the Nurse Case Manager will meet with the Veteran and/or caregiver in their hospital room to introduce themselves and the C-TraC program. At this time the Veteran and/or caregiver will be given a brightly colored half sheet of paper with some key information, including red flags (signs that condition is worsening), follow-up appointments, and contact information for the C-TraC nurse and the VA triage service with instructions to call if red flags or other concerns arise. Working with the Veteran, a telephone appointment will be scheduled for 48–72 hours after discharge.

At the prearranged time, the C-TraC nurse case manager will call the Veteran and/or caregiver to reinforce the four goals of transitional care which are to educate and empower the Veteran/caregiver in medication management, to ensure the Veteran/caregiver has medical follow-up, to educate the Veteran/caregiver on red flags, and to ensure the Veteran/caregiver knows whom to contact if questions arise. The majority of this phone contact will be spent completing a patient-led medication reconciliation. Calls will continue on a weekly basis until the Veteran is seen by their PCP or appropriate specialty provider, the Veteran and C-TraC nurse agree that no additional calls are necessary, or four weeks pass. All communication between the Veteran and the transitional care nurse is documented using templated progress notes and copied to the PC outpatient provider and nurse case manager.

Replicability

C-TraC has become part of routine care at the Madison VA over the past six years for many reasons. It is fiscally responsible showing a net cost avoidance of $1,225 per Veteran enrolled. It reduced the number of readmissions within 30 days of hospital discharge by one-third resulting in increased bed capacity. It brings care to the Veteran in their home thereby reducing distance barriers. Veteran and caregiver satisfaction with services has been consistently reported as good or excellent.

C-TraC has been successfully replicated at several VA and non-VA facilities over the past couple of years utilizing a modified Replicating Effective Programs (REP) model to guide standardize adaptation to local context.

Recognition

Alan Bridges, Becky Kordahl, John Rohrer, Christine Kleckner, VACO GRECC leadership, GEC leadership, Madison VA GRECC leadership and staff, Marilyn Bazinski, Michele Pawlowsky, Jennifer Anderson-Ott

Reducing Readmissions Through Improving Care Coordination at the VA Caribbean Healthcare System

Claudia Rosales, MD, Merida Colon, MD, Chair

VA Caribbean Healthcare System, San Juan, PR
claudia.rosales@va.gov

The Coordinated Transitional Care (C-TraC) program contributed to a significant decrease of 48 percent in 30-Day Readmission Rates (30 DRRs) at the pilot unit. This program provided patient-centered management and coordination of care. VA Caribbean Healthcare System (VACHS) is in the process of spreading this program across all the Internal Medicine wards.

Introduction

An elderly man, dependent on family for his daily living activities, was admitted with a diagnosis of aspiration pneumonia. The patient was bedbound and fed through a gastrostomy tube. His acute condition improved during hospitalization for which discharge planning was initiated promptly. At the time of admission, the health care team determined he had a high risk for readmission. The team reviewed and reconciled his medications at admission and at the time of discharge. His caregiver received education about red flags, care at home, and nutrition. The team scheduled an appointment with his primary provider prior to discharge. He enrolled in C-TraC, an innovative program through which he received weekly calls from the discharge advocate nurse until seen by his PCP. During the first post-discharge phone call, the C-TraC team determined the caregiver was having difficulty feeding the patient due to gastrostomy malfunction. The nurse immediately coordinated an appointment for evaluation and tube exchange. The patient was evaluated as outpatient and within 48 hours the feeding tube was endoscopically replaced. The relatives appreciated the prompt intervention. This action prevented patient deterioration and readmission.

This case resembles one of many patients who continue to be positively impacted by this program, which not only provides close follow-up to discharged patients, but includes patient and caregiver education, medication review, and properly coordinated transition of care.

Key Information

VA Pittsburgh Veterans Engineering Resource Center (VERC) partnered with the Office of Patient Care Services (PCS) to determine if bundling strategies reduces 30-Day Readmission Rates (30 DRR) and improves care transitions. The Readmission Reduction Bundle is a structured model connecting In-Hospital Care Coordination strategies to Post-Discharge Care Coordination strategies. The readmission risk prediction model identifies patients at risk for readmission at 30 days in three distinct groups: high, moderate, and low. This initiative was piloted in eight different institutions, but we were the only site with remarkable results.

The pilot unit was a 28-bed Internal Medicine ward. All diagnoses were included in the focus. Stakeholders included all patients admitted to the selected acute medicine ward and leadership. Internal Medicine Service led the implementation of this effort in collaboration with nursing, pharmacy, social work services, and leadership support.

The Bundle Strategy was implemented at the VA Caribbean Healthcare System (VACHS) (VISN 8, station 672) from April 2015 through September 2015. Our aim was to reduce the 30-day risk-standardized readmission (30DRR) rate by 5 percent by September 30, 2015, from 18.68 percent to 17.7 percent by improving transition of care. We obtained a 40.7 percent reduction in 30 DRR within four months after the implementation of the Bundle Strategy, including the C-TraC program for high-risk patients. The estimated cost avoidance was $123,675. The total number of admissions to the pilot unit during the four-month period was 289 patients. Due to the success attained, our leadership embraced the Readmission Reduction Bundle as the standard operation strategy to improve the transition of care and reduce avoidable readmissions. These efforts have continued at the pilot location and are in the process of expansion to all acute Medicine wards.

Context

The VACHS is a complexity level 1A facility, with 209 approved medicine beds, of which 154 are operational. During FY 2015, there were 6,185 admissions to Medicine. FY 2014 IPEC reports an 18.68 percent all-cause 30D RSRR (this was our challenge). Our objective was to improve care transitions, adjusted length of stay, patient satisfaction, access, and to reduce readmissions, standardized mortality rates, and adverse events. Our barriers included time-consuming telephone calls and the fact that it has been difficult to overcome high demand for pertinent clinical staff, who are key players in the process.

Practice Description

Risk prediction stratification was applied to all patients admitted to pilot unit. The team decided that all patients would receive in-hospital and Post-Discharge Care Coordination, including strong discharge practices; high-risk patients would be included in the new C-TraC program. Inpatient care coordination included a multi-disciplinary team approach: medication reconciliation led by a PharmD at admission and upon discharge, and patient and caregiver disease-specific education provided by dietitian and nurse staff. We introduced a new Hospital Transition of Care tool: a template and hand out with the identification of Red Flags (signs or symptoms of pathological worsening).

Outpatient care coordination included scheduling follow-up appointments with PC/PACT prior to discharge; following up with C-TraC program until first face-to-face evaluation (reinforcement in red flags, medication reconciliation, and assessment of social problems at each call).

Replicability

This new Bundle Strategy and C-TraC program was applied to all our high-risk patients since May 2015. The practice was adopted with the purpose of decreasing all-cause readmission rates, which had reduced by 40 percent at the end of the collaborative. Having achieved favorable results, leadership has decided to adopt and replicate this effort across acute care wards. For this initiative, we need to realign, recruit, and retain the staff required, such as the discharge advocates (RN) and the PharmDs. Currently, team members already experienced in the bundle are helping to champion the effort in sister wards for a seamless and sustainable transition to this new model of care.

Recognition

Margarita Figueroa, Evelyn Velazquez, Margarita Hernandez, Ivette Morales, Marcos Cruz, Arleen Llamas, Cynthia Viera, Yarmine Nieves, Jenny Vera, Lourdes Tirado, Brenda Urbina, Ivelisse Medina, DeWayne Hamlin, Antonio Sanchez, Doris Toro, Jose Acevedo Valles, Carlos Tirado, Naomi Rivera

Reducing Readmissions Through Improving Care Transitions

Kathryn Sapnas, PhD, RN-BC, CNOR, Director, Clinical Strategic Planning and Measurement
VACO, Washington, DC
kathryn.sapnas@va.gov

Reducing Readmissions Through Improving Care Transitions (RRTICT) is a novel, evidence-based, collaborative, Veteran-centric method to reduce 30-day readmissions and improve care transitions. RRTICT's risk stratification and tailored intervention bundles reduced 30-day readmissions at multiple VHA pilot facilities.

Introduction

One of the main goals of Reducing Readmissions Through Improving Care Transitions program has been to enhance cooperation among members of the multi-disciplinary team. This collaboration ensures that our Veterans get the best possible care both in the hospital and following discharge. A recent case illustrates the dramatic success of our approach.

A 59-year-old Veteran with a history of bladder cancer with metastases to his brain was admitted to the Pittsburgh VA due to inability to care for himself at home. He was receiving home hospice services, but had no family in the area and had become unable to care for his ileostomy due to progressive weakness. The multi-disciplinary team of doctors, nurses, case managers, and social workers met with the Veteran during his admission, at which time he shared that his final wish was to travel to Florida to be with his family.

At first, the case managers, social workers, and our patient advocate considered arranging a commercial flight for him, but determined that he was too medically unstable to travel without medical support. The team then began searching for alternative travel options, ultimately identifying an agency called "Grace on Wings" that could fly him to Florida via air ambulance. The team also solicited donations from local Veteran organizations and from VA to pay for the flight. After five days in the hospital, the Veteran was flown to Florida where his family and staff from his new home hospice agency met him. Through the multi-disciplinary care team collaboration established by working together in the RRTICT program, this Veteran received the highest quality of care that would rival the best care delivered anywhere.

Key Information

The RRTICT program began as a field-led pilot at the VA Pittsburgh Healthcare System (VAPHS). It is a program tailored to the needs of the Veteran and designed to improve Veteran experience and have a positive effect on employee engagement. The results of the VAPHS pilot combined with evidence-based best practices found in the literature and field-based promising practices submissions from 32 VAMCs led to the development of a bundled approach aimed at reducing 30-day all-cause readmissions. Central to the application of RRTICT was a synthesis of a novel readmission prediction model and the clinical judgment of the care team. Based on risk stratification and clinical review, pilot teams were able to efficiently and appropriately tailor their interventions. For high and moderate risk patients, clinical teams implemented all in-hospital care coordination strategies. In addition, high-risk patients received a tailored post-discharge care coordination strategy. Low risk patients received at least one in-hospital care coordination strategy.

The RRTICT program was piloted on select inpatient medicine wards at seven VAMCs from April 2015 to September 2015. The seven sites are located across VISN 2, VISN 8, and VISN 23 and include Albany Stratton VAMC, Bay Pines C.W. Bill Young VAMC, Gainesville Malcom Randall VAMC, North Florida/South Georgia Veterans Health System (NF/SGVHS), Miami VA Healthcare System, Omaha VA Nebraska-Western Iowa Healthcare System, San Juan VA Caribbean Healthcare System, and Sioux Falls Royal C. Johnson Veterans Memorial Medical Center.

The Office of Patient Care Services (PCS), VA Pittsburgh Veterans Engineering Resource Center (VERC), and care teams from the seven VAMCs collaborated to implement RRTICT. PCS and VERC facilitated inter-site communication while VERC and the care teams implemented the RRTICT strategies and predictive model.

Readmissions negatively affect access to inpatient care, increase the burden on patients and family members during care transitions, and increase the potential for adverse events. Readmissions reduce value at the patient level by increasing bed utilization, increasing inappropriate use of hospital services, and affecting quality, safety, and cost. They negatively affect Veteran experience and quality of life. RRTICT also has a clinical connection with the MyVA goal of improving hospital discharge and it is consistent with the Under Secretary for Health's strategic priorities to improve Veteran quality of care and to find a consistency of best practice. The project aligns with VHA strategic objective for Innovation and Improvement, the overall strategic goal to be patient-driven, personalized, and proactive, the theme of the Blueprint for Excellence to Improve Performance, and improvement of ORYX Core Measures for Congestive Heart Failure (CHF), Acute Myocardial Infarction (AMI), and Pneumonia as measured by the Joint Commission. Overall, RRTICT provides a best practice framework and readmission prediction support tool that improves the employee experience through enhanced team coordination and facilitates provision of the best care for the Veteran.

Context

Following a national invitation for VAMCs to voluntarily participate in the RRTICT program, the VERC and PCS selected seven sites based upon their organizational readiness. The site teams, with VERC and PCS support, implemented RRTICT onto one to two medicine wards for a six-month pilot. Veterans were identified by a statistically reliable and sensitive readmission risk predictive tool, in coordination with care team independent clinical judgment, to receive care tailored by risk assessment.

Practice Description

By implementing RRTICT, teams were able to assess readmission risk and implement an improved Veteran-centric discharge process that started upon the first day of admission. RRTICT involved ward staff nursing, pharmacy, medicine providers, social workers, and case managers. The care team would provide feedback in huddles regarding which Veterans were ready for discharge, with all team members needing to concur on the discharge. After there was agreement, a formalized and tailored process to appropriately discharge the Veteran would be initiated.

Replicability

The RRTICT program is highly replicable across wards within a facility and into new facilities. By empowering the care team to implement best practices and providing a predictive tool to facilitate application of those practices, six of the seven sites reduced readmissions by an average of 28 percent when compared to previous FY data. The Miami VA Healthcare System implemented their own custom decision support tree in lieu of the RRTICT model. This has limited their comparison to the other pilot sites, but demonstrates the flexibility of RRTICT to be implemented at a medical center. Overall, to best replicate this work, RRTICT requires a proactive multi-disciplinary staff who can work in a team environment with the Veteran.

Recognition

Kathryn Sapnas, Maureen McCarthy, Rajiv Jain, Heather Woodward-Hagg, Robert Monte, Ashley Ketterer, Terrence Hubert, Michael Kennedy, Emily Rentschler, Sara Paronish, Brianna Scott, Ali Sonel, Gaetan Sgro, David Alston, Tom Bassett, Lisa Denk, Brittany Littlejohn, Beth Marciniak, Maggie Mizah, Megan Sanchez, Patricia Kidder, Dr. Anna Paszczuk, Laura Ackerman, Michael Kelley, Ray Rush, Mabel Labrada, Regina Wieger, Deborah Shimerdla, Claudia Rosales, Merida Colon-Caban, Carlos Tirado, John Mills

Pharmacist Managed Telephone Tobacco Cessation Clinic

Timothy Chen, PharmD, BCACP, CGP, Director

VA San Diego Healthcare System, San Diego, CA
timothy.chen@va.gov

The Pharmacist Managed Telephone Tobacco Cessation Clinic (PMTTCC) is designed to provide long-term follow-up for at least one year, providing intensive tobacco cessation behavioral treatment and pharmacotherapy, the key components of effective tobacco cessation treatment.

Introduction

The PMTTCC is modeled after the California state quit lines, but differs significantly in delivery as health care providers (pharmacists) with full prescriptive authority deliver a behavioral intervention integrated with pharmacotherapy. The PMTTCC is designed to provide long-term follow-up for at least one year, providing intensive tobacco cessation behavioral treatment and pharmacotherapy, the key components of effective tobacco cessation treatment. The chronic, relapsing nature of Tobacco Use Disorder (TUD)/nicotine dependence is often forgotten; however, this model provides for an evidenced-based practice that addresses the chronic nature of the disorder while removing barriers to pharmacotherapy access and lack of behavioral treatment as identified by the 2010 VHA "Smoking and Tobacco Use Report."

Tobacco cessation programs traditionally consist of face-to-face groups; however, many Veterans are unable to come to VA facilities for group meetings. Since implementation at VA San Diego, about 60 percent of patients treated (greater than 500 annually) in an intensive tobacco cessation program are now enrolled in the PMTTCC. In addition, the PMTTCC created a toolkit to assist other sites in developing a similar program: http://vaww.publichealth.va.gov/docs/smoking/pmttc-toolkit.pdf

Key Information

The PMTTCC first started at VA San Diego with a reactive model, where Veterans initiated the calls (average calls for abstinent Veterans were 2.27 total calls versus 1.4 for non-abstinent Veterans). This was compared to Standard of Care (SoC) (receiving pharmacotherapy from PCP) and the quit rates were 16 percent at six months for the PMTTCC group versus 10 percent for the SoC group (p < 0.001). Consistent with literature, the number of calls was key to their success. Since 2010, the PMTTCC adapted a proactive, evidence-based model which is designed to provide telephone treatment at Baseline, one to two weeks following the smoker's identified Target Quit Date (TQD), every month for six months, then at three-month intervals (nine and 12 months) and, as needed, thereafter (total of ten calls and more if needed after one year). This proactive model addresses the chronic, relapsing nature of the disease. Abstinence rates increased to over 30 percent at six months with this model, demonstrating the efficacy and importance of having intensive behavioral interventions for tobacco treatment and nicotine dependence.

Context

VA San Diego Healthcare System (VASDHS) is part of VISN 22 and serves about 60,000 unique Veterans annually. Within the health system, traditionally, the facility provided only outpatient tobacco cessation groups which were not accessible to all and therefore many Veterans who desired to stop smoking were not able to receive intensive treatment. After implementation of the telephone clinic, our reach to Veterans has increased dramatically and allows our VA to provide intensive tobacco cessation behavioral treatment and medication to all Veterans who would like to receive treatment.

Practice Description

Clinical pharmacists worked with the Chief of Pharmacy to ensure that the clinic met the goals of the 2003 VHA directive to provide the highest quality of care. The Chief of Pharmacy, medical staff, and ambulatory care pharmacy supervisors supported the pharmacy initiative. This led to the development of the PMTTCC in 2005. It was later adapted to a proactive clinic in 2009 and now consists of the following chronic sessions: baseline, one to two weeks post-TQD, every month for six months, and then at nine and 12 months.

Replicability

The results show PMTTCC is a valuable part of the chronic, intensive tobacco cessation programs for VASDHS. Since being introduced in 2005, the program has received national attention culminating in a PMTTCC toolkit. The model continues to enroll a large number of patients annually with relatively minimal staffing cost relative to workload (approximately one FTE was able to manage this clinic over a course of 1 year), and continues to increase in enrollment annually. In addition, several VA facilities, including VA Long Beach, Minneapolis VA, and Dallas VA, have adopted this model and added to the validity and replicability of this model.

Recognition

Binh Lee, Jessica Harris, Khanh Nguyen, Stacey Nguyen, Jeanna Detwiler, Marisol Downing, Mark Myers, Dana Christofferson, Kim Hamlett-Berry, Mark Bounthavong

The Gateway to Healthy Living Program

Karen Cayce, RN, Health Promotion and Disease Prevention Program Manager

Southern Arizona VA Health Care System, Tucson, AZ

karen.cayce@va.gov

The Gateway to Healthy Living program (Gateway) combines healthy living messages, tools, and resources in one place. Veterans participate in a 90-minute group session, followed by two phone calls with a facilitator, who provides self-management support, assistance setting a Specific, Measurable, Achievable, Relevant, and Time-bound (SMART) goal, problem solving, and connection with their program of choice.

Introduction

A Veteran enrolled in the Gateway to Healthy Living program knowing he wanted to make changes in his life. After exploring what was important to him and why, he recognized that he did not have a routine in his day-to-day life, was staying up late, and sleeping in. He felt like his only purpose was to take care of his day-to-day needs. After being engaged in Gateway, he was motivated to enroll in Healthy Living classes and the Mindfulness-Based Stress Reduction workshop. He and his wife attended both, and went on to develop Specific, Measurable, Achievable, Relevant, and Time-bound goals and action plans to achieve those goals. Ultimately, he become a volunteer and lay leader for some of the facility Health Promotion/Disease Prevention (HPDP) program offerings. Another Gateway participant, discussing the choice to lead a healthy lifestyle, said, "I didn't know it was MY choice to make!"

A survey of participants immediately following Gateway revealed that 100 percent of respondents were satisfied with their Gateway session (83 percent "very satisfied" and 17 percent "somewhat satisfied"). In preparing for potential barriers to achieving their health goal, the majority also said that Gateway helped (57 percent) or somewhat helped (42 percent). A qualitative analysis of responses to the open-ended question, "What was most helpful about your Gateway session?" revealed three main themes: that it 1) was engaging and supportive; 2) helped the individual set a goal for change; and 3) provided new knowledge and information. One participant shared that, "Not what I 'should do,' but the 'importance to me' approach made the difference."

Sixty-three percent of the participants who completed follow-up call two self-reported successfully linking to a program or resource, which was a primary outcome for the pilot. Forty-two percent of participants were linked to programs for weight management, while others chose to focus on nutrition, physical activity, diabetes management, tobacco cessation, or stress reduction. Overall, 89 percent of staff thought Gateway was of moderate to high value for Veterans. Fifty-four percent thought that it was "helpful" and 32 percent "somewhat helpful," in connecting Veterans to programs and resources; 56 percent thought that Gateway was very helpful for supporting health behavior change. One comment shared by staff was, "I really think this is a no-brainer. It truly opens the door to unlimited opportunities that otherwise may go missing." Gateway facilitators also benefitted from the program, which allowed them to strengthen their Motivational Interviewing and health coaching skills. They collaborated with PACTs to develop marketing and educational materials to help guide Veterans to Gateway. Now, when staff asks Veterans about their health goals and barriers, they can offer Gateway to help Veterans proactively develop a plan for better health and well-being and make the link to ongoing support.

Key Information

Gateway was designed by the VHA National Center for Health Promotion and Disease Prevention (NCP) with help from a national workgroup that included program office staff, field clinicians, and Veterans. It serves as an entry point to engage Veterans seeking information, motivational support, and collaborative goal setting in support for healthy living, and empowers them to develop a personalized, proactive, patient-driven plan. Gateway provides evidence-based HPDP guidance, strategies, links to existing clinical programs, and self-management tools to help decrease risky health behaviors and the burden of chronic disease. With VHA prevention staff as leads, Gateway was piloted at six sites: Bronx, NY, Gainesville, FL, Indianapolis, IN, Murfreesboro, TN, Richmond, VA, and Tucson, AZ, facilities. Clearly, Gateway aligns with VA's Blueprint for Excellence Essential Strategies, specifically Strategy 6, "advances health care that is personalized, proactive, and patient-driven and engages and inspires Veterans to their highest possible level."

Context

Southern Arizona VA Health Care System (SAVAHCS), located in Tucson, and seven CBOCs, serve over 171,000 Veterans in Southern Arizona and Western New Mexico. Decreasing risky health behaviors (i.e., obesity, inactivity, unhealthy eating, and/or drinking, smoking) in Veterans is an important strategy to reduce the burden of chronic disease. Clinicians struggle to engage Veterans in positive health behavior change. Gateway is an efficient and effective intervention to engage Veterans in health behavior change, develop a personalized, proactive, patient-driven plan, and improve their overall health and well-being. As Veterans leave Gateway, they take with them a completed action plan and a plan for follow-up with their health care team.

Practice Description

Gateway brings together Healthy Living messages, tools, and resources in one place. It connects Veterans who are considering a health behavior change to existing support within VA and/or the surrounding community. In the pilot, Veterans participated in a 90-minute, face-to-face group session, followed by two phone calls with the session facilitator (HPDP Program Manager, MOVE! Coordinator, Health Behavior Coordinator, or Veterans Health Education Coordinator), who provided self-management support, assistance setting a SMART goal, problem solving, as needed, and connection with their program of choice.

Replicability

SAVAHCS HPDP and PACT teams were excited to participate in the Gateway pilot to address an identified need: enhancing Veteran engagement in HPDP/self-management programming. We saw Gateway as an opportunity to meet this need using relatively few resources. We had the support of our PACT leadership and a strong HPDP team who took the lead on educating staff, engaging Veterans, and implementing the program. We also had well-developed HPDP programming that included MOVE! and tobacco cessation. We were able to arrange adequate space to conduct the group sessions, and leadership supported our needs for staff time. NCP provided initial training, ongoing support for facilitators, and materials needed for staff and Veterans. Gateway was highly effective relative to the resources needed to implement it. The success demonstrated in the pilot created interest from other services, and a decision was made to continue offering Gateway after the pilot ended, with no break in services. This allowed the team to capitalize on momentum and support, which has translated into continued success and satisfaction among Veterans and staff alike.

Recognition

Tucson, Bronx, Murfreesboro, Indianapolis, Gainesville, and Richmond HPDP teams; NCP Development team, Gateway Veteran participants

EMPLOYEE ENGAGEMENT

Using External (Non-VA) Comparative Data to Achieve Excellence and Engage Employees

Jill Stephens, Health Care Analyst

Mountain Home VA Medical Center, Mountain Home, TN

jill.stephens@va.gov

Expands non-VA benchmark data to provide indicators of how Veterans and caregivers view VA care and services in relation to other health care choices in their region. This results in higher performance and employee engagement.

Introduction

In 2008, Mountain Home VA Healthcare System (MHVAHCS) submitted our first Baldrige-based Carey Award application. We received our feedback report indicating that while our results were "better than average," we had not proved we were "the best." In 2012, we submitted a new application. This time we asked staff to find benchmarks that proved they were "the best." The clinical benchmarks came mostly from the Strategic Analytics for Improvement and Learning Value Model (SAIL), but the administrative benchmarks were a bigger challenge. We engaged process owners in identifying their own benchmarks, and discovered that not only did we win the Carey Trophy, but we also increased our employee engagement scores, as demonstrated in SAIL Best Places to Work and the Federal Employees Viewpoint Survey. Our employee satisfaction, as measured in SAIL, was in the third quintile in 2010–2011, the second quintile in 2012, and the top quintile in 2012–2015. Our VA FEVS Employee Engagement Scores topped VA and government wide rankings in 2014 and in 2015 in the employee engagement categories: "Overall," "Leaders Lead," "Supervisors," and "Intrinsic Work Experience."

Key Information

Executive leadership, Quality Management and Improvement Service, and process owners at MHVAHCS conceived this practice. Our goal was to prove our process results were in the top 10 percent as evidenced by the Baldrige Criteria in the Carey award application. Our efforts generated a foundation of 18 non-VA benchmark sources. Should VHA use this foundation to establish a formal list of non-VA benchmarks and provide them to all VHA sites, anyone seeking to measure the efficacy of similar processes will benefit. VHA should encourage sites seeking Carey Award recognition to contribute their non-VA benchmark sources to expand the list so that it becomes more inclusive, allowing other locations to identify processes that excel as well as opportunities for improvement.

Context

MHVAHCS serves the needs of Veterans in east Tennessee, southwest Virginia, and southeast Kentucky. It consists of 11 care sites, including one tertiary care level 1C medical center, one large outpatient clinic, six CBOCs, and three rural outreach clinics. All sites offer PC, and many sites offer specialty care, including specialty care via telehealth. The medical center offers acute care (114 hospital beds), geriatric and rehabilitation services (120-bed Community Living Center (CLC)), and a variety of treatment options, including a homeless inpatient treatment program (150-bed domiciliary). MHVAHCS is part of VISN 9, serves approximately 54,000 Veterans, and has over 2,200 employees.

Our practice addresses the issues of identifying and locating new benchmarks that are not currently included in SAIL performance measures, and motivating and engaging all employees to strive toward providing quality, safety, and value in every product and service we provide. This enables us to prove to Veterans, their caregivers and families, and to other stakeholders, that we are committed to excellence and providing the best care anywhere.

Practice Description

To determine where improvements are possible and to identify the criteria necessary for measuring process outcomes, we needed to find best practice benchmarks. Measuring our process outcomes against these benchmarks allows us to evaluate the success of our endeavors. This is a difficult task, particularly for non-clinical processes. As part of the Carey/Baldrige, employees reviewed the current results of their processes and identified related targets/benchmarks in the top 10 percent of their professions. We focused on processes that impacted the end user, customer, and/or the Veteran. Process steps included:

1. Leadership identified the need for a benchmark and tasked staff to locate the appropriate benchmarks.

2. Staff used the Internet, professional relationships, and peer-reviewed industry publications to locate and identify benchmarks.

3. Staff compared current process performance to these benchmarks to validate whether data definitions between current process and benchmark were comparable. If comparable, staff used the newly identified benchmarks to determine best practices and opportunities for improvement.

4. Staff notified leadership of the newly identified benchmarks, and leadership approved these benchmarks for use in Carey/Baldrige applications.

   – Staff evaluated how current practices compared to newly identified benchmarks.

   – Staff could now compare data to the newly identified benchmarks/best practices and include the comparison in the Carey/Baldrige application.

5. Staff celebrated, knowing they had correctly identified which processes were truly "the best."

Replicability

Through participation in Carey/Baldrige, MHVAHCS recognized that workforce engagement is paramount to achieving excellence. Engagement begins at new employee orientation and is strengthened through clear communication, employee empowerment, and pride in the role employees' play in the MHVAHCS mission and performance. Key factors for this successful mission included systems redesign, recognition and career development, teamwork/communication, and meeting Veteran and customer needs. A culture of Process Improvement (PI) exists across MHVAHCS.

The key elements that enabled our performance improvement to evolve from single service level or quality management responsibility to an organizational interdisciplinary team of engaged employees collectively promoting and participating in improving outcomes through process improvement are:

- Leadership commitment to transparency, systems redesign, and empowering employees to initiate change
- Employee commitment to our mission and their desire to be "the best"
- Clearly established and measurable targets
- Ongoing training and education on PI and systems redesign tools, including lean
- Taking time to celebrate success and to recognize all those responsible

Conditions under which it would be possible for others to reproduce or replicate this practice in their facilities are:

- A culture of improvement and a desire to be "the best"
- Leadership willingness to identify the root cause of poor performance versus placing blame for poor performance
- Employees who want the best for their customers
- Supervisors willing to help employees identify and locate benchmarks that measure what matters

Recognition

MHVAHCS staff, Charlene Ehret, Dan Snyder, David Hecht, Linda McConnell, Baldrige Application Writing team members, Pam Bergbigler

Unit Tracking Board, Where We Stand at a Glance

Michael Finch, MSN, RN, CNL Quality Management Specialist
C. W. Bill Young VA Medical Center, Bay Pines, FL
michael.finch3@va.gov

The Unit Tracking Board (UTB) is an easy-to-read, low-cost, customizable tool that presents unit data and drives performance improvements. It provides a solution to the often-chaotic problem of distributing data to the nursing staff.

Introduction

The primary impact of Unit Tracking Board (UTB) practice is getting useful data into the hands of bedside nurses to help them provide excellent Veteran care, unit level improvement, and staff engagement. Through data, RNs can identify and address trends, nursing metrics, and outcomes, leading to improved outcomes for Veterans.

Key Information

The initial implementation was in the Surgical Intensive Care Unit (SICU). After this, a new board was created for the inpatient mental health units. Medical Intensive Care Unit (MICU) and SICU clinical nurse leaders then collaborated to update the UTB for each Intensive Care Unit (ICU) to improve outcomes and collaboration between ICUs. After a Clinical Nurse Leader National Call presentation, other VA facilities requested boards for their units, which we provided. After a presentation at the VISN 8 Process Improvement Forum, additional facilities began requesting UTBs. This is significant because it gives nurses vital information in a format that allows rapid assimilation and use.

Context

Bay Pines VA Healthcare System serves the needs of America's Veterans in West Central and Southwestern Coastal Florida. Bay Pines is a complexity level 1A facility that provides comprehensive health care to more than 100,000 Veterans. Services include primary and various specialty care services, inpatient (medical/surgical/psychiatric) care, inpatient nursing home and hospice care, inpatient domiciliary care, inpatient and outpatient mental health services, and women's programs. We offer services through our Cape Coral outpatient clinic, and seven community-based outpatient clinics.

Practice Description

In today's health care systems, data collection can lead to significant process improvement, better patient outcomes, greater fiscal responsibility, and improved health.

Nevertheless, communicating this information to frontline staff can be challenging. Unit data can be difficult to interpret, and staff often struggle to convert data into a usable form. As a result, important information can be overlooked or neglected by those who are best positioned to positively affect patient outcomes. To address this issue, the C.W. Bill Young Medical Center created a reusable UTB of core metrics. The UTB is easily accessible by all direct care staff. UTB data is presented in its simplest form, contrary to the percentage format for most data. For example, the National Database of Nursing Quality Indicators (NDNQI) presents data on falls as 0.6 percent. This appears to be a very low percentage, and it is not clear that this figure is calculated per 1,000 patient days. Instead, the UTB states: "one fall since November 23." This allows the staff to quickly understand and apply these numbers in their daily practice. When no new data is available (or there are no new falls or infections), the board shows the "Days since_____," as "432 days without Central Line Associated Blood Stream Infection (CLABSI)."

The UTB also displays Veteran satisfaction scores for Bay Pines VAHCS, VISN 8, and VHA; admission, discharge and daily census for the unit; and the number of alerts responded to per month (customizable for each type of unit). Staff can track and take pride in their success, which reinforces their commitment to providing the best care possible. It also enhances staff collaboration and the goal to utilize evidence-based practice in providing excellence in care. Laminated boards allow staff to use dry erase markers to record current data and to add new tracking points to the chart.

Providing information to staff is challenging, as is communicating the importance of core measurements. A UTB is an inexpensive tool that can share and sustain outcomes, while spreading the word about nursing excellence. Every unit can customize a template to include any type of data. For example, nurses can benefit from useful, time-sensitive data and reminders of the importance of utilizing evidence-based practice. The UTB is about providing easily applied information on where a unit currently stands. Armed with this data, frontline staff is empowered to improve Veteran care. When used as a huddle or debriefing tool, the board also allows rapid and blame-free learning and discussion to occur in a "Just Culture Environment."

Replicability

This practice is extremely replicable. Using a standardized template and inputting data points that are relevant to a specific unit, a board can be created in a few hours. Staff input is extremely important to capture metrics that are important to the unit and overall Veteran care. After the board is created, it can be printed and laminated by a local reproduction department or print shop. The board can then be placed in an area where it can be seen by all staff every day. Staff members can each "own" a metric, such as falls, and update the information, as needed. This also allows staff to notice trends and take action when needed, such as providing additional training to colleagues. With leadership buy-in, a UTB can be used during care/executive rounds to evaluate a unit's overall standing, engagement, and current improvement projects.

Recognition

Staff and managers of Bay Pines SICU, Suzzette Seril, Lorraine Kaack, the Clinical Nurse Leader community

Teaching and Learning Together to Foster Excellence in Team-Based Care

Amber Fisher, PharmD, BCACP, Co-Director, Boise VA Center of Excellence in Primary Care Education

Boise VA Medical Center, Boise, ID
amber.fisher3@va.gov

Our inter-professional noon conference allows trainees to learn from, with, and about each other in a familiar setting. It also teaches inter-professional trainees how to offer team-based, patient-centered care in our PACT training clinic.

Introduction

We believe that team-based care is improved when people from different backgrounds learn and teach together. Our Boise VA inter-professional training program, the Center of Excellence in Primary Care Education (CoEPCE), strives to integrate our professional trainees from pharmacy, psychology, nursing professions, and Internal Medicine (IM) into inter-professional education and practice experiences. Based upon literature and our own experience, we understand the importance of defining roles and responsibilities in any inter-professional practice. To improve role clarity among our inter-professional trainees, we transformed our single profession IM program called "Ambulatory Noon Conference" (ANC) into an inter-professional ANC (iANC).

The overall impact of the new iANC was very positive for participants. In response to the statement "The content was useful for my professional work," participants' average score on a five-point Likert scale (1 - Strongly Disagree, 3 - Neutral, and 5 - Strongly Agree) was 4.5; 95 percent of respondents agreed or strongly agreed that the program was useful.

Key Information

The iANC was implemented at the Boise VAMC in Boise, ID, via the Boise CoEPCE. The Co-Directors of the CoEPCE and Associate Director for Evaluation led the implementation, along with program directors and senior trainees from each professional program. We have held an iANC every week since our first meeting on September 2, 2015. Our data and anecdotal experience shows that this conference provides staff with valuable professional knowledge and fosters role clarity via the inter-professional co-presentations.

Context

The Boise VA is a small academic hospital (40 inpatient acute beds) that serves a large, primarily rural geographic area. Our patient population of more than 26,000 Veterans spans 40,000 square miles, which includes parts of Idaho, eastern Oregon, and northeastern Nevada.

As an academic hospital supporting first and second year post-graduate pharmacy residency programs, an IM residency program that is part of the University of Washington, post-graduate psychology trainees, NP and nursing students, and residents from schools around the US, we have the challenge of providing efficient and effective clinical training. We found that many common ambulatory topics were being taught in multiple programs with little cross-teaching and learning. To take advantage of the knowledge and expertise of our various faculty members, we developed a didactic series that combines these intersecting training areas.

Practice Description

Because the pre-existing conference was well established with the IM residency and managed by the IM chief residents, we began with several stakeholder meetings that included faculty and senior trainees from all the participating professions. The involvement of the IM chief resident was a key step in obtaining buy-in for the transformation to an inter-professional conference. Multiple discussions resulted in the creation of an academic year calendar that was populated with key speakers, topics, and dates. In addition to professional programs taking ownership of specific topics and dates, each program requires trainees to conduct an inter-professional presentation to the larger group. The process owners are the CoEPCE Co-Directors and Associate Director for Evaluation. The steps that occurred during the iANC included:

1. Compiling a list of 100 ambulatory topics that was reviewed in a meeting with each profession and vetted for suitability for inter-professional training; each selected topic was then assigned to a profession to "own," with the profession responsible for presenting that topic and finding a co-presenter from another profession.

2. Obtaining commitments from program directors and the IM chief resident for conference transformation, which included a commitment that each trainee would have a program requirement to complete at least one co-presentation during the academic year.

3. Conducting a series of stakeholder meetings to plan the transformation to an inter-professional conference.

4. Populating and assigning topics on calendar by senior trainees after decisions were made about the structure and processes.

5. IM chief resident in charge of conferences posted the calendar to their website.

6. Program directors ensured assigned trainees found a co-presenter for their designated topics and posted names to the website.

7. First four conferences were co-presented by inter-professional faculty or senior trainees who appropriately role-modeled the expectations for future conferences.

8. CoEPCE process owners checked with speakers weekly to make sure presenters prepared.

9. CoEPCE process owners ensured trainees given post-conference feedback from mentors and each conference evaluated for quality.

Replicability

The transformation to an inter-professional conference was successful because the key stakeholders were able to agree that the change was desirable. The IM chief resident, individual professions' program directors, and CoEPCE leaders committed their support, time, and expertise, and enforced the requirement that all trainees participate. Frequent communications between CoEPCE process owners helped find specific programs to "own" a topic and individuals willing to co-present on their assigned date. The process owners also found inter-professional mentors to give trainees feedback and evaluated each conference.

Other teaching facilities where multiple professions are present could adopt this practice to help streamline trainee education. The noon hour is a common shared learning time, and we have found that this time is generally available to most professions. It is important for stakeholders to discuss the logistical barriers and benefits associated with establishing an inter-professional conference. Each stakeholder must understand how this transformation would benefit participants. Having experienced faculty and staff who can advocate for the transformation is also very important. Lastly, having process owners who are able to commit weekly time and energy to maintain the conference is critical. We have found that it takes about one hour per week to maintain this conference, along with several hours each week in May and June (prior to the new academic year) to plan the upcoming conference schedule.

Recognition

India King, William Weppner, Danielle Ahlstrom, Chris Schamber, Christine Henesh

Mandatory Training Expo

Peatchola Jones-Cole, MD, Chief of Employee Education

Memphis VA Medical Center, Memphis, TN

peatchola.jones-cole@va.gov

A mandatory training expo through the Memphis VAMC Education Service that addresses the training needs of employees and patients, increasing participant and Veteran satisfaction.

Introduction

The Mandatory Training Expo (MTE) is the most popular training activity organized by the Education Service for Memphis VAMC. It allows for an increase in the esprit de corps of the facility, with employees from all services working and learning together. The expo is innovative and efficient, saving hundreds of hours of employee work time, and increasing the ability of staff to meet organizational goals and improve patient-centered care and services. This further enhances customer satisfaction among employees, which directly impacts patient satisfaction among Veterans. Each year, employees are required to access our Talent Management System (TMS) to complete their mandatory training. Education Service observed several gaps that prevented employees from completing the required TMS training, including:

- Not all employees have ready access to a computer (i.e., canteen employees, housekeeping, and nutrition and food employees to name a few).

- We have groups/segments of employees with low or no computer skills who are intimidated when operating a computer.

- We have a segment of employees whose time is consumed with providing health care and treatment for our patients and completing notes/charts (i.e., medical and nursing staff).

Context

The VAMC in Memphis, TN, consists of a 33-acre campus and includes an onsite 60-bed Spinal Cord Injury (SCI) unit, and nine offsite CBOCs. Memphis VAMC is a tertiary care facility classified as a Clinical Referral Level I Facility and one of the most complex medical centers in the VA system. It is also a teaching hospital that provides a full range of patient care services with state-of-the-art technology, as well as extensive education and research programs. Comprehensive primary, secondary, and tertiary health care are provided in the areas of medicine, general cardiovascular and neurological surgery, psychiatry, physical medicine and rehabilitation, spinal cord injury, neurology, oncology, dentistry, and geriatrics. Specialized outpatient services are provided through general, specialty, and subspecialty outpatient clinics, including a women's health center.

Practice Description

To address gaps in training and employee requests, the education service implemented the MTE. Both leadership and employees supported this initiative as an alternative for meeting and completing required training.

Quick facts about the expo:

- Every local, mandatory, all employee training course is covered.

- Storyboards are created by the subject matter experts for each of the 13 mandatory training courses.

- Several multiple-choice questions are featured on each storyboard, along with key information relating to each subject.

- The storyboards are deployed for the expo running for four (12-hour) days.

- Volunteers from all the services help manage the storyboards, distribute the answer sheets, and provide refreshments.

- Employees enter the theater and are immediately given a no. 2 lead pencil, clipboard, and a Scantron-compatible answer sheet to mark the appropriate answers to the 153 test questions.

- Employees usually take anywhere from 45–90 minutes to complete the test.

- The results are tabulated immediately using a Scantron scoring machine, with greater than or equal to 80 percent considered passing. Remedial training is provided on the spot, and employees must readdress the missed questions if they don't have a passing score.

- A TMS training specialist credits employees in TMS as having met the mandatory training requirements for the courses.

- Since 2008, participation in this method of training has increased 20 to 25 percent.

- MTE supports the Workforce Development policy in providing training and development and utilizing various modalities and methods for meeting adult learning needs.

Although the expo started back in the early 2000s, with an attendance of slightly over 300 employees, the use of the expo (storyboard) method has consistently increased over the years. For FY 2016, there were 1,180 completions using the MTE.

Recognition

Education Service staff, other employee volunteers

Caring for Our Veterans by Putting Training First

Renée Sperling, MS, HIS, Lead Clinical CPRS Trainer, Clinical Informatics Service; Justine Koshes, MSN, RN, CAC, Clinical Informatics Service
North Florida/South Georgia Veterans Health System, Gainesville, FL
renee.sperling@va.gov

This clinically focused, targeted, and interactive online CPRS training program delivers the most crucial information for new providers to successfully navigate within the CPRS chart. It has a positive impact on the VA Culture and, most importantly, provides more rapid clinical access to our Veterans.

Introduction

It is important to provide timely CPRS training to new students and clinicians in VHA. In fact, all clinicians must complete the CPRS computer training prior to caring for our Veterans, but the North Florida/South Georgia Veterans Health System (NF/SGVHS) has limited capacity for in-person training sessions. Realizing this capacity was an issue, Renée Sperling, who has responsibility for training over 700+ incoming medical students, interns, residents and fellows, as well as training permanent clinical staff, came up with an innovative solution: implementing an online CPRS training program that allows students and new clinicians faster access, which can benefit the Veteran by allowing for earlier medical intervention. The numbers tell the story. Creating new and innovative ways to deliver education either virtually or online is important to VHA because we are the nation's largest provider of graduate medical education, with over 118,000 health professions trainees and 25,000 affiliated medical faculty.

An online "Student CPRS Training" was created that did not require face-to-face interaction (the direct link is https://mix.office.com/watch/178ci6muswx86). The program is specifically designed for students, taking into account only the most crucial information needed for successful navigation within the CPRS chart. This online format presents full demonstrations, includes realistic voice-overs, and requires student interaction through intermittent quizzes. The North Florida/South Georgia VHS Information Security Officer (ISO) and Privacy Officer approved the program, which complies with all Continuous Readiness in Information Security Program (CRISP) initiatives.

A pilot program implemented between October 2014 and October 2015 showed a 55 percent increase in CPRS training of students, and a 32 percent increase among new clinical providers. In addition, the training received "positive reviews" on the VA Pulse online site, a collaborative platform for staff to share best practices, solve problems, and discover ideas to help improve the Veteran experience.

Key Information

The NF/SGVHS team researched training methods that would increase the supply of qualified practitioners, without sacrificing quality. Office Mix, a free add-on to MS PowerPoint2013, was used to record video demonstrations, insert quiz questions, and upload trainings to the internet. Feedback was solicited on format and ease of use. In addition, the URL link was added to intake paperwork for all new university medical students rotating to VA. Collaboration with partnering universities made it possible to implement the new process for students, and the upgrades to the CPRS training program increased the volume of clinical interactions with Veterans.

Context

NF/SGVHS is a large system encompassing hospitals in Gainesville, FL and in Lake City, FL, with three outpatient clinics, and nine CBOCs between Georgia and north central Florida. This system serves more than 135,500 Veterans and employs more than 4,000 clinical and administrative staff. Historically, due to a shortage of CPRS training computers, students, interns, residents, fellows, and new clinical staff had to wait until a space was available to receive CPRS training. At times, this translated into a few weeks wait, which caused delays in providing clinical care to Veterans. To address these challenges, NF/SGVHS created an online training program that is accessible on mobile or desktop, and anywhere with internet.

Initial feedback from clinical staff, process holders, and the university has been overwhelmingly positive. More importantly, we now have a way to train clinicians more quickly, resulting in more timely and comprehensive care for our Veteran population.

Practice Description

With a clear goal of providing excellent medical care to Veterans, we used the Define-Measure-Analyze-Improve-Control (DMAIC) cycle model from Six Sigma to create a new virtual training process. In the initial phase, we outlined the problems and opportunities facing our organization. We recognized the need to reduce time constraints placed on CPRS training for providers and students, especially during the months of June and July. The intent was to reduce wait times for students, while providing more comprehensive education to licensed clinicians and improving quality of Veteran care. Accurate measurement is vital for effective interdisciplinary communication and Veteran medical intervention. We collected data in the measurement phase that was used to evaluate current processes.

As demand for CPRS student training increased, the number of training computers and time slots remained the same. Analysis showed increased wait times and shorter training sessions. After examining the issues and possible solutions, we began developing procedures aimed at improving the CPRS training process and providing quicker access to care for Veterans.

Initially we created a PowerPoint presentation with voice-overs, but we quickly realized more viewer interaction was needed to keep the students' attention. We turned to an online program called "Office Mix," which allows for more engaging voice-overs, video demonstrations, and multi-formatted quiz questions. This software made it possible to produce a high-quality, one-hour online training tool specific to NF/SGVHS. We recorded demonstrations of tabs, menus, notes, etc. that students would be expected to understand and utilize at the start of their clinical rotation. We also intermittently inserted interactive questions to reinforce topic areas. Before release, we used the presentation in several classes to solicit feedback on format and ease of comprehension. After making minor modifications, the file was uploaded to Microsoft Office Mix online and to the university's website, and the URL link was added to intake paperwork for all new Medical Students rotating to VA.

By using this online training tool, students receive CPRS instruction prior to beginning their VA rotation, which enables them to spend more time caring for VA patients rather than having to wait for face-to-face classes. To limit regression and maintain improvements in the control phase of the project, we monitor student logins, analyze student responses, and review wait times for CPRS face-to-face training.

Replicability

This method would be helpful to all VA sites with affiliated universities that provide clinical rotations to students. Online student training has been successful at NF/SGVHS because it can be customized to suit the site-specific needs of CPRS students, and it can be updated, as needed, with new information. Because Office Mix is free with Microsoft PowerPoint 2013, other VAs can use this tool without additional cost. This virtual training method also benefits educators, freeing them up to provide CPRS training to other employees.

At the VISN Improvement Forum, several Administrative Officers and Directors were excited to hear about our Online Student CPRS Training. The online aspect of the training allows students to revisit specific lessons, as needed, on any computer or mobile device. When they return in the future as licensed clinicians, a more detailed, practice-specific training is available.

Recognition

Leadership and colleagues within the Clinical Informatics Service of NF/SGVHS and other services involved throughout all phases of creating online CPRS training

Geriatric Scholars Program

Josea Kramer, PhD, Associate Director for Education/Evaluation, and Director of the Geriatric Scholars Program

VA Greater Los Angeles Healthcare System, Los Angeles, CA
bettyjo.kramer@va.gov

The Geriatric Scholars Program, a national project based at the VA Greater Los Angeles Healthcare System Geriatric Research Education Clinical Center (GRECC), is a resource for VA providers who work in rural CBOCs or are focused on rural home-based PC.

Introduction

The Geriatric Scholars Program addresses the shortage of geriatrics skills and knowledge in VA clinical settings by offering participants a tailored educational experience aimed at building competencies specific to aging Veteran populations, particularly individuals with multiple co-morbidities and functional decline. LCSW Janelle Brock and her colleague Dr. Marjie Heier participated in the Geriatric Scholars Program to learn how to better treat geriatric patients in rural areas. Their focus was oral care among aging Veterans living in rural America. They knew that the cost of dental care and a shortage of dental services providers in rural areas were significant barriers for older Veterans. After taking part in the intensive geriatric training, they formed a team at the Grand Island CBOC in central Nebraska to improve access to dental care for more than 10,000 older rural Veterans.

The Grand Island CBOC Geriatric team partnered with local agencies that provide dental care to low-income individuals. Together, they disseminated information about local dental care resources to Veterans and established a referral system within the VA electronic medical record. The Grand Island CBOC staff also collaborated with local churches and volunteers to assist patients with transportation. They created a system to ensure the provision of relevant medical records, such as medical imaging and medication lists, so that dental care could be provided efficiently within community dental clinics. Within six months of launching this care coordination project, more than 150 Veterans had received referrals to community resources for dental care. This Grand Island Geriatric Scholars project demonstrated the effectiveness of care coordination with non-VA community providers, as well as the creative approaches that care teams can devise to treat rural Veterans in areas with shortages of specialty care providers. The project is currently being expanded to other rural VA clinics within Nebraska. This is just one example of a clinical CBOC improvement project that resulted from the Geriatric Scholars training.

Key Information

The Geriatric Scholars Program is a national project based at the VA Greater Los Angeles Healthcare System Geriatric Research Education Clinical Center. It is a resource for providers who work in rural CBOCs or who are focused on rural home-based PC. Training clinicians within target communities greatly improves older Veterans' access to and quality of care. VISNs nominate all learners, who commit to implementing systematic changes in personal and clinic practices to improve the quality of care for older Veterans. This effort involves collaboration between sixteen

GRECCs, many CBOCs, every VISN, VA's Employee Education System (EES), the Office of Geriatrics and Extended Care, the ORH, VA's National Quality Scholars Program, community partners such as Area Agencies on Aging, and academic affiliates, including Harvard Medical School, The Icahn School of Medicine at Mount Sinai, UCLA, the University of Wisconsin School of Medicine, and the Wisconsin College of Medicine.

Context

There are too few clinicians trained in geriatrics and gerontology practicing in rural areas to address the needs of America's growing population of aging Veterans. Although about half of the Veterans who seek health care annually at VA are over the age of 65, VA has a lower ratio of geriatricians in comparison to the nationwide average. This is even more problematic in rural areas where there are fewer specialists and the patient population is older, on average, than in urban areas. Surveys of past participants in the Geriatric Scholar Program indicate that 66 percent of rural CBOC patients are elderly Veterans, yet few care providers have any training, even in residency rotations, in geriatric medicine. Currently there is insufficient training in geriatrics across health care professions, too few geriatricians, and poor incentives to recruit and retain professionals who have developed competencies in geriatrics.

Practice Description

The underlying philosophy of the Geriatric Scholars Program is continuous professional development to tailor educational experiences to each learner's stage of knowledge and skill, providing additional relevant learning activities over several years to build competency. With funding from the ORH, this multi-modal program adheres to principles of adult learning. The longitudinal Geriatric Scholars Program is designed to integrate state-of-the-art geriatrics into PC practices in rural CBOCs as well as into clinical practices of key disciplines that support the PC team (e.g., pharmacy).

The basic program involves intensive didactic education and implementation of a quality improvement project to demonstrate application of new knowledge to the needs of older Veterans in the rural CBOC. The program funds the cost of support personnel, development of new materials and resources, external educational event tuition, and travel. In addition, each learner has a tailored education program, which also involves distance education, clinical practicum experiences, mentorship, and coaching and interdisciplinary team training. After completion of a quality improvement project, alumni are eligible to continue developing geriatric competencies and leadership roles in geriatrics through additional educational courses, clinical practice, mentorship, and other educational opportunities that are available at the request of scholars. The program encourages peer-to-peer teach-back, as well as the sharing of clinical practices. Since September 2009, 287 VA employees who work in rural CBOCs or CBOCs that serve rural populations have participated in the Geriatric Scholars Program. VA administrators in all 21 VISNs are invited to nominate participants for the Geriatric Scholars Program, including PCPs (physicians, NPs, and Physician Assistants (PAs)), clinical pharmacists, Social Workers (SWs), and psychologists (PhD, PsyD, and registered MA level). Plans exist to expand the program to include rehabilitation therapists. Subject areas and disciplines included in the program continue to expand to meet the evolving needs and challenges of rural care providers.

In addition to providing these resources to participants directly, the Geriatric Scholars Program also creates monthly toolkits, covering different geriatric issues, and distributes them to VA's network of hundreds of CBOCs. This step ensures that geriatric knowledge extends beyond those selected as scholars. More than 60 percent of rural clinicians (including non-scholars) self-report changing one or more clinical processes after exposure to the Geriatric Scholar Program Toolkit.

Replicability

To earn the designation of Rural Promising Practice from the ORH, this program demonstrated 1) improvement in access to care; 2) evidence of improved direct program impact or clinical results for Veterans; 3) patient, provider and/or caregiver satisfaction; 4) return on investment via reduced cost of care, but not at the expense of quality; 5) operational feasibility and replicability at other facilities or service sites; and 6) strong partnerships or working relationships that maximize efficiency or effectiveness.

The Geriatric Scholars Program grew from 20 rural CBOCs at its inception in 2008 to more than 170 in FY 2015. This model also expanded beyond VA sites of care and is used by community facilities in Western and Central New York; is used to educate care providers of the Indian Health Service; and inspired the spinoff online learning community, GeriScholars.org. Coordination of the many-faceted program and collaborative activities is essential and requires strong leadership, vision, management skills, and sufficient funding.

Recognition

Administrators, practitioners, and partners who continue to serve Veterans using this rural promising practice

Geriatric Research, Education and Clinical Center Community-Based Outpatient Clinic Connection

William Hung, MD MPH, Associate Director for Clinical Programs (Acting); Lauren Moo, MD; Thomas Caprio, MD; Michelle Rossi, MD; Cathleen Colon-Emeric, MD; Steve Barczi, MD; Kimberly Garner, MD; Sara Espinoza, MD; Stephen Thielke, MD

James J. Peters VA Medical Center, Bronx, NY
william.hung@va.gov

Older Veterans living in rural areas often do not have access to specialized geriatric care. Through the Geriatric Research, Education and Clinical Center (GRECC) Connect program, established geriatric teams at the GRECC serve as clinical resources connecting with providers at rural clinics, where Veterans are assessed remotely.

Introduction

An older, rurally-located Veteran with multiple chronic diseases has experienced a decline in his health. Although his PCP would like him to visit a geriatric specialist, the nearest facility where these services are available is too far for the Veteran to travel. Through the Geriatric Research, Education and Clinical Center Connect program, which connects the geriatrics team at the GRECC with rural clinics, this Veteran can be assessed remotely. Through telemedicine, practitioners are able to diagnose and treat the physical and cognitive problems that elderly Veterans often experience and can help assess a Veteran's living situation and social support network. At GRECC, providers and frontline staff participate in monthly conferences, which allow for ongoing discussion of issues related to the care of older Veterans. Frontline employees learn about how to assess and manage complex conditions, such as cognitive decline and functional impairment.

In FY 2014 and FY 2015, the GRECC Connect program provided education and support to numerous providers and staff across a network of nine hub sites as well as consultations to Veterans living in rural areas. We estimate that by participating in our program, Veterans saved, on average, 80–100 miles of travel.

Key Information

Older Veterans living in rural areas often do not have access to specialized geriatric care, the availability of which is critical to improving the quality of care among older adults, who often suffer from multiple chronic diseases, geriatric syndromes, or have functional limitations. Rural providers and staff often lack opportunities for education on how to manage the elderly and are challenged to address more medically and psychosocially complex cases that require the real-time input of an interdisciplinary geriatric team. GRECCs, located at urban tertiary medical centers, have established geriatric teams and can serve as clinical and educational resources for providers at rural clinics where geriatrics expertise is lacking. Because the need is so great, we have developed a network of specialists to support rural providers using the resources of GRECCs across multiple states.

Context

Rural Veterans are, on average, older than their urban counterparts. These individuals often lack access to specialized geriatric care, which is usually concentrated in urban medical centers. This project provides access to geriatric care and consultation that rural Veterans would not otherwise have and promotes the development of geriatrics skills and expertise of rural providers, while enhancing their clinical competency through the discussion of cases that the providers encounter. For Veterans who might otherwise need to travel to see a geriatric consultant, there is significant mileage avoided, thereby overcoming a significant barrier for rural Veterans with or at risk for functional impairments that make travel difficult.

Practice Description

GRECCs in VISN 1, 2 (VAMC), 3, 4, 6, 12, 16, 17, and 20 have established links with rural CBOCs within their VISNs to provide clinical and educational support through a number of modalities, which vary by site based on GRECC resources and rural needs. These modalities include:

- Regularly scheduled case-based conferences: This educational initiative allows geriatric specialists to share their expertise with rural PCPs who are caring for older adult Veterans age 65 and over. The format of these sessions includes a clinical case presentation, a brief didactic portion to enhance knowledge of participants, and an open question/answer period. The focus is on challenging clinical case discussions, addressing common problems like driving concerns, and the assessment/management of geriatric syndromes (e.g., cognitive decline, falls, and polypharmacy).

- Electronic consultation: Geriatric teams from GRECCs provide electronic consultation to rural providers to address clinical needs by clinical referral and also condition-specific case finding.

- Virtual meetings with PCPs and staff (telehuddle): Rural providers review care plans with GRECC teams for medically-complex older adults who may benefit from an interdisciplinary approach to geriatric care, such as those with polypharmacy, recent or multiple falls, increased care utilization (ED, hospital and/or clinic visits), a diagnosis of dementia or cognitive impairment, and recent functional difficulties or social issues.

- Clinical Video Telehealth (CVT): GRECC teams provide geriatric consultation to rural Veterans via telemedicine so that Veterans only need to travel to their local rural CBOCs to be seen. Via CVT, the team can help identify cognitive decline, determine if there are any interventions that may improve cognition, educate caregivers about the disease and services that can ameliorate caregiver burden, and provide assistance with disturbing behaviors that can develop in later stages of the illness. Ongoing support is provided to Veterans and caregivers over the course of the disease.

Replicability

The program has been established and expanded to nine sites in FY 2015. We have seen evidence of improved access, clinical impact, and satisfaction, which is encouraging. In considering expansion to other sites, it is important to consider the existing resources that sites can leverage to develop educational and clinical interventions within their region. For centers that do not have an existing educational or consultative relationship with rural clinics, one of the challenges of implementing successfully the project is achieving buy-in on the local level and building relationships with rural providers and staff. Rural providers are full-time clinicians, and finding time to participate in an educational program is a challenge. Other significant barriers include hiring delays and administrative steps needed to set up a particular clinical modality; each facility has unique established policies that impact how these modalities can be set up.

Recognition

Greater LA GRECC, Josea Kramer, ORH, the Office of Geriatrics and Extended Care, VISN leadership

Use of Multi-Modal Education Including Simulation to Enhance Delirium Education

Denise Kresevic, RN, PhD, GRECC AD Education

Louis Stokes Cleveland VA, Cleveland, OH

denise.kresevic@va.gov

This multi-modal multi-disciplinary program used simulation education and bedside rounds and computerized templates to improve assessment and management of Veterans with delirium.

Introduction

Mr. X was a patient on a general medical-surgical ward following repair of a hip fracture he sustained as a result of a motor vehicle accident for which he was cited. He was an 86-year-old Veteran who served in the Pacific during World War II (WW II). After four years in the service, he started a realty company. He recently retired due to memory problems. His first postoperative day, he denied pain and continued to drop off to sleep when awakened. On this second post-op day, Mr. X was found trying to climb out of bed and became agitated with efforts to calm him. Following a family discussion, he was placed on alcohol withdrawal precautions.

During rounds with the delirium team on post-op day three, Mr. X was again agitated and clearly unable to focus. He denied pain but was not able to complete physical therapy. Risk factors for delirium were reviewed and included alcohol withdrawal, PTSD, dementia, depression, pain, and infection. Chest X-ray and head Computed Tomography (CT) scan were negative for acute changes. The surgical wound was healing. Urine culture was positive for <100,000 bacteria and + leukesterase.

The medical team and family developed a plan of care that included: round-the-clock acetaminophen, laxatives, antibiotics for a urinary tract infection; restarting pre-op medications, including antidepressants; consistent use of glasses and hearing aids; volunteer and family visitors to play cards and offer food and fluids during the day; and dim lights and uninterrupted sleep at night. Mr. X summoned his nurse and said "I thought I was dead, I saw snakes on my arms (IV tubing) and people in white coats all whispering, but I could not talk; what happened to me?" After reassurance, pain medication, and increased mobility, Mr. X, on day five, was alert, cooperative, and ready for discharge to rehabilitation.

Key Information

This project, led by the VISN 10 Geriatric Research, Education and Clinical Center (GRECC), was part of a quality improvement initiative that included simulation education, bedside rounding, pocket clinical cue cards, and an activity cart for patients. Following the intervention, participants demonstrated significant improvements in pre-and-post delirium knowledge scores, 84 to 91 percent. Post-intervention surveys indicated that participants had improvements in assessment and non-pharmacological management of Veterans with delirium. Patient charts (N=107) were reviewed for documentation of Confusion Assessment Method (CAM) and patient management. Patient outcomes included increased non-pharmacological interventions (<10 percent at baseline to 43 percent, p=.003). Simulation training in conjunction with bedside rounding appears to be a robust intervention to enhance caregiver's delirium knowledge and management skills.

Context

The Louis Stokes Cleveland VAMC in Cleveland, OH, houses 183 acute care beds and 155 beds in the Community Living Center (CLC) services for Veterans. Baseline reports of delirium were low, with inconsistent documentation of CAM and increasing use of "sitters."

Practice Description

Using a simulation center and standardized patients, teams of interdisciplinary care providers were able to "practice" communication techniques and recommend treatment strategies with the help of a delirium "coach." Interactions were guided by a checklist to provide targeted feedback to over 100 participants. These education sessions were followed up with bedside rounding by a delirium team member who distributed pocket cue cards to all staff, including sitters, and advocated for assessment of risk factors and targeted interventions, such as pain management or distraction. A multi-disciplinary delirium work group has been convened and is addressing guidelines for assessments, documentation, medication use, and patient activities, such as early mobility.

Replicability

This intervention was initially supported by a T-21 grant from VA to decrease institutionalization and promote patient-centered care and was led by the GRECC interdisciplinary group, which partners with nursing, geriatrics, medicine, psychology, and social services to develop didactic education and simulation training for education. The intervention is now being expanded to the Community Living Center and Intensive Care Unit (ICU) clinical areas as part of a quality improvement education project. The GRECC developed and continues to update a manual.

Findings from this quality improvement project support the usefulness of multi-modal education, including simulation, bedside coaching, and pocket cue cards to enhance clinical practices for care of patients with delirium. These methods helped facilitate team collaboration, patient family communication, and synthesis of a large amount of information in a relatively short period of time. Clearly, didactic education alone may be insufficient to adequately enhance clinical care for delirium. The impact of a multi-modal strategy, including a delirium resource consultation team that was able to provide bedside mentoring, encourage the use of pocket cue cards, and support evidence-based non-pharmacological interventions, cannot be underestimated. In addition, the use of simulation education provided a unique opportunity for health care teams to "practice" assessment, communication, and collaboration skills in a supportive setting with real-time feedback. While not all facilities have access to a simulation laboratory, many may have the ability to implement the use of videos, case studies, and role-playing to enhance didactic education in an effort to achieve improved outcomes for patients with delirium. Enhanced clinical management of complex syndromes, such as delirium, may be most influenced by a combination of multiple methods of education, practice, and mentoring. The use of simulation as an adjunctive teaching method is a promising learning strategy that may enhance the care of individuals with delirium. This quality improvement project demonstrated positive educational and clinical trends in a VA setting.

Recognition

Denise Kresevic, Barbara Heath, Elizabeth Fine

Chicago Veterans Association Community Employment Coordinator Collaborates with Salute Incorporated to Connect Veteran with Data-Center Industry

Beatrice Smith-Redd, Community Employment Coordinator, Vocational Development Specialist
Chicago-Jesse Brown VA Medical Center, Chicago, IL
beatrice.smith-redd@va.gov

The primary goal of this program is to provide a range of employment-related services to Veterans who are unemployed, underemployed, or at risk for becoming unemployed, in order to mitigate factors related to a current episode of homelessness and/or to prevent a future episode of homelessness.

Introduction

Mr. X, a once-homeless Veteran, was among the many Veterans nationwide looking to secure gainful employment. Like his fellow servicemen, Mr. X possessed the core skills necessary to fill roles in the data industry but needed hands-on experience to launch his career. Although his homelessness was resolved about a year prior, he had fallen behind in his electric payments and sought immediate employment to sustain his housing and utilities.

Mr. X was referred, through his social worker, to Beatrice Smith-Redd, a Community Employment Coordinator (CEC) with the Jesse Brown VAMC. Smith-Redd, who is among the nearly 150 VA CECs working at VAMCs nationwide to help homeless Veterans, found that Mr. X possessed "great leadership skills," and she worked to find a job placement matching Mr. X's skills and career goals.

Smith-Redd was contacted by a Chicago-based company called Salute Incorporated (Salute), which was interested in learning more and potentially partnering with the CEC. Col. Robert Lee Kirby (Retired) and Technology Consultant Jason Okroy founded Salute in 2013 to build Veteran careers in the data-center industry. Smith-Redd found a potential candidate in Mr. X, and the feeling was mutual. For Mr. X, "the job was exactly what [he] wanted to do. It was a godsend."

After a positive interview process, Salute hired Mr. X to work in the data center. According to Sonda Kolodzinski, Salute's director of operations, Mr. X "was enthusiastic from our first conversation. He did everything he said he would, from minute one." A representative for the facility where Mr. X now works said, "He is a shining example of Salute's mission in action. As a Veteran myself, supporting [Mr. X] and watching him grow is gratifying on so many levels."

Mr. X advises other Veterans looking for work to find their niche and pursue it. "Salute is helping me live the life I want to live," he said.

Key Information

VA CECs across the country lead efforts to establish a local employment collective, collaborate with VA and non-VA partners to identify local gaps in current competitive employment services for homeless Veterans, and develop opportunities to engage with community partners and local employers who are also committed to ending and preventing homelessness among Veterans.

To locate Veteran recruits and train them in the fundamentals of the data-center field, the Salute team contacted Beatrice Smith-Redd, the CEC at Jesse Brown VAMC, to form a unique collaborative in 2015 using a recovery-oriented holistic approach to drive success. These two entities fostered a partnership with the aim of empowering Veterans to start or advance their careers. Salute provided an outlet for Veterans to do so in the data industry.

Context

The VHA Homeless Program Office developed the CEC position to coordinate and maximize the impact of employment resources across VA and the community. Currently, Jesse Brown VAMC provides care to approximately 58,000 Veterans who reside in the City of Chicago and Cook County, Illinois, and in six counties in northwestern Indiana. As of January 2014, there were 725 homeless Veterans residing in and around the Jesse Brown VAMC. Smith-Redd is focused on collaborative initiatives to connect Veterans to resources that address their employment needs, impacting their ability to sustain permanent housing.

Salute seized an opportunity to assist in reducing the high Veteran unemployment rate, and prepare for the anticipated 20 percent staff shortage in a field that requires a steady stream of recruits to fill open positions. Veterans of all stripes, including those exiting homelessness, possess great potential for these high-demand jobs. The challenge was in connecting the two.

Practice Description

Upon first contact, Salute and Smith-Redd came to understand and align the needs of the data industry with the needs and skills of the Veterans seeking jobs in the Chicago area. In the case of Mr. X, when Smith-Redd found that Mr. X would be a viable candidate for the job, she worked with him to identify and address potential barriers to employment. This included employment-readiness training consisting of enhancing self-confidence, resume development, and interview preparation as well as assessment and counseling of vocational knowledge, skills, and abilities. Before hire, Salute made sure to lay out a clear blueprint of what the job would entail. After being hired, Mr. X's supervisors set the expectations and vision they had for him. They gradually reintroduced him into the workforce and agreed to initially pay him on a per-day basis so he could get a handle on his bills.

Beyond the Veteran's outstanding work ethic, Salute's flexibility in payroll practices was a big help. The Veteran used his daily salary to catch up on bills and secure transportation to and from work, overcoming a common roadblock to successful employment of Veterans exiting homelessness. "Steady performance reports were essential, too," said Smith-Redd. Ms. Smith-Redd receives regular progress updates from the Veteran's Salute supervisors about his job performance. "Supervisors and co-workers are also building one-on-one relationships with him so he feels part of the team." Mr. X now advises other Veterans looking for work to find their niche and pursue it. VA and Salute both agree that Mr. X's success is due to his preparation, commitment, skills, and dedication to a job well done.

Smith-Redd shared that, "When companies (are involved in the performance and progress of the Veteran hire and integrate them into the team), it engages (the Veteran) that much quicker, which increases retention and sustains their employment." According to Smith-Redd, "this is probably the most effective and cost-efficient way to onboard a new employee, particularly one who's experienced homelessness and/or chronic unemployment." Smith-Redd and Mr. X still meet every one to two weeks for job coaching sessions. Structured intervention techniques are used to help him learn the professional and interpersonal skills required to be a successful employee and to sustain employment, such as workplace communication and conflict resolution strategies.

Replicability

Employment is one of the key elements in helping Veterans climb out of homelessness permanently or avoid it all together. Employment provides an improved quality of life, increased self-confidence and independence, opportunities for socialization, and a decreased reliance on institutional care. With nearly 150 CECs hired at VAMCs across the country, the CEC is a central figure within the Homeless Program for ongoing education on the importance of employment, and for matching a Veteran to the right job with the appropriate level of supports. The CEC is a change champion that promotes the development of community employment opportunities and partnerships to end Veteran homelessness.

Through development of strong community employer collaborations, Veterans are afforded the opportunity to return to competitive employment at a functional level that aligns with their skills and preferences, while also taking into account their support needs. This model can be duplicated in both rural and metropolitan locations, as well as with national and regional employers.

Recognition

Jason Okroy, Sondra Kolodzinski, the employees of Salute Incorporated, Beatrice Smith-Redd, Homeless Program, vocational programs at the Jesse Brown VAMC

Specialty and Inpatient Nurse Practitioner Practice: Time as a Resource

Rochelle Carlson, MS, RN, GNP-BC, CRRN, Nurse Practitioner Manager, Specialty & Inpatient NPs

William S. Middleton Memorial Veterans Hospital, Madison, WI
rochelle.carlson@va.gov

Self-reporting by NPs, using a time tracking tool, is an effective method to describe NP practice. The time tracking data can be used to improve the accuracy of NP productivity measures and labor cost accounting.

Introduction

NPs straddle the worlds of medicine and nursing but are increasingly held to the productivity and performance standards of physicians. PC NPs working in the VA system are measured by patient panel size, as defined by specific outcome indicators. However, there are few defined productivity expectations or outcome benchmarks for NPs working in specialty or inpatient settings.

The 2014 Madison VA All Employee Survey scores indicated that NPs working in specialty and inpatient settings feel more burnout and are less engaged as compared to NPs working in other areas. In addition, other staff members had questions and misconceptions about how specialty and inpatient NPs spend their time because their practices look different than PC NPs.

Key Information

Twenty-nine NPs that practice in a specialty and/or inpatient role at the Madison VA self-reported work tasks using a Time Tracker form for five days in December 2014. This project was led by Rochelle Carlson, NP Manager Specialty, and Inpatient NPs in collaboration with Joyce Feller, Analyst. All the NPs working in specialty or inpatient roles participated in collecting data. The information gathered helped better understand the time NPs spent in different activities and described the different roles carried out by the specialty and inpatient NP group. This baseline information helped correctly map NPs for cost accounting purposes, develop realistic productivity expectations, and evaluate additional resources in specialty and inpatient areas.

Context

The William S. Middleton Memorial Veteran's Hospital in Madison, WI, is an 87-bed acute care facility and a 26-bed Community Living Center (CLC) that provides tertiary medical, surgical, neurological, and psychiatric care, and a full range of outpatient services. This facility serves 130,000 Veterans who live in 15 counties in South Central Wisconsin and in five counties in northwestern Illinois. The Madison VA is also the specialty care referral center for an additional 57,000 Veterans who reside in a neighboring VA service area. Because Madison VA is affiliated with the University of Wisconsin School of Medicine and Public Health, many specialty physicians practice at both facilities. Because specialty physicians are part-time providers at the Madison VA, the Madison VA specialty NPs are usually the full-time continuity providers for the services and function as the central resource for the specialty. The inpatient NPs work as a "hospitalist" group, managing an inpatient population and the CLC patient population. Both the specialty and inpatient NPs function autonomously in highly specialized roles with limited ability to cross-cover or back each other up.

Practice Description

When completing the Time Tracker form for five days, the NPs identified work tasks as either inpatient or outpatient. NPs also indicated the type of practice role: clinical, administrative, or educational for each activity. The amount of time spent in inpatient versus outpatient activities was used to "map" each NP to the appropriate area for internal cost allocation. Next, the NPs were categorized into like groups for data analysis, including: medical outpatient, surgical outpatient, medical/surgical inpatient and outpatient, and inpatient/hospitalist. While all NP groups spent about 90 percent of time in clinical activities, only 39 percent of clinical time was spent "face-to-face" with patients. Outpatient surgical NPs spent the most time in "face-to-face" type tasks, while the Inpatient/Hospitalist NPs spent the most time in post-appointment tasks, including documentation. Differences in time spent with appointment and pre- and post-appointment tasks were also noted based on years of experience as a NP.

Replicability

This practice indicates that self-reporting by NPs using a Time Tracker tool is an effective method to describe specialty and inpatient NP practice and time use. This practice was successful because the specialty and inpatient NPs recognized the need for better reporting and were willing to objectively describe their practice to improve understanding of their roles within the organization. Results from the time analysis have increased the accuracy of labor cost accounting, which is a key element in determining NP and specialty service workload and efficiency. Nursing Service provided the analyst and data input necessary to make this project possible.

Support by administration for assistance with data management is necessary, and willingness by staff to have their practices examined closely is imperative. This practice could be replicated by NPs in other facilities and by other types of clinicians (i.e., physicians, pharmacists, social workers, etc.) or by interdisciplinary clinics who want to more fully describe their practice in an objective manner.

Recognition

Joyce Feller, the specialty and inpatient NPs at the Madison VA, Becky Kordahl, Dave Murray, Matt Updike, Michelle Lucatorto

Nursing Assistant Schedule Flow Template

Katherine Dufresne, Nursing Assistant

Albuquerque Vet Center, Albuquerque, NM
katherine.dufresne@va.gov

The Nursing Assistant Patient Flow Template can facilitate attention and consistency within a department and can improve outcomes. The template is the perfect size to fit in a badge holder and makes a great reference tool for new or temporary employees.

Introduction

When I was completing my Nursing Assistant orientation with my Preceptor, I found myself taking numerous notes and filling out many evaluation forms. After a few days, I came to the conclusion that a printable and wearable daily schedule of tasks and duties for the Nursing Assistant's position would be very helpful. The Nursing Assistant Template is especially useful considering our department has several shifts, and each shift has varying duties and responsibilities. It is also an excellent guideline for new employees as well as floating employees who serve on our floor from different departments and unfamiliar with our work flow, procedures, and schedule.

In addition, it can help facilitate more consistent and accurate measurement of patients' fluid intake, resulting in better Veteran care.

Key Information

In November 2015, I introduced the Nursing Assistant Template to our inpatient Telemetry department, where we monitor Veterans' cardiac activity. A Veteran's intake and output of fluids can play a very important role in his or her health and recovery. The Nursing Assistant Template is a great way to keep track of this information.

Context

The New Mexico Veterans Affairs Health Care System (NMVAHCS) serves Veterans in New Mexico, southern Colorado, and West Texas. The NMVAHCS is part of the Southwest Healthcare Network, VISN 18. That network is based in Mesa, AZ, and includes Prescott, Phoenix, Tucson, Big Spring, Amarillo, and El Paso. The Nursing Assistant Patient Flow Template serves as a reference tool for employees and provides quick information and facilitates better and more consistent care for Veterans.

Practice Description

With the help and input of a few of our day, evening, and night shift employees, I designed and created three badge holder-sized templates. Two of the templates together cover a full 24 hours of a Nursing Assistant's timeline of duties on our unit. The Fluid Intake measurements have their own template.

I originally created these forms in Excel so I could update or change them, as needed. To reduce the cost of printing and laminating, I designed a small template that fits in a badge holder. Also, instead of trying to fit everything on one or two sides of paper, there are three separate print-outs:

day shift, night shift, and a side that has fluid intake amounts, as well as a quick go-to list of when to take Blood Sugars and Vitals.

Replicability

The Nursing Assistant Patient Flow Template can be changed and adapted to meet a department's specific needs. The idea is to use it as a guide for anyone who would like to utilize it; the template helps bring attention and improved consistency to a work area and improve its outcomes. The Excel document can be changed or updated, as needed.

Recognition

Jessica A., Heather G., Ray M., Carla D.

VISN 16 Nurse Leader Mentoring Program

Amy Smith, DNP, FAANP, VISN 16 Deputy CMO/VISN Chief Nursing Officer
South Central VA Health Care Network, Ridgeland, MS
amyw.smith@va.gov

This formalized mentoring program supports the professional development of emerging nurse leaders, equipping them with skills to provide transformational leadership to support Veterans and frontline staff.

Introduction

Nursing staff play a critical role in caring for our Veterans and providing quality health care. The interaction that nursing professionals have with our Veterans impacts the way Veterans perceive our VA health care system. Nursing provides the human touch to our Veterans across the care continuum.

Approximately 22 percent of current VA nursing professionals are eligible for retirement. The majority of the nurse leaders in VISN 16 are nearing retirement eligibility. VISN 16 recognized the need to "grow our own" and support the professional development of the next generation of nurse leaders across VISN 16. As part of succession planning, VISN 16 developed a formalized Nurse Leader Mentoring Program, including a robust curriculum focused on developing the knowledge, skills, and experiences necessary for successful nursing leadership.

Since implementation of the program, nurse leader mentees from across the VISN have expressed appreciation for the investment in their growth and development. On the most recent RN satisfaction survey, the majority of sites across VISN 16 showed improvement in the RN manager and RN-MD relations categories as well as an increase in overall satisfaction.

Information about the Nurse Leader Mentoring Program has spread informally to other VISNs. Another VISN recently imported the program, and a second expressed interest in doing the same. Mentoring our emerging nurse leaders will support efforts to retain and empower the frontline nursing staff and, in doing so, will improve access and quality of care for the Veterans we serve.

Key Information

VISN 16 implemented a formal mentoring program to support the professional development of nurse leaders across the network. After comprehensive program development, the VISN deployed the program at the beginning of FY 2016. Dr. Amy Smith, Deputy CMO/Chief Nursing Officer for VISN 16, collaborated with a project team that included nurse leaders from various levels at all ten facilities across VISN 16. The focus of the program is to develop nurse leaders, to promote effectiveness and retention. This program empowers and develops future nurse leaders by equipping them with the skills necessary to succeed.

Context

According to the VHA Workforce Succession Strategic Plan, nurses are ranked as the second highest occupation needed for recruitment and retention. Although nearly 5,200 nurses practice in VISN

16, there is a recognized need for seasoned nurse professionals to advance into leadership roles. Recognizing the cost of RN turnover to the organization and the nearly 700,000 Veterans we serve, VISN 16 took action to develop nurse leaders at all levels, with a focus on frontline nurse managers.

Practice Description

The project team conducted an extensive literature review, benchmarked with mentoring programs within VA, outside of VA, within nursing, and across other disciplines. The team incorporated best practices from successful programs into the development of the program, developed a conceptual framework, a marketing plan, a process to identify participants and match mentees with mentors, and a robust curriculum, along with processes for monitoring and evaluating the program.

After the program was developed, it was presented to VISN leadership, who approved it for implementation across the VISN. Although the initial plan had been to pilot the program, leadership requested a full and immediate implementation. The facility nurse executives identified a program coordinator for each facility, and the coordinators were trained during a two-day face-to-face meeting. An implementation toolkit was developed and disseminated. The VHA Core Mentor Training was leveraged for training, and the mentors were also trained on the Nurse Leader Mentoring Program curriculum. The VISN holds monthly calls with the coordinators and receives quarterly updates. VISN recognition of participants is an important aspect of the program.

Replicability

The success of this program is driven by the desire to improve nurse succession planning at each of our sites. We have received support from facility leadership, and marketing of the program has been successful. The two-day training for program coordinators got the program off to a strong start, and the monthly calls are valuable.

The program can easily spread to other sites. We are collaborating with two other VISNs to make the program available for their facilities. The development of the program includes an implementation toolkit that makes it easy to roll out at the local level and promotes replication. The content is valuable to all nurse leader audiences.

Recognition

Amy Smith, Angelica Hawkins, Salena Wright-Brown, Sheila Cox-Sullivan, Donna DeLise, Deatosha Haynes, Joyce Smithling, Laurie Mitchell, Karen Scott

Angels Food Pantry

Jeff Soots, CLO, Angelia Scott, CFO

William Jennings Bryan Dorn VA Medical Center, Columbia, SC
jeffrey.soots@va.gov

The Angels Food Pantry, one of ten in VHA, was established in 2015. It is the only 24/7 VHA food pantry and is supported through community affiliations like Harvest Hope Food Bank and the Gary Sinise Foundation. Angels Food Pantry feeds over 30 Veterans a month and provides basic life necessities.

Introduction

Dorn VAMC identified a need to provide Veterans with the basic life necessities, including food and toiletries. In the past, when Veterans arrived at our facility for an appointment and requested food, we would have to send them downtown to the local food bank.

Dorn is one of only ten VA hospitals with a food pantry and the only facility with a food pantry that is open 24/7. Our food bank is a separate room with organized items, including food, toiletries, refrigerated items, clothing, blankets, utensils, and laundry items. Every Social Work (SW) provider has access to our food pantry. Every Veteran that visits the pantry completes a referral form with the SW provider for tracking and awareness. We have created a single stop where Veterans visiting our facility can acquire additional items, if needed.

Since getting permission from the Office of Special Counsel to operate a food pantry nine months ago, Dorn has served over 500 Veterans, with increasing numbers each month. Weekly inventories are completed to ensure no food items are close to expiring, but due to the tremendous volume of Veterans visiting the food pantry, none of the items remain in the pantry for more than two weeks.

Dorn leadership partnered with the local food bank, Veteran Service Organizations VSOs), and the Gary Sinise Foundation to help ensure the food pantry is stocked to meet the needs of our Veterans.

Key Information

Dorn VAMC had an increasing number of Compensated Work Therapy (CWT) patients that were in need of food items. This inspired us to create a pantry. Thanks to community donations, we quickly outgrew the drawer we had been using to store food items and decided to repurpose an empty office. The facility CFO and CLO maximized resources on hand, as well as donations from community members, to make this possible. They partnered with the Gary Sinise Foundation to ensure the pantry was successful and supporting the Serving Heroes initiative.

Context

The Dorn VAMC opened in Columbia, SC, in 1932 at its current location and consists of seven CBOCs located in upstate, Midlands, and Pee Dee areas of South Carolina. Dorn VAMC is a level 1C, tertiary care teaching hospital, providing a full range of patient care services, with state-of-the-art technology, education, and research. Dorn VAMC provides comprehensive health care, from PC through hospice care, in areas of medicine, surgery, psychiatry, physical medicine and rehabilitation, cardiology, neurology, oncology, dentistry, geriatrics, and extended care. As one of the Teague-Cranston Act medical schools, University of South Carolina, School of Medicine is located on the campus of Dorn VAMC with 48 residency positions between USC/VA. Dorn VAMC is growing rapidly, as an increasing number of military and Veterans move into the area. In FY 2014, Dorn processed the highest number of Compensation and Pension (C&P) examination requests in the nation. For FY 2013, Dorn VAMC gained 2.8 percent in enrolled patients and has continued to increase in enrolled patients every year since.

Practice Description

The challenge was to determine where and how to provide a food pantry with 24/7 access for Veterans in need. We reutilized an unwanted office and partnered with our Social Work providers to provide access to the pantry. Any Veteran can visit the pantry with an authorized team member. We ask Veterans to complete a referral form, which is used to track the number of visitors. SW providers complete follow-up checks on Veterans who need additional assistance. Several key stakeholders were involved in making this program a reality, including Dorn leadership.

Replicability

There is a vital need to provide Veterans with the basic necessities of life. Most of the Veterans who visit our facility don't have transportation and, in the past, their only other option was to go to the local food bank downtown. Now we provide them with food, clothing, utensils, toiletry items, and other basic necessities. Every facility must be creative when it comes to serving Veterans in need.

Recognition

Gary Sinise Foundation

Lean Transformation Plan

Ester Visser, Systems Redesign Coordinator & Crystal Bayless, Program Analyst

Mountain Home VA Medical Center, Mountain Home, TN

ester.visser@va.gov

The Lean Transformation Plan provides a successful roadmap to engage and immerse employees in the lean culture. The plan can be used at any point during a facility's lean journey to jump-start the interest and participation of employees at all levels.

Introduction

The main goal of the Mountain Home VA Healthcare System's (MHVAHCS) Lean Transformation Plan is to create a culture where staff at all levels of the organization feel empowered to make a positive difference for both Veterans and staff by reducing waste or improving the process flow.

The very first lean project that we received was submitted by a staff member from our sterile processing service. He was responsible for cleaning IV poles, pumps, and other equipment that would be put back in service. Part of his role was to maintain a tracking system for inventory so he could locate equipment if needed. In the past, when the equipment was cleaned, he used a two-part inventory tag as the tracking mechanism. The tag was perforated, and one part would go on the equipment, while the second stayed in the "equipment locker." When the process was computerized, the equipment locker became obsolete, but the service continued to order the two-part tags. Every time a piece of equipment was cleaned, the staff member would tear the tag apart and put one-half on the equipment and the other in the trash. You can almost hear him saying, "what a waste."

When this employee learned about the Lean Corporate Goal, he had the idea to look for a one-part tag for this process. Turns out, there is a one-part equipment tag that is less expensive than the original. This small change has saved the facility $1,200 a year for the last four years. Of equal value, it is only one of hundreds of examples of employees finding ways to save resources or improve the process flow in our system.

Key Information

MHVAHCS developed and implemented a three-year System Redesign/Lean Transformation Plan to promote system-wide, high-reliability processes and to reduce waste, in support of the facility's strategic plan. This initiative provided MHVAHCS' more than 2,300 employees with a framework for identifying opportunities to improve processes and save resources. The plan addresses training, project identification, improvement, and sustainment, while promoting a culture where respect for staff and Veterans is the foundation of all actions, and improvement is a vital part of everyone's job. With tremendous teamwork, the three-year plan produced 704 projects with a cost avoidance of over $3.8 million and time equivalent of 36 FTEs.

Context

The MHVAHCS is a comprehensive health care system serving the needs of Veterans in east Tennessee, southwest Virginia, and southeast Kentucky, consisting of 11 sites of care. The main campus offers PC, inpatient care (114 acute care beds), domiciliary care, nursing home care (120 beds), home health care, and outpatient specialty care in an environment of teaching, research, and emergency preparedness. The MHVAHCS serves approximately 54,000 Veterans and has over 2,300 employees. The Lean Transformation Plan challenges all sites of care to identify waste and improve processes. Removing waste, wherever it is found, allows us to redirect resources to additional services for the Veteran, or toward the purchase of vital equipment or supplies. Improving the flow of work processes boosts staff morale by fostering a sense of accomplishment, teamwork, and effective productivity.

Practice Description

In FY 2011 we contracted with the Veterans Engineering Resource Center (VERC) to provide lean training, initially for leadership and then for staff from all departments. We specifically looked for volunteers and created a core group of advocates to lead at all levels. The plan was rolled out in phases, which made it more acceptable and less overwhelming. At its core, lean is respect for our Veterans, our stakeholders, and each other while we strive to eliminate waste. There are three types of waste identified, and we introduced one waste type each year with specific tools to eliminate that type.

We also encouraged two levels of projects. One followed the basic Plan-Do-Study-Act (PDSA) methodology and was reported on the Lean Brag Sheet. These projects were completed by anyone who had control over a waste that was identified. The second level included service-level team projects led by a facilitator who attended at least Green Belt Training, or a facility level team project led by a facilitator who attended Black Belt Training. These projects were documented on the A3 form.

Replicability

Training is the spark for igniting the interest in lean. The more people who are trained and train others through active team facilitation, the stronger and more sustainable the program. The majority of staff must be involved, not just the quality department.

The executive leadership team made lean thinking the corporate goal. The vision was for each staff to receive lean training, and for each work area to complete a certain number of improvement projects. In addition to the money and time savings, we've received many comments about the enthusiasm and engagement of staff.

Improving the Delivery of Services to Veterans with Post-Traumatic Stress Disorder

Kathleen Sherrieb, DPH, Program Coordinator and Evaluator

White River Junction VA Medical Center, White River Junction, VT
kathleen.sherrieb@va.gov

This education and training project uses an Academic Detailing (AD) approach to improve the quality of care delivered to Veterans with PTSD. A mental health clinical pharmacist promotes evidence-based treatments by meeting with clinicians and "detailing" key messages that highlight best practices for PTSD treatment.

Introduction

Our practice is funded by the VA ORH to provide education and training to promote evidence-based treatments for Veterans with PTSD. One goal of our project is to reduce the use of psychiatric medications not recommended for PTSD which may be harmful, especially when prescribed concurrently. For example, Veterans with PTSD may also have chronic pain and be prescribed multiple sedative medications, including opioids. The therapists in our VA medical center and clinics voiced frustration about opioid use, as they had limited alternatives to offer Veterans. We organized and sponsored a training for therapists called, Cognitive Behavioral Therapy for Chronic Pain, which was conducted by a national expert in the field. Clinicians who started using this therapy in the field reported that participating Veterans were doing well and reducing opioids.

Key Information

This project supports clinicians through education and training, and offers in-person and telehealth clinical expertise on effective treatment practices for patients with PTSD. We use an Academic Detailing model to help clinicians improve the quality of care delivered to Veterans with PTSD in the rural states of Vermont and New Hampshire. In AD, a mental health clinical pharmacist promotes evidence-based methods by meeting with clinicians and "detailing" the key messages that highlight accepted treatments for PTSD. For example, we will review clinical data related to a clinic or a prescribing clinician and use the data to discuss methods for change. The pharmacist can play a role in facilitating change, such as developing a taper schedule for a patient on benzodiazepines, a medication not recommended for PTSD, and providing follow-up with that patient. The pharmacist can also assist the psychotherapist in that clinic in providing education and cognitive behavioral therapy to Veterans going through a benzodiazepine taper. The customized outreach and education to clinicians related to prescribing practices also addresses barrier resolution strategies for clinicians and patients, case consultations, and case reviews that can highlight common significant problems across clinic settings in our catchment area.

These interventions are augmented with project-developed educational tools to help the Veteran and the clinician make informed and shared decisions about a course of treatment. Currently, we are sharing our educational tools with clinicians treating Veterans in rural areas throughout the national VA system. Although this project specifically targets VA mental health and PC clinicians and their trainees, implementation of the Veterans Choice Act has expanded the project to include community-based clinicians who partner with VA and may be treating Veterans. The ultimate goal is to reduce morbidity and mortality connected to inappropriate use of mental health medications and underutilization of psychotherapies by Veterans with PTSD in rural areas.

Context

There is a significant shortage of mental health professionals across the mental health industry, including VA's health system. Many rural VA facilities in northern New England struggle with psychiatric support for rural clinics. This deficit particularly impacts Veterans with PTSD, as approximately 34 percent of VA mental health patients in our catchment area have a diagnosis of PTSD. Furthermore, many of these afflicted Veterans are receiving medications that are not recommended, instead of evidence-based psychotherapies for PTSD. For example, nearly 10 percent are receiving benzodiazepine medications, which the VA Clinical Practice Guidelines (CPGs) caution against using to manage core PTSD symptoms due to increased safety concerns. Those at high risk include Veterans with chronic use, over 65 years old, or taking concomitant sedatives, especially opioids. Overall, more than 330 Veterans with PTSD in our bi-state area are currently prescribed benzodiazepines, and over 90 percent of those fall into high-risk categories. One-third of these Veterans have no documented treatment with psychotherapies and/or antidepressants, which are the evidence-based treatments for PTSD. These challenges are reflected in the goals of our project, which seeks to facilitate 1) a decrease in the use of benzodiazepines particularly for at-risk Veterans with PTSD, 2) a reduction in off-label use of atypical antipsychotics for Veterans with PTSD and no confirmed psychotic disorder, 3) greater use of prazosin to target PTSD-related sleep disorders, 4) promotion of increased referrals to evidence-based psychotherapies (cognitive behavioral therapies for PTSD, insomnia and anxiety), and 5) an increase in the use of patient-level measurement-based care for PTSD, using the PTSD Checklist.

Practice Description

Educational presentations address specific topics that focus on the goals and learning needs of clinicians serving Veterans with PTSD, as previously noted. These include but are not limited to: 1) pharmacological innovations in PTSD, especially as they relate to evidence-based medications; 2) pharmacological treatments for PTSD and co-morbid disorders; 3) pharmacological management of PTSD and substance use disorder; 4) guidance in the use of alternatives to opioids to treat chronic pain. Our needs assessment survey identified these topics as the top four learning needs. We conducted the survey during the first year of the program. Ongoing assessments will capture additional education needs.

AD training and educational strategies include: 1) educational module training; 2) face-to-face contact with clinical staff, followed by telehealth; and 3) material development to promote key messages and detail professional behavioral changes to improve patient outcomes. This proactive model promoting evidence-based practice has shown promising results in VA VISNs on the West Coast. Our project interventions have already led to a discussion about initiating a benzodiazepine tapering clinic in our medical center that will standardize and institutionalize the goal of reducing benzodiazepine use.

Replicability

This project aims to change the medication prescribing culture through learning programs that develop capacity and capability for improvement. A strength of this project is its timing. The issue of inappropriate prescribing in mental health is a timely issue and a major health challenge for VA. Given what we have learned through our own research efforts and clinical data, we know that prescribing clinicians are often not adhering to the CPG recommendations (Bernardy et al., 2012). An innovative aspect of our project is the use of AD to change clinicians' prescribing behaviors when the medications do little to improve the health and quality of life of the patients. We have shared our project model and educational materials with VA leadership, clinicians, and the clinical pharmacists serving a rural CBOC with the West Palm Beach, FL, VA. We continue to collect data to track among clinicians receiving "detailing" messages and clinical pharmacist interventions. We plan to standardize components of our interventions in the development of the benzodiazepine tapering clinic so that protocols and outcome data will be available at a later date for replication.

Recognition

Nancy Bernardy, Macgregor Montaño, Kathleen Sherrieb, ORH, the National Center for PTSD

The Veterans Affairs New York Harbor Healthcare System 17 North Unit's Employee Influenza Vaccination Program

Linda Kaplan, RN, MSN, Patient Care Team Coordinator

VA NY Harbor Healthcare System, New York, NY

linda.kaplan@va.gov

The staff on the 17 North unit at the VA New York Harbor Healthcare System (NYHHS) realized that an important part of providing "The Best Care Everywhere" was to receive the flu vaccine themselves. They achieved a 100 percent compliance rate with a voluntary influenza program.

Introduction

The VA health care system still embraces a voluntary flu vaccination program for their staff, unlike their private sector counterparts. It is a challenge each year to have staff "willingly" accept the flu vaccine for a multitude of reasons. But in order to provide first-rate care to both our internal and external customers, it is imperative that our staff at the VA New York Harbor Healthcare System be fully immunized against influenza. Flu can be a very serious illness, even causing death. Health promotion of staff equals health promotion for our mental health patients on the 17 North acute inpatient psychiatric unit. Mental Health employees need to be role models for their patients.

The staff on 17 North realized that an important part of providing "The Best Care Everywhere" was to receive the flu vaccine themselves. It was so important to the staff on 17 North that they made this one of their unit-based performance improvement initiatives. A "Flu Champion" was selected on the 17 North unit and, in collaboration with the patient care team coordinator and the staff on 17 North, the staff achieved a 100 percent immunization rate, including all clinicians and support staff that work on this unit. As a health care provider, getting a flu shot is an excellent health care practice and protects you, your co-workers, and importantly, the Veterans we serve.

Key Information

The evidence-based literature supports the benefits of health care workers receiving influenza vaccinations. Research indicates that influenza, a vaccine preventable illness, is a frequent cause of death. The CDC and Association for Professionals in Infection Control and Epidemiology (APIC) both recommend the vaccination of health care workers to limit the spread of influenza and promote safety for patients and colleagues. There are numerous debates regarding the pros and cons of voluntary versus mandatory vaccination programs (Poland, Tosh & Jacobson, 2005). The 17 North staff achieved a 100 percent immunization rate within the acute care unit (in comparison to the VA NYHHS Hospital rate of 32 percent). The Flu Champion analyzed the reasons why staff did not accept a flu vaccine, as cited during FY 2014 (achieved 85 percent), and then provided extensive education to staff and designated staff to immunize the colleagues right on the 17 North unit, making it more convenient. The champion also kept a data sheet of who accepted the vaccine, attended VA NYHHS staff meetings to discuss strategies and new evidence-based research, and shared information back with the 17 North employees.

Context

The VA NYHHS is an A1 facility, serving Veterans in a metropolitan area, with facilities in Manhattan, Brooklyn, St. Albans, and various CBOCs. This initiative took place in an acute inpatient psychiatric unit, serving Veterans with acute mental health needs and focused on the staff serving these Veterans. The VA NYHHS still has a voluntary Influenza Vaccination program, unlike their private sector counterparts, which have mandatory flu vaccination programs that require either accepting the flu vaccine or wearing a mask. This makes getting staff to willingly accept the flu vaccine challenging. The overall VA NYHHS rate for staff receiving their flu vaccine in FY 2014–2015 was 37 percent; the 17 North unit had a compliance rate of 85 percent. The acute inpatient psychiatric unit decided to make this their performance improvement initiative and worked to achieve 100 percent compliance. Peer support between disciplines was a strong motivator.

Practice Description

The 17 North Flu Champion conducted a SWOT (Strengths, Weaknesses, Opportunities, and Threats) Analysis as part of its unit's performance improvement initiative and as a method to explore new ideas and enhance support. We educated and encouraged employees to receive their vaccinations for 2015–2016 and drilled down on reasons staff refused the vaccine in 2014–2015 (85 percent of employees vaccinated). The result was that 100 percent of staff working on 17 North received the flu vaccine for FY 2015–2016, compared to the VA NYHHS Hospital-wide rate of 32 percent.

Replicability

The 17 North team encouraged colleagues to receive their flu vaccination, and conducted surveys on the importance of increasing vaccination compliance. They sent facility-wide e-mail blasts to all staff encouraging vaccinations and attended bi-weekly NY Harbor HCS meetings to brainstorm ways to increase compliance. 17 North was recognized at different forums for their achievement. For example, they were acknowledged for their 100 percent flu vaccination compliance at the Director's Morning Report, Harbor-wide Flu Champion Meeting, Patient Services Key Staff meeting, and Chief of Staff's Clinical Service Chief's meeting.

Recognition

Cynthia Caroselli, Karel Raneri-Vitale, Jacob Herzog, the 17 North acute inpatient "team" at the VA NYHHS

B.R.E.A.T.H.E. Staff Resilience Training

Karen Wall, EdD, PMHRN-BC, BSN, Geriatric/Dementia Care Coordinator

VA Palo Alto Healthcare System, Palo Alto, CA
karen.wall2@va.gov

This interactive training provides a supportive and empowered way to practice "self-soothing" when dealing with difficult family members, and sometimes residents. The skills are also transferable for stress management.

Introduction

"Met with Veteran's spouse to discuss behavioral expectations for respectful communication. This meeting was called in response to unit staff reports that on multiple occasions Ms. 'X' has expressed her frustration by shouting and choosing words to express her anger that are insulting and demeaning to staff. Returned phone call and spoke with Mr. X. Resident's wife began to raise her voice over the phone, expressing dissatisfaction with overall care. She used inappropriate words (i.e., 'stupid') and became very argumentative, so the provider needed to end the call."

The application of positive psychology principles to help nursing staff avoid deflation of their "zest" for work has been shown to increase feelings of sense of self-worth, and to restore professional enthusiasm, even in the presence of challenging family members or residents (Seligman, et al, 2005). In the book FISH (Lundin, Paul, & Christensen, 2000), love of work is linked to enjoyment and commitment. Recently, the author visited Menlo Park Division of the VA Palo Alto HACS to give a presentation on the principles of self-care and empowerment at work. As part of this talk, he introduced staff to the acronym B.R.E.A.T.H.E., which represents the seven components of resilience.

Verbal feedback from attendees was positive. They reported trying to apply positive psychology principles during interactions with difficult family members and residents. Community Living Center (CLC) staff also reported heightened awareness of their own internal triggers, as well as an increase in their ability to use positive psychology principles to refocus themselves during moments of conflict. Staff members reported a decrease in negative interactions with challenging family members, because they are more comfortable referring that person to nursing management.

Key Information

Nursing leadership approached the author of FISH in December 2015 about a training program to help staff on one CLC unit cope with verbally and emotionally abusive family members. In response, the author developed a class to teach resiliency.

Context

The Menlo Park Division of the VA Palo Alto HCS operates a number of CLCs for long-term residential care of Veterans living with dementia and other neurocognitive disorders. Caregiving staff in the VA CLCs often report high levels of stress when caring for these residents. While trying to provide safe, compassionate, and thorough care, they struggle with challenging family members of residents. Frontline staff is often the target of anger, hostility, and verbal and emotional abuse. As a result, they are reluctant to care for certain residents. Under these conditions, staff begin to lose sight of the meaning in their work, eventually leading to burnout and a "just making it through the day to get their pay" attitude (Frankl, 1959). This sense of lost dignity affects residents, who will suffer from decreased engagement, suboptimal care, or worse. The use of positive psychology principles has been shown to restore zest for work, even in the face of the challenges (Seligman, et. al., 2005).

Practice Description

The author of FISH developed a training program to help CLC nursing staff cope with difficult family members and residents. The author created the acronym B.R.E.A.T.H.E. to represent the seven components of caregiver resilience, which are based on a review of positive psychology literature, as well as extensive personal experience as a student and teacher of mindfulness, resiliency, and self-care. Training the staff on how to retain dignity and sense of self has a major impact on Veterans, as staff can communicate with residents and their family members in a therapeutic and collaborative way.

Using an experiential approach to learning, the author developed a PowerPoint presentation outlining the principles of self-care at work. Attendees were introduced to the concept of self-care and empowerment, as well as to the acronym B.R.E.A.T.H.E., which represents the seven principles of resiliency:

1. B: BE present
2. R: REMEMBER your smile
3. E: ENGAGE your heart
4. A: ANSWER the call
5. T: TAKE time for yourself
6. H: HEAL from within
7. E: EMBRACE the moment

This acronym was used, in part, to teach the students about B.R.E.A.T.H.E work. The breathing technique demonstrated during this presentation was tactical breathing, which is based on an easy-to-use mobile app of the same name from the Center for Telehealth and Technology (T2) and the National Center for PTSD. After each segment of the presentation, the class was lead in a round of tactical breathing. This provided the opportunity for attendees to practice the technique and commit it to muscle memory. At the end of the class, attendees were led through a final breathing exercise and provided with encouraging thoughts and plans for follow-up by the author.

Replicability

The initial program was so successful that the author has been invited back to provide positive psychology training to all CLC staff. The initiative was also highlighted in February 2016 at the monthly Nursing Grand Rounds as part of an effort to share resources for staff self-care. The author will be scheduling regular trainings for the CLC staff (nursing and non-nursing) and will submit the training for continuing education credit. The author recently submitted the training as a promising practice in the VA Pulse project. This training could potentially become part of VHA-wide staff resiliency training. It could be replicated, as it does not require extensive instructor training, nor does it require special certification. The author has been approached with requests from other VISNs, as well as by the National Center for Organization Development (NCOD), to provide the training.

Recognition

Ann Narciso, Cherina Tinio, Jennifer Santos, Maria C. Alba, the nursing staff of the Menlo Park CLC

Whole Health for Employees: Caring for VA's Greatest Resource

Marc Castellani, PhD, Health Behavior Coordinator and Clinical Champion for Patient-Centered Care

W.G. (Bill) Hefner VA Medical Center, Salisbury, NC
marc.castellani@va.gov

By providing Whole Health retreats for all VA employees, our staff learn skills to better care for themselves and are motivated to use the approach with Veterans.

Introduction

At the start of every Whole Health retreat, participants are asked what they've heard about the session, what their co-workers have said, and why they chose to attend. In one session, a nurse shared that her colleagues, "Said I had to go. They said it would change my life."

When the team from the University of Wisconsin presented the Whole Health approach at Salisbury, we recognized this should be shared not only with the Veterans we serve, but also our colleagues. We believed that helping staff identify their personal mission, learning about self-care, and developing a change plan would result in happier, healthier employees who are more engaged at work, have a more positive view of our VA, and provide a higher level of care to our Veterans. Feedback from the 300-plus attendees supports this, with comments, such as:

- "You made me aware that all things are possible."
- "I realized that I matter and need to provide for and take care of ME!"
- "The presentation cut to the heart about what this is all about, what life is all about."
- "I'm glad to be part of an organization that provides such a focus on employee health. [It] helps me feel valued, when often employees do not feel valued."

Key Information

Following the "Whole Health: Change the Conversation" course at Salisbury in June 2014, a steering committee was formed to develop and implement our vision of a Whole Health retreat for staff. Our steering committee included physicians, psychologists, nurses, and others located in PC. Using information from the University of Wisconsin, we developed a one-day retreat focused on helping staff members learn about Whole Health. The day closed with each person developing a personal change plan. We recognize that our employees are VA's most valuable resource and that having an engaged and healthy workforce is essential for providing our Veterans with quality of care. We also believe that clinicians experiencing Whole Health will be more likely to offer this approach to Veterans. Our leadership attended the first sessions in January 2015 and found the program beneficial, and further authorized every staff member the opportunity to attend a session. Currently, a faculty of 16 clinicians is divided into teams that offer the retreat twice a month, with additional sessions facilitated in affiliated outpatient clinics.

Context

The Salisbury VA is a Level 1C Hospital that serves 95,000 unique Veterans with close to 70 PACTs. Primary and secondary inpatient health care are available to more than 287,000 Veterans living in a 24-county area of the Central Piedmont Region of North Carolina. This includes over 100,000 Veterans in the Charlotte area, and 65,000 Veterans in the Winston-Salem area. This retreat was developed to raise scores on the All Employee Survey, and improve employee morale and well-being.

Practice Description

The University of Wisconsin, through a contract with the Office of Patient Centered Care and Cultural Transformation, developed a 2.5-day workshop on the Whole Health approach to care. Our steering committee created a one-day program focused on self-care, and how each person can apply Whole Health principles in their everyday lives. The course was piloted before being offered to leadership. Publicity is generated through emails, the weekly bulletin, flyers, staff meetings, and word-of-mouth; every participant is asked to invite a colleague to a future session.

The retreat combines PowerPoints and brief lectures, videos, and small-group and large-group exercises. Participants consider their personal mission for life, learn the value of mindfulness, explore the eight components of self-care, and discuss how they can make changes. We close the day with the opportunity to write a personal change plan.

Replicability

There are two specific elements that helped this program become as success: support from leadership and a faculty with a vision and dedication to develop the program and facilitate the sessions twice a month. This combination of administrative support and staff dedication is necessary for our program to be replicated, and others are already taking steps to bring the Whole Health retreats to their facilities.

Recognition

Kaye Green, the entire Salisbury pentad, Parag Dalsania, Dave Rakel, Christine Milovani, Randall Gehle, Kathy Hedrick, Cecilia Novitt, Sudip Roy, Jennifer Terndrup, Shanyn Aysta, Bruce Eads, Scott Emsley, Penny Greer-Link, Ellen Leonard, Paras Mehta, Keri Obric, Camille Robinette, Christy Robbins, Melissa Yost

Managerial Cost Accounting Tiger Team

Rochelle Jones, Management Analyst; Angela Scott, CFO; Danielle Terrell, Health System Specialist; Angela Donald, MCA&DM Site Liaison; Courtney Murray, VERA Coordinator

William Jennings Bryan Dorn VA Medical Center, Columbia, SC
rochelle.jones@va.gov

Executive leadership worked with five facility subject matter experts to implement a workgroup of representatives from different service lines to outline a process to educate staff on managerial cost accounting and decision-making components, trend data, and service line productivity.

Introduction

Managerial Cost Accounting and Decision Making (MCA&DM) system is used in many facets and functions of VA to assist with budgeting, resource allocation, and to provide statistical data on clinical services. Additionally, this system is used to measure overall productivity of department resources. The application and monitoring of MCA&DM data to ensure proper utilization of resources and effective management of department functions is a critical responsibility.

Key Information

The VISN 7 MCA&DM productivity goal is for all MCA&DM direct departments to be between 80 and 100 percent. Dorn VAMC has 23 direct departments associated with our service lines. As a result of consistently low MCA&DM monthly scorecard ratings, leadership worked with five facility subject matter experts to implement a workgroup to outline a process to educate staff on MCA&DM components, trend data, and monitor service line productivity. The goal of the workgroup is to ensure data quality with an increase of MCA&DM scorecard ratings. In an attempt to grow MCA&DM subject matter experts in each service line, the section chief designated a primary and secondary point of contact to work with the workgroup. Once this was accomplished, the workgroup provided training on MCA&DM data, data retrieval, and analysis.

Context

The Dorn VAMC opened in Columbia, SC, in 1932 at its current location and consists of seven CBOCs located in the upstate, Midlands, and Pee Dee areas of South Carolina. Dorn VAMC is a level 1C, tertiary care, teaching hospital, providing a full range of patient care services, with state-of-the-art technology, education, and research. We provide comprehensive health care, from PC through hospice care in areas of medicine, surgery, psychiatry, physical medicine and rehabilitation, cardiology, neurology, oncology, dentistry, geriatrics, and extended care. As one of the Teague-Cranston Act medical schools, University of South Carolina, School of Medicine is located on the Dorn VAMC campus with 48 residency positions between USC/VA. Dorn VAMC is growing rapidly with an increasing number of military and Veterans moving into the area. In FY 2014, Dorn processed the highest number of Compensation and Pension (C&P) examination requests in the nation. For FY 2013, Dorn VAMC gained 2.8 percent in enrolled patients and has continued to increase in enrolled patients every year since.

Practice Description

The workgroup developed a 90-day review period to allow the appropriate amount of time for service line changes to have an impact on the scorecard data. Of the 23 departments, 13 departments were below the 80 percent productivity goal and were placed in the 90-day review period.

The workgroup worked with colleagues from each service line to ensure understanding of the MCA&DM data components. The workgroup assisted service lines with retrieving data, identifying reports to monitor service line operations, assisting with tracking and trending data, and explaining business operations of MCA&DM.

At the end of the 90-day review period, there was a 62 percent positive result rate, and eight of the 13 departments showed potential increases in productivity. Three of the 13 departments increased their overall productivity score to 80 percent. Five the 13 departments have action plans in place that should result in improved productivity as we move into the second quarter of FY 2016. The program also boosted service line awareness around the importance of MCA&DM. 100 percent of the staff reported learning about the impact of MCA&DM on our business and clinical operations. We expect to achieve a 15 percent improvement in overall productivity by the first anniversary of the project.

The Dorn VAMC successfully developed MCA&DM subject matter experts within service lines, increased productivity scores, assist in building data integrity, and brought an overall awareness of the MCA&DM system importance.

QUALITY AND SAFETY

Flu Self-Reporting Desktop Icon to Capture Employee Flu Vaccinations Received Outside VA

Vanessa Coronel, RN, VA Boston Flu Fighter and Patient Safety Nurse

VA Boston Healthcare System, Boston, MA

vanessa.coronel@va.gov

A simple desktop icon allows employees to self-report when they have received a flu vaccination outside of VA.

Introduction

The best protection against the flu is getting vaccinated. By promoting flu vaccination among employees, VA Boston takes a proactive approach in reducing Veterans' risk of flu exposure. With the Flu Self-Reporting Icon (Flu Icon), which facilitates the quick, easy reporting of non-VA flu vaccinations, more employees are encouraged to get vaccinated. As more employees are vaccinated, the risk of Veterans being exposed to the flu is lowered. This is the core mission of the multi-disciplinary flu vaccination committee, VA Boston Flu Fighters.

When first utilized in 2013, VA Boston employees fully embraced the Flu Icon due to its convenience and simplicity. They no longer have to go to Occupational Health and fill out the paperwork to report their flu shots. Occupational Health and the Flu Fighters also save time since they no longer have to obtain and hold on to the paperwork. Time saved can be used on vaccinating more Veterans and employees.

By 2020, a Joint Commission initiative recommends that the employee flu vaccination compliance rate should be at 90 percent. Since VHA does not yet mandate employee flu vaccination, reaching the 90 percent compliance rate is a huge undertaking. With the Flu Icon, externally obtained flu vaccination data can be easily captured. With more accurate data, better strategies can be formulated and implemented to increase flu vaccination uptake among VA employees.

Key Information

The brainchild of System Redesign, Occupational Health, and Infection Prevention, the Flu Icon simplifies and standardizes the reporting process of externally obtained flu shots by employees. Accessible anytime and on any desktop or laptop workstation, employees complete flu vaccination reporting within 30 seconds or less. The Flu Icon has improved the capture of non-VA flu vaccinations, and helped VA Boston to achieve its highest flu vaccination compliance rate ever in 2013.

Practice Description

This simple, straightforward, and time-saving innovation requires no funding, no position description changes, and no policy changes. System Redesign built the InfoPath form and linked it into SharePoint. Only Occupational Health has the secure access to protect employee information. The Information Resource Manager (IRM)/IT uploads the Flu Icon to all workstations before the start of the flu season. With a click of the Flu Icon, employees are directed to the secured

SharePoint, and enter their information quickly and safely in no more than five mouse clicks or 30 seconds. Occupational Health gets the report and documents it into the Occupational Health Reporting System.

Public Affairs promotes the Flu Icon through blast emails, screensavers, and intranet articles. The Flu Fighters (Occupational Health, Nursing, Infection Prevention, and Patient Safety) help spread the word when they vaccinate the front line. In summary, the success of the Flu Icon was achieved through teamwork and collaboration.

Replicability

The Flu Icon is free, simple, and quick to implement. In two easy steps, it can be set up in any facility within half a day. The InfoPath form has already been designed by System Redesign and is available for sharing with other VAs. Linking the InfoPath form into the secured SharePoint software takes 2–4 hours. The second step, IRM/IT uploading the Flu Icon image into all workstations, takes 1–2 hours.

Nine of the 36 VAs that have tried to replicate it have been successful. The major deterrent is gaining upper or regional clearance. The Flu Fighters have shared this innovation for the past two years through numerous teleconferences sponsored by VACO Infection Don't Pass It On (IDPIO) and the National Center for Patient Safety (NCPS). Before the start of the 2015–2016 flu season, NCPS endorsed the Flu Icon nationwide. The ninth and most recent replication was made possible by the innovation platform, VA Pulse.

Recognition

Boston Flu Fighters, Robert Sprague, Tom Young, Judy Strymish, Sucheta Doshi, Denise Dulude, Anne Marie Fredericks, Suzanne Mosesso, Pallas Wahl, Pam Bellino, Troy Knighton, Pamela Hirsch, Keith Trettin, Caryl Lee, Beth King

Planning for Future Medical Decisions via Group Visits: "My Life…My Choice"

Kimberly Garner, MD, JD, MPH, FAAFP, Associate Director for Education and Evaluation
Central Arkansas Veterans Healthcare System, Little Rock, AR
kimberly.garner@va.gov

This interactive and patient-centered group visit approach to engaging Veterans in planning for future medical decisions allows patients' wishes to be honored while reducing unwanted treatments.

Introduction

We conducted one of our advance care planning group visits at the Central Arkansas Veterans Healthcare System (CAVHS) VA Day Treatment Center, which houses an addiction treatment program and other resources for homeless Veterans. At this group visit, a Veteran explained that he had been very worried about what would happen to him if he ever had to go to the hospital and was unable to talk or express his wishes. He was not familiar with advance directives or a living will until he attended our group visit. He stated, "I want to do this right now!" With the assistance of the group leader, he completed a living will at the conclusion of the group visit. His living will provided clear guidance for his medical providers if ever he was in a situation where he could not speak for himself. He thanked the project leader over and over for assisting him.

Key Information

The program, which we call "My Life…My Choice," helps Veterans plan for the possibility that in the future they may become very ill and not have the ability to communicate their wishes for care. A central component of the program is the use of group visits to interact with the Veterans and promote open discussion about the meaning and relevance of advance care planning. In this supportive atmosphere, leaders encourage Veterans to think about planning for future medical decisions on a personal level while using the group dynamic to foster open dialogue and alleviate anxieties.

"My Life…My Choice" was implemented at the CAVHS in August 2012. At that time, only 16 percent of enrolled Veterans in VISN 16 had an advance directive in the CPRS. When we talked to Veterans, few understood and had engaged in advance care planning even if they had an advance directive. We also found that Veterans received little help in this area from their health care providers. Many providers indicated that they wanted to talk to their patients about advance care planning, but they just did not have time.

Context

This project was developed to address the concern that few Veterans enrolled at the CAVHS had an advance directive and even fewer appeared to understand the process of advance care planning. This is likely because few of them had received the education they needed to fully understand the purpose and importance of an advance directive or what they needed to do to become fully engaged in the advance care planning process.

Practice Description

"My Life…My Choice," educates Veterans about advance care planning in a non-threatening, Veteran-centric manner using group visits.

This program has two mechanisms for making these groups available to Veterans: the first is to conduct advance care planning discussions with established groups (such as PACT Shared Medical Appointments). The second is to conduct advance care planning group clinics that are open to all Veterans, especially those with appointments at the facility on the same day. Letters are sent out in advance notifying Veterans of these group clinics.

Group discussions are led by one or two specially trained health professionals; as the primary leader, we have generally used a social worker and/or a nurse. Some Veterans are ready to fill out an advance directive by the end of the group visit. If needed, we provide one-to-one assistance for completing the document. Two weeks following the group discussion, the group leader calls each Veteran to discuss whether his or her next step was completed and to assist with problem solving and/or setting an additional next step in the advance care planning process.

Replicability

This program was successful due to the convergence of several key factors. Foremost, as a physician trained and certified in geriatrics and palliative care, Dr. Garner was fortunate to have a full-time position in the Geriatric Research Education and Clinical Centers (GRECC). This position allowed her the time to develop the program and gave her the opportunity to work with a number of health professionals who were very enthusiastic about promoting advance care planning. Together they implemented, evaluated, and refined the program and then developed a standardized program curriculum and toolkit that could be used to promote program dissemination.

Using the aforementioned tools, any facility could implement this program with minimal cost and the use of existing FTEs as it increases the effectiveness and efficiency of employees responsible for assisting Veterans with advance care planning. The program only requires identifying employees willing to take on these responsibilities and to complete the training curriculum. The extensive knowledge and experience gained in developing this program and addressing barriers to implementation has been incorporated into our training programs and toolkit.

Recognition

Geriatric Research Education and Clinical Center, Mental Illness Research Education Clinical Center, VISN 16, Geriatrics and Extended Care, ORH, National Center on Ethics

Code Tray Redesign

Kristine Gherardi, CPhT

VA Boston Healthcare System, Boston, MA
kristine.gherardi@va.gov

This simple and compelling solution was designed to reduce the time it takes to find a certain drug within a code tray (a tray containing medications which have been organized and labeled). This easy-to-implement, low-cost strategy reduces medication distribution errors, improving outcomes for Veterans.

Introduction

My thought process behind the tray redesign was that it needed to be functional for the end user: the code team.

Most of the vials in the tray are of similar size and shape, making it difficult to quickly identify specific medications. I designed the medications to be placed in a foam grid, in alphabetical order, with the labels facing up, making it faster to locate and identify vials. The time this process saves could be life-saving.

Key Information

This design was first implemented about a year ago at the Jamaica Plain, MA, campus. It received so much positive feedback that it was then implemented by the West Roxbury and Brockton campuses. I was the sole collaborator for this best practice. The design makes it more efficient for the trays to be updated and checked by pharmacy staff, saving time and money.

Context

VA Boston serves Veterans from PC and specialty clinics to surgical patients and long-term care.

Practice Description

This practice aimed to make the code tray user-friendly for all parties involved. By processes of elimination, I created an efficient and intuitive design.

Replicability

This practice is easily replicable with very little cost and personnel time. It was replicated at the VA Loma Linda Healthcare System in Loma Linda, CA, as part of the Diffusion of Excellence initiative. VA Boston code cart committee asked for pictures of the redesigned code tray and decided that my design would be implemented at all three sites (Jamaica Plain, West Roxbury, and Brockton). Any site that uses code carts or crash carts at their facilities could easily duplicate this simple practice, at a minimal cost.

Recognition

Roy Daley, John Donovan, Robert Henault

Design the Anesthetic to Meet the WAKE© Score

Brian Williams, MD, MBA, Director, Acute Pain Medicine/Regional Anesthesia, Ambulatory Anesthesia, and Preoperative Optimization

VA Pittsburgh Healthcare System, Pittsburgh, PA
brian.williams6@va.gov

The WAKE© Score replaces a previous anesthesia recovery scoring system, which would often leave patients with nausea/vomiting, lightheadedness, and pain. The WAKE© Score takes a "zero tolerance" approach to anesthesia side effects, improving the Veteran patient experience and outcomes.

Introduction

By transitioning from traditional Aldrete-based recovery room discharge criteria to WAKE©-based discharge criteria in 2011, VA Pittsburgh Healthcare System (VAPHCS) was able to decrease unplanned hospital admissions and improve overall patient satisfaction and outcomes. The WAKE© Score prompts practitioners to consider patients' pre-procedure condition in determining discharge readiness. To enhance patient safety, the WAKE© Score has "zero tolerance" for anesthesia-related complications.

Historically (2010 and prior), Veterans at VAPHCS had undergone surgery exclusively utilizing general anesthesia. This typically involves inhaled gases and intravenous medications for pain, such as fentanyl. Following surgery, all general anesthesia patients were transferred to the Phase 1 Post-Anesthesia Care Unit (PACU) recovery room for a minimum of one hour, and remained there until they met Aldrete Score-based discharge criteria. Phase 1 entails "emergence from anesthesia." Typical side effects of inhaled gases and fentanyl include Postoperative Nausea and Vomiting (PONV). Even though inhaled gases and fentanyl are inexpensive, PONV (an expensive and labor-intensive symptom to treat) was experienced (historically) by 31 percent of patients in our Phase 1 PACU recovery room following general anesthesia. The WAKE© Score addresses the entire patient condition, and not just PONV.

Key Information

In late 2010, VAPHCS pioneered (within VHA) the use of the WAKE© Score for all anesthesia and Moderate Sedation Procedures, prior to later national directives. To maximize patient safety while providing a Veteran-centered and family-centered care experience, VAPHCS eliminated Aldrete-based recovery discharge scoring criteria from all institutional policy and procedure.

The implementation team was created by Director of Ambulatory Anesthesia and the Preop Optimization Clinic Dr. Brian Williams, and Toby Nalepka, RN, PACU. This multi-disciplinary team consisted of PACU RNs, physician anesthesiologists, pulmonary and sleep-lab physicians, respiratory therapists, biomedical engineering, and nursing informatics. Changes to practice were first implemented in partnership between the Pre-op Clinic and the Phase 1 PACU recovery room. We incorporated multi-modal analgesia/anesthesia in tandem with evidence-based practices and cultural changes. After being established as a new policy, we used the WAKE© goals as "targets" to then ultimately "design the anesthetic to meet the WAKE© Score."

The effect the WAKE© Score had on patients with Obstructive Sleep Apnea (OSA) was important. In 2008, our Anesthesia and Pulmonary Services at VAPHCS identified OSA as critical risk factor for perioperative complications. The initial VAPHCS response to this realization was "unplanned" overnight admissions with pulse oximetry monitoring for all patients undergoing general surgery with a diagnosis of OSA. The stopgap practice of routine overnight admission, purely for observation of their OSA and not as a result of the actual surgical procedure, and in the absence of a published safe alternative, led to an increase in unplanned hospital admissions.

With the WAKE© Score, patient pre-procedural health status was taken into account, along with OSA history and/or risk factors, to ensure anesthetic planning and discharge scoring were considered in tandem to alleviate the risk of complications. By applying the WAKE© Score to our OSA population, for example, we safely reduced unplanned hospital admissions for OSA patients from "all" to less than 30 percent by 2012.

Another multi-disciplinary workgroup was formed to create a standardized recovery process throughout the facility for procedures that were not technically "surgery." The WAKE© Score would ultimately be incorporated into the policies that governed all areas that recovered patients from anesthesia or sedation. To do so, the Phase 1 PACU recovery room team leaders formed a group of four content experts to educate designated unit champions in each of the relevant areas. Staff education sessions were conducted, posters/placards were created for display in each of the areas, laminated pocket reference cards were distributed, and electronic documentation templates were revised. Ultimately, a standardized WAKE©-centered peri-procedural continuum was achieved, starting with the initial pre-procedural evaluation and flowing through post-procedural disposition (for surgery, Gastrointestinal (GI) lab, and all other procedures requiring anesthesia or moderate sedation).

Workgroup members then audited each unit's incumbent sedation score documents to ensure that WAKE's parameters were sufficiently similar, working in collaboration with the nurse managers for each moderate sedation unit. Over time, the team designed a WAKE© Score CPRS template that satisfied the needs of every unit. The WAKE© Score electronic template and paper contingency form were submitted through the VA Forms process and received formal approval to be substituted for all incumbent documents that referred to the Aldrete Score (or any other incumbent scoring systems). The group then worked with the Clinical Information System/Anesthesia Record Keeper (CIS/ARK) and VA National coordinators through numerous revisions to create a WAKE© Score template that was applied to the newly-acquired Picis electronic charting package. Picis is utilized in all critical care units, the Phase 1 PACU recovery room, and in the Operating Room (OR) suites.

Educational rollout began in November 2011, and was completed after only three weeks. Then, WAKE© was formally instituted hospital-wide. Ongoing chart audits were performed for a period of three months after rollout to ensure compliance. Areas found to be non-compliant were re-educated, and additional follow-up was completed.

Context

VAPHCS provides both minor and complex operative and procedural services to the western half of Pennsylvania in VISN 4 (including much of Pennsylvania, West Virginia, and eastern Ohio, in an approximate 120-mile radius of Pittsburgh). We also provide liver and kidney transplant services for the national VHA network. The age demographics of the Veterans we serve are 65–79-year-olds comprising 40 percent of the patient population, 46–64-year-olds at 30 percent, 80+ at 20 percent, and 19–45-year-olds at 10 percent.

Replicability

The WAKE© Score was adopted because there was a need for a discharge scoring tool capable of incorporating multiple factors that the traditional Aldrete Score did not address. Specifically, the Aldrete Score did not account for the zero tolerance criteria. The WAKE© Score is built first on its Zero Tolerance Criteria, followed by application of its five scored criteria. VAPHCS leadership wanted specific action plans for OSA patients, as previously described. Ambulatory anesthesia patients (scheduled for same-day discharge) required care plan "goals" provided within the WAKE© Score structure, such that when these goals were met, the Veterans did not necessarily require routing to the Phase 1 PACU recovery room after time in the OR. This "PACU Bypass" reunites Veterans with their families sooner, and decreases the chance of Veterans missing the departure time of VA-provided transportation. Regional anesthesia patients had their own unique circumstances not applicable for Aldrete Score evaluation. The WAKE© Score also allows for a clear distinction between Phase 1 recovery (emergence from anesthesia in PACU) and Phase 2 recovery (preparation for homegoing after same-day surgery). This Phase 1/Phase 2 distinction allows for both maximum efficiency and safety. With education of bedside staff, designation of "superusers," policy revision, reference material, and documentation revision, rapid transition to success was achieved. Given that the primary necessary resource is education, WAKE© Score implementation is easily reproducible. Once the WAKE© Score is implemented as policy, then facilities can progress actively toward the next cultural change of "designing the anesthetic to meet the WAKE© Score."

Recognition

Allison Schanck, Toby Nalepka, Jody Kulas, Kylie Cermenaro, Michael Mangione, Charles Atwood, Visala Muluk, Mark Wilson, Sally Ollio, Gail Bader, Catherine Thompson, Tim Shapiro, Alissa Kmatz, Jamie Vaughn, Steve Herman, Marcos Lopez, Jeff Wagner

Diabetes Nurse Case Management: Improving Glucose Control

Sharon Watts, Diabetes NP

Louis Stokes Cleveland VAMC, Cleveland, OH

sharon.watts@va.gov

This practice of utilizing RN case managers in diabetes increases customer satisfaction and access. The nurses utilize advanced training and protocols to accomplish safe and efficient results.

Introduction

For the past ten years, Veterans have been familiar and comfortable in working with their nurse case managers in diabetes management. These RNs have gone on to obtain additional training and certification as Certified Diabetes Educators (CDE). The Veterans have an excellent rapport with the nurses. For example, when the Veterans go to Endocrine Clinic, they often request to review a proposed new plan with their "Diabetes Nurse" first. As the NP who trained the RNs, I explain to the Veteran that I initially trained their RN in diabetes management and then they are more likely to agree to the revised plan.

Key Information

Registered Nurse Case Managers (RNCM) have a long tradition of intervention particularly for the high-risk diabetes chronic disease population with an A1C of 9 percent or more. This 10-year-old RNCM program was started by the Diabetes NP to reduce wait times in the Endocrine Clinic. RNs interested in diabetes were trained in the basics of case management for diabetes and supported by the NP.

There was a large population (N=3,956) of high-risk Veterans with a baseline A1C of 9 percent or more (Mean=10.6 percent) seen by the RNCMs. Paired T-tests of A1C after the last RNCM visit showed a statistically significant reduction (P<0.001) in A1C (Mean=8.5 percent) after 14–26 months of intervention. A large sample of high-risk Veterans with diabetes seen by RNCMs demonstrated significant reductions (~2 percent) in A1C overall, demonstrating the clinical effectiveness of RNCMs in improving A1C in this population. Chronic diabetes disease management can be labor-intensive for the primary provider, and access in PC can be improved by team care. With the implementation of RNCMs, high-risk diabetes Veterans can be treated by the Nurse, thereby freeing up provider time as well as reducing consults to endocrine.

Context

Over 23,193 Veterans with diabetes are enrolled in the Louis Stokes Cleveland VA Medical Center (LSCVAMC) and are active patients in VISN 10 (i.e., have had a PC visit or diabetes medication dispensed within the past 18 months). The best practice review indicated that 5,022 Veterans had an A1C greater than 9 percent.

Travel to the Endocrine Clinic can take two hours, and our Veterans often did not want to travel, especially during inclement weather. Additionally, local diabetes education and nutrition augment

248

diabetes outcomes. The availability of consistent providers who are knowledgeable about a Veteran's particular likes and dislikes can enhance success.

Practice Description

An experienced CDE who is a NP in the Endocrinology Section of the LSCVAMC trained each RNCM in weekly sessions that included review and discussion of patient charts and glucose data. The CDE mentored each Nurse Case Manager (NCM) in the core principles of diabetes self-management education (DSME) and glucose pattern management, including medication safety. The PCPs made medication adjustments and the RNs monitored results and provided teaching and assessments about adherence. RNCMs were encouraged to study for the CDE exam 16 and were given time to attend an annual day-long Cleveland VA retreat on DSME. Although the targeted population was patients whose A1C levels were 9 percent (secured from a registry), the NCMs also worked with any patients as requested by PCPs.

Replicability

This process is successful because: 1) the Veterans do not have to travel; 2) they develop local ongoing relationships with the nurse CDEs; and 3) a population health approach to seeking out these Veterans is utilized. Support is provided by the endocrine diabetes NP, endocrinologist, telehealth, and Specialty Care Access Network-Extension for Community (SCAN-ECHO) Diabetes. A national manual has been created to assist RN care and case managers in PACT with diabetes chronic care management.

Other sites can replicate this successful intervention by providing support and training for nurses (especially in rural areas) who are interested in becoming CDEs. Local endocrine services and SCAN-ECHO Diabetes programs are available nationally. Additionally, the Office of Nursing Services has established and supported a national SCAN-ECHO training site for RNs who are interested in diabetes management.

Enhanced Early Response Team

William Alt, BSN, RN, VHA-CM, Clinical Performance Improvement Specialist

North Florida/South Georgia Veterans Health System, Gainesville, FL

william.alt@va.gov

The changes in Early Response Team (ERT) composition and extended response areas have increased early intervention and led to a decrease in non-Intensive Care Unit (ICU)/ED Cardiopulmonary Arrest Events (CPE).

Introduction

In 2008, an ERT was implemented at the Malcom Randall VAMC in Gainesville, Florida. The formation of the ERT was initiated by Patient Safety in response to National Patient Safety Goal 16.01.01 which in 2010 evolved into The Joint Commission standard PC.02.01.19: "The hospital recognizes and responds to changes in a patient's condition, and informs the patient and family how to seek assistance when they have concerns about a patient's condition."

Key Information

During early 2013, the North Florida/South Georgia Veterans Healthcare System (VHCS) Emergency Effectiveness Committee took on the task of restructuring the Malcom Randall VAMC ERT. Based on feedback from stakeholders, the committee decided change was necessary to better meet patient and staff needs, thereby leading to improved patient outcomes. In the first full year following implementation, there was a 125 percent increase in ERT requests, a 12.5 percent reduction in non-ICU/ED CPE, and a decrease in ERT responses that converted to CPE (from seven CPE per 100 ERT to one CPE per 100 ERT) through FY 2015. These trends have been sustained through the end of Quarter 1 FY 2016 with an 11 percent decrease in non-ICU CPE and a 61 percent increase in ERT responses. Based on the data, the new enhanced ERT has led to an increase in early interventions with a subsequent decrease in the number of non-ICU/ED CPE.

The North Florida/South Georgia VHCS Emergency Effectiveness Committee led by co-chairmen Dr. Eloise Harman, Medical Director of Medical Intensive Care Unit (MICU), and William Alt, RN in collaboration with Patient Safety, MICU, and the Surgical Intensive Care Unit (SICU), implemented the changes described in June 2013. The most significant change was moving from an ED to a MICU/SICU-based response team that includes a MICU/SICU physician. Inclusion of a physician on the team has allowed for treatment orders to be placed more rapidly and facilitation of transfer in level care, if indicated. ERT response has also been extended to include the Community Living Centers (CLCs) on the Malcom Randall campus providing the same timeliness in delivery of needed resources to the Veterans and staff at those facilities. An update currently in process will identify family members as ERT requesters. Once finalized, the new process will provide information to patients and their families on how to access and request an ERT for any concern(s) they may have. The intent is to include such information in the admission packet and in each patient room.

Context

Malcom Randall VAMC is a large 1a facility affiliated with The University of Florida College of Medicine. Due to the large geographic area of the system, a highly diverse Veteran population is served. The ability to quickly and efficiently provide immediate care and transfer to a higher level of care, if indicated, were the primary challenges leading to the changes described.

Practice Description

The Emergency Effectiveness Committee is made up of representatives from all areas involved in the delivery of emergency and resuscitative care. This includes clinical units (both inpatient and outpatient), adjunct services, support services, and administrative services. Prior to adoption, the process was reviewed by all parties who, in turn, provided input on how to best implement the changes. Prior to the "go live" date, education was provided to all clinical areas involved. During the education campaign, further input was solicited from bedside clinical staff and those staff members who would be assigned to the ERT. A fluid approach to the process has been maintained with issues and concerns being addressed as they arise to provide the highest level of service to Veterans, families, and staff.

Replicability

The success of this practice can be attributed to the patient-centered approach to care within our system. All of the parties involved have supported and sustained the practice. No one is ever criticized for initiating an ERT. The ERT members work collaboratively with one another as well as with the requesting staff. This process could be replicated and adapted for use by any sized facility that has identified similar needs. A key to implementation would be to engage all parties, in particular frontline staff, early in the process and listen to them. In addition, we need to continuously seek out opportunities for improvement while maintaining a responsive and flexible approach to improvement.

Recognition

Ileana Koerner, Amy Manna, Denise Cochran, Julie Whitney, Brenda Brinkley, Nestor Santiago, Carrol Graves, Amado Diaz

Enhancing Quality of Prescribing Practices for Elderly Veterans Discharged from the ED

Melissa Stevens, MD

Atlanta VA Health Care System, Decatur, GA

melissa.stevens2@va.gov

Enhancing Quality of Prescribing Practices for Elderly Veterans Discharged from the Emergency Department (EQUiPPED) is a multi-component quality improvement initiative designed to improving medication safety for older Veterans in the ED. EQUiPPED provides ED clinicians with education, clinical decision support tools, and individual feedback to reduce the use of potentially inappropriate medications.

Introduction

Problems with prescribing Potentially Inappropriate Medications (PIMs) for older patients have been described in a number of ED-based studies. There is accumulating evidence that inappropriate medication use is associated with increased risk of hospitalization and that hospitalization is associated with a risk of continued institutionalization in older adults. In a study of 942 Veterans discharged from the ED at the Durham VAMC, suboptimal pharmacotherapy was common and was associated with a 32 percent greater risk of repeat ED visits, hospitalization, or death. Avoiding the use of inappropriate and high-risk drugs is an important, simple, and effective strategy in reducing medication-related problems in older adults.

Not only is there a need for better quality prescribing, but VA ED providers indicated in a needs assessment conducted by collaborators from multiple Geriatric Research Education and Clinical Centers (GRECCs) and VA Emergency Medicine Field Advisory Council in 2012 that they welcome education in this area.

Initial data from the first four sites to complete implementation of EQUiPPED show a significant and sustained reduction in the average monthly proportion of PIMs prescribed to older Veterans at the time of ED discharge.

Key Information

EQUiPPED is an ongoing multi-disciplinary quality improvement initiative aimed at changing prescribing practices of ED providers to decrease the use of PIMs, as identified by the Beers List, in older Veterans discharged from the ED. The Beers List was developed by Dr. Mark H. Beers in 1991 to identify medications that are potentially inappropriate in older patients because the risk of adverse drug events outweighs the potential benefits of the drug. The Beers List is widely used by government agencies and supported by research in various settings.

Atlanta VAMC serves as the lead site for this eight-site collaborative that started in FY 2013 and is currently in its fourth year. Current sites include the Atlanta VAMC, Durham VA Medical, Tennessee Valley Healthcare System (TVHCS) (Nashville & Murfreesboro sites), Birmingham VAMC, Bronx VAMC, Central Alabama Veterans HCS (Montgomery and Asheville VAMC).

Context

EQUiPPED started as a collaborative among the Birmingham/Atlanta VAMC, Durham VAMC, and TVHCS GRECCs, with Atlanta serving as the lead site. In the first year EQUiPPED was implemented in three urban VAMC EDs, the second year two additional urban sites were added, and in the third year three rural sites were added. EQUiPPED targets ED providers at these sites and aims to improve the quality of prescribing for Veterans 65 and older treated and released from the ED. In the first year EQUiPPED impacted 6,665 unique Veterans at the first three implementation sites. In the second year 14,700 unique Veterans at five VAMC sites were impacted, and in the third year, over 16,000 Veterans at eight VAMC sites were impacted.

Practice Description

EQUiPPED was developed by an interdisciplinary team comprised of ED physicians, geriatricians, gerontologists, clinical pharmacists, quality improvement nurses, and clinical applications coordinators using the Vision-Analysis-Team-Aim-Map-Measure-Change-Sustain (VA-TAMMCS) model of process improvement. At each site, key stakeholders, including facility leadership, ED providers, and clinical pharmacists were involved in implementation.

Interventions include: 1) provider education in the form of didactic lectures and journal club; 2) informatics-based clinical decision support with electronic medical record embedded geriatric pharmacy order sets and links to online geriatric content; and 3) individual provider education, including academic detailing, audit and feedback, and peer benchmarking.

Replicability

EQUiPPED has been successfully implemented in eight VA EDs, and the team is currently developing a toolkit to make resources available to other medical centers for implementation. Using the EQUiPPED implementation framework and EQUiPPED toolkit, it is possible to replicate the program in virtually any other VA ED. Additionally, the EQUiPPED team has been awarded a grant by the Agency for Healthcare Research and Quality (AHRQ) to implement EQUiPPED at three non-VA University-Affiliate sites.

The team is also adapting the EQUiPPED model for the Atlanta VAMC Mental Health ED and exploring options for implementing EQUiPPED in the inpatient medical setting at the Atlanta VAMC.

Recognition

Camille Vaughan, Anna Vandenberg, Katharina Echt, Anita Schmidt, Ted Johnson, S. Nicole Hastings, William Bryan, Jason Moss, James Powers, Alayne Markland, Gerald McGwin, Ula Hwang, William Hung, Molly Mcgaughey, Carolyn Clevenger, Lawanda Kemp, DeWayne Cross, Christine Jasien, Purvi Patel, Gerald Thomas

VA's Mobile Health Provider Program Equips VA Care Teams with On-The-Go Technology

Dr. Deyne Bentt, Clinical Director of Mobile Health Deployment and Evaluation; William Cerniuk, Co-Director, VA Mobile Health Provider Program
Washington DC VAMC, Washington, DC
deyne.bentt@va.gov

The Mobile Health Provider Program delivers mobile devices (tablets) to VA care teams, equipping them with the tools they need to operate while on-the-go.

Introduction

They say that a picture is worth a thousand words. For Dr. Leslee Davis, who received a VA-issued mobile device, that adage stands true. As a PCP and the Women's Clinic Medical Director at the Orlando VAMC, the integration of a mobile device into her clinical practice has enabled her to enhance patient education at the point of care.

"I recently used my [device] with a patient who thought she had a certain dermatological condition. I brought up the dermatology app, showed her some pictures, and thanks to the clear visual, she quickly realized that she was going to be okay. This is a great tool," said Dr. Davis, who was among the first 1,000 providers to receive a mobile device as part of VA Mobile Health Provider Program.

Likewise, Dr. Sarah Niles at the Tomah VAMC places instant orders with her device while remaining at her patient's bedside. "If I'm bedside with a patient who is not stable and I don't want to leave them, I can now use my device to send orders directly to the laboratory, radiology, or pharmacy," said Dr. Niles.

Key Information

Launched in 2014, the Mobile Health Provider Program delivered mobile devices (tablets) to more than 12,000 VA care teams at 40+ geographically diverse VA Medical facilities, equipping them with the tools they need to operate while on-the-go. For VA care teams involved in the program, this means easier access to the resources they need to treat their Veteran patients. For Veterans and their families, it means enhanced care and communication with their VA physicians and health care teams.

VA-issued tablets provide care teams with immediate access to VA email, real-time clinical information, and easy access to medical tools and applications (apps). Public and VA-developed apps offer a variety of resources when looking up medications, prognoses, patient education materials, and other medical references. The devices are equipped with access to VA network through Virtual Private Network (VPN) capabilities in the medical center as well as offsite.

Context

The Mobile Health Provider Program has fostered many innovative ways for mobile devices to address unique challenges in the 40+ medical facilities in the pilot. For example, the Orlando

VAMC piloted a Community Inpatient Care Team model at non-VA hospitals to better serve rural Veterans in their region. A key to the success of this pilot is ensuring VA care teams at non-VA hospitals have access to VA information, including patient history, records, and more.

"The Community Inpatient Care Teams use their devices as an essential tool in non-VA hospitals to provide overall supervision of the Veteran's quality of care, facilitate processes, coordinate follow-up care, and look up patient records," said Dr. Angel Colon-Molero, National Director for Specialty Care Services at the Orlando VAMC and founder of the Community Inpatient Care Team pilot.

Dr. Colon-Molero believes the success of this pilot could expand to other parts of the country, as long as VA-issued devices are available. The mobile devices enable the Community Inpatient Care Teams to improve productivity, workflow, accessibility, and communication with the Veterans, even when providing care at a non-VA facility.

Practice Description

The VHA Product Effectiveness team surveyed more than 1,800 program participants at 18 different VA locations, and found that 91 percent of users like that VA is offering new and innovative tools. Also, nearly 70 percent of users feel their VA-issued mobile devices have made them more productive in their daily work routine. VA care teams are most enthusiastic when the device fills a specific gap in functionality or saves them time. For example, Christopher Mastriano, a speech pathologist at VA Boston Healthcare System (HCS) said, "My office is in one building, but I see patients in three different buildings. Sometimes finding a work station and logging on can take me 30 minutes to get access to a patient's chart, but now with my device, I can do this in minutes."

Replicability

The success of the Mobile Health Provider Program allows VISNs and VA National Program Offices to purchase mobile devices for use in clinical care through the Connected Care National Mobile Health Provider Program contract. As the program evolves, so will opportunities. VA is developing and releasing a series of VA-developed web and mobile apps that will enable VA care teams to write progress notes, enter a subset of orders, complete clinical tasks, and support specific common workflows.

Recognition

Neil Evans, Kathleen Frisbee, Deyne Bentt, William Cerniuk, Kevin DeOrsey, DJ Kachman, Stacy Washington

CPRS Documentation and Workload Capture Enhanced by a Macro

Joseph Beraho, MD, PCP

Greenville Clinic, Greenville, SC

joseph.beraho@va.gov

This Windows Script executes a series of preprogrammed CPRS actions for quick and accurate pairing of a clinic location and a note title. This ensures proper capture of workload credit and encourages use of non-face-to-face encounters by simplifying documentation.

Introduction

You just got off the phone with one of your favorite Veterans and you realize that you spent over 20 minutes trying to improve his diabetes management. You start to document this encounter and realize that a simple addendum to a previous note is not appropriate, as it would cheat you of clinical workload. Therefore, you decide to enter a "proper" telephone note.

You also realize that this requires laboriously picking the correct "telephone clinic" location (configured to accurately reflect phone clinic code) and an appropriate telephone note title (preferably configured to contain the elements needed to reflect the clinical decision making that just occurred).

A typical clinic location name is long and unintuitive, and is usually buried deep among other similarly cryptic names. Having to pick this and the note title every time you make a phone call is arduous. When the Macro is installed on the task bar and clicked, it takes control by typing in the preconfigured clinic location and opening the proper telephone note, leaving it ready for the note to be entered.

"I could get used to this," you tell yourself. Many CPRS users have been able to shave valuable seconds off the time it takes to document, while ensuring that workload capture is enhanced.

Key Information

The CPRS Macro is a small text file that contains information that is needed to load a clinic note. It sends instructions to CPRS in the same sequence as the user would when preparing to document a phone encounter. This includes simulated mouse clicks, tabbing, and typing, akin to the well-known commercial Program "Dragon Medical."

The Macro was developed by Joseph Beraho, MD and first implemented at the Greenville, SC, VA Clinic. After review by his supervisor Ramoth Cox, MD, she recommended it for all her CBOCs. In mid-2014, the chief of staff at the main hospital in Columbia, SC, Bernard Dekoning, MD, recognized its potential and asked that it be installed on as many computers as possible across the DORN VAMC and its CBOCs. This enormous task was taken on by Clinical Informatics Supervisor, Cheryl Crouse, RN, BSN, CCM along with her team of Clinical Application Coordinators (CACs).

Context

Good access to health care is more critical now than ever, especially with such a high number of Veterans being served. Care delivered through non-face-to-face encounters needs to be integrated more. The ability to capture this type of workload is critical.

Practice Description

After recognizing that this repetitive sequence of actions can be replicated by Windows for free, a JavaScript-powered macro generator was built that would accept: 1) the clinic location name; and 2) the note title. The generator would then create the Macro code needed to send these to CPRS every time it was accessed.

Computer savvy users can install this without much effort, but others may need help from a CAC.

Replicability

The practice was adopted at this facility because of a need to encourage and improve proper documentation of non-scheduled telephone clinic encounters, capture the entire workload, and positively influence financial bottom lines. It is hoped that future versions of CPRS with have this functionality built in.

Recognition

Ramoth Cox, Bernard Dekoning, Cheryl Crouse, John Demchak, Jennifer McFaddin, Kipton Garrett, Roger Depra, Bliss Webb, Karen Minner, Tiffany Frialde, Kristie Eisenbrei

Clinical Reminder for Hepatocellular Carcinoma Surveillance

Lauren Beste, MD MSc, Staff Physician

VA Puget Sound Health Care System, Seattle, WA

lauren.beste@va.gov

The electronic clinical reminder increased the rate of liver cancer surveillance at our facility for a vulnerable and complex group of patients with cirrhosis. It was supported by collaboration between primary and specialty care, radiology, medical informatics, and our national VA program office.

Introduction

"How long do I have, doc?" is the most common response I hear when I deliver the all-too-common news that one of my cirrhosis patients has developed Hepatocellular Carcinoma (HCC), or liver cancer. My answer varies, but the statistics are devastating; the median length of survival after diagnosis of HCC is about nine months. Effective treatments for HCC exist, but only when the cancer is detected at an early stage. Studies show that treatment can be offered in only half of cases, typically because the cancer is so advanced at the time of diagnosis that there are no available treatment options. Even more worrisome is that HCC is the fastest growing cause of cancer death in US males.

Unlike breast cancer or colon cancer, there are no glamorous celebrities touting liver cancer screening and there are no national advertising campaigns reminding patients to talk to their doctors about it. My cancer patients are usually individuals with cirrhosis or viral hepatitis, and often their life paths have been dogged by substance use disorders, poverty, and other barriers to health care. Patients with risk factors for liver cancer are not necessarily followed by specialists. Given the complex needs of such patients, it is far too easy for liver cancer screening to fall through the cracks for busy PCPs trying to juggle patients' many competing necessities.

Puget Sound VA Healthcare System (HCS) was the first station in the country to implement a clinical reminder to promote screening for HCC in patients with cirrhosis by liver ultrasound every 6 months, as recommended by the American Association for the Study of Liver Diseases (AASLD). After using the reminder for 18 months, our HCC surveillance rate improved 51 percent over baseline and our rate of HCC detection was significantly better compared to other regional stations, even after adjusting for patient characteristics and HCC risk factors.

Key Information

The HCC Clinical reminder was developed by Dr. Lauren Beste and implemented in VA Puget Sound HCS as a multi-disciplinary collaboration between Hepatology, PC, Radiology, and Medical Informatics at our facility, as well as VA Office of HIV, Hepatitis C, and Public Health Pathogens. The reminder was deliberately designed to be simple, efficient, and easy to integrate into routine PC practice—all features that evidence shows improve the uptake of clinical reminders by health care providers. We have shared the reminder with other stations by request, including facilities in San

Francisco VAMC, Eastern Colorado HCS, White City VA Rehabilitation Center, El Paso VAMC, and Long Beach HCS.

Context

VA Puget Sound HCS is an urban, tertiary care facility located in western Washington state. We serve as a referral site for liver subspecialty care for Alaska, Washington, and parts of Idaho. We found that only 46.2 percent of cirrhosis patients at our facility and 31.8 percent of those in our VISN are followed in Gastroenterology or Hepatology clinic for liver disease. However, almost 90 percent are seen in PC each year. Therefore, our clinical reminder was specifically designed for use in PC settings in order to increase screening among patients not followed in specialty care.

Practice Description

The HCC Surveillance Clinical Reminder functions by electronically identifying patients with cirrhosis using their CPRS problem list. If the patient has not undergone liver imaging in the preceding 6 months (i.e., ultrasound, computed tomography, or magnetic resonance imaging) the clinical reminder automatically generates a pre-populated liver ultrasound order for the provider to sign. With the approval of PC leadership in Puget Sound HCS, the HCC Surveillance Clinical Reminder was piloted by a volunteer group of providers who contributed guidance and feedback before release to all Puget Sound clinics, including CBOCs.

Replicability

The HCC Surveillance Clinical Reminder was successful because it was a true collaboration between PC and specialty care, with strong support from our national VA program office. Stakeholders from multiple levels, including end-users and both national and hospital leaders, were involved in the conceptual design and contributed to the finished product. It would be feasible to implement in other facilities in VA system, or even non-VA facilities that utilize electronic medical records.

Recognition

Jason Dominitz, Michael Chang, Connie Morantes, Chris Vanderworker, David Ross, Carol Achtmeyer

Assisted Early Mobility for Hospitalized Older Veterans

S. Nicole Hastings, MD, MHS

Durham VAMC, Durham, NC

susan.hastings@va.gov

"Assisted Early Mobility for Hospitalized Older Veterans" (STRIDE) is a supervised walking program for hospitalized older adults, designed to address the important clinical problem of immobility during hospitalization, and its negative consequences, including hospitalization-associated disability.

Introduction

Here is an example of how STRIDE helped a Veteran:

Ural Kincaid, Army Veteran and Recreation Therapy Assistant at the Durham VAMC, recently took fellow Army Veteran Mr. X on a walk as part of STRIDE. Mr. X was an Army Corporal who served during the Korean War and Kincaid served during the Vietnam War. They bonded instantly. "My goal is to get back on my feet," Mr. X said. He was joined by his wife of 53 years, and they were positive and motivated to go for a walk on the inpatient unit. His wife supported the work being done by the STRIDE team, and joined the walk just steps behind her husband and Kincaid.

Kincaid is passionate about his work at VA helping Veterans, and he wishes that a program like STRIDE existed shortly following his time in service, as it would have benefitted the recovery process.

Key Information

STRIDE was initiated by a physician and health services researcher at the Durham VAMC and funded through operations by the VHA Office of Geriatrics and Extended Care (GEC). STRIDE was designed to address the important clinical problem of immobility during hospitalization and its negative consequences, including hospitalization-associated disability. Although the dangers of immobility in the hospital have been recognized for more than two decades, sustained solutions to this problem have been elusive. Developed by a team of Physical Therapists (PTs), physicians, nurses, exercise physiologists, recreation therapists, and clinical service managers, STRIDE consists of a one-time gait and balance assessment conducted by a PT, followed by daily walks supervised by a Walk Assistant (non-licensed therapy aide) for the duration of the hospital stay.

To examine program impact, we compared STRIDE participants (n=92) to patients referred but not enrolled, because the program was at capacity or they refused (n=35). These two groups were similar according to all demographic and clinical characteristics examined; however, we found a significant difference in post-discharge destination among those who participated in the walking program compared to those who did not. Overall 92 percent of STRIDE participants were discharged to home compared to 74 percent from the usual care group (P=0.007); the remainder went to skilled nursing or rehabilitation facilities. Based on these positive outcomes and high program satisfaction from both Veterans and staff, STRIDE was made a permanent clinical service in 2013, and now serves more than 600 Veterans annually.

Context

The Durham VAMC is a 271-bed referral, teaching, and research facility providing tertiary and extended care. The Durham VAMC offers services to more than 200,000 Veterans living in a 26-county area of central and eastern North Carolina. STRIDE was designed to combat the epidemic of immobility among hospitalized older Veterans. Hospitalized older adults spend only 3 percent of their time standing or walking. Immobility during hospitalization leads to loss of muscle mass, de-conditioning, and overall weakness which in turn contribute to inpatient complications, such as functional decline and falls, longer hospital stays, higher rates of discharge to skilled nursing facilities, and increased risk of readmission to the hospital. Older Veterans are especially vulnerable to the adverse physical effects of immobility and their resultant consequences.

Practice Description

Patients are eligible for STRIDE if they are age 60 or older and admitted to the General Medicine Service of the Durham VAMC. Veterans with admitting conditions that limit their ability to ambulate safely (e.g., new neurological deficit or unable to follow one-step commands) are excluded. Patients are referred to STRIDE by their treating physician. Next they are evaluated by a PT who assesses their safety for walking and provides an assistive device (e.g., walker) if needed. After the PT evaluation, patients begin daily supervised walks that continue for the duration of the hospital stay (with a goal of 20 minutes, divided into two sessions). Daily walks are supervised by a recreation therapy assistant who works with each patient's nurse to determine the best timing for the walk and follows established protocols for offering rest breaks as needed, and monitoring vital signs.

Replicability

STRIDE is safe and well received by Veterans: 90 percent of STRIDE participants reported feeling better immediately after their walk. STRIDE participants had shorter hospitalizations (4.7 days compared to 5.7 days) and were less likely to be discharged to a nursing home: 92 percent of STRIDE participants went home after hospitalization, compared to 74 percent of patients who were eligible but did not participate. STRIDE is cost-saving: taking all program personnel costs into account, we anticipate annual cost savings of $958,348 based on reduced inpatient bed-days-of-care alone.

Based on these data, previous research in other settings, and positive feedback on the program from staff and Veterans, STRIDE was made a permanent clinical service at the Durham VAMC in June 2013, just 20 months after initial funding. STRIDE now serves over 600 Veterans annually at the Durham VAMC, and the VHA Office of GEC has funded a dissemination grant to launch the program at another medical center. The rapid evolution of this project from clinical demonstration to permanent clinical service was a direct result of clinicians, researchers, and managers working together to develop and implement a program that was tailored for local conditions, had a rapid data collection and analysis plan, and was responsive to the needs and interests of Veterans and hospital leadership.

Recognition

VHA Office of GEC, Karen Massey, Kenneth Shay, Deanne Seekins, Daniel Hoffmann

CART Coronary Major Adverse Event Program

Candice Gillmann, National Program Manager

Office of Analytics and Business Intelligence (OABI), Denver, CO
candice.gillmann@va.gov

This national peer review program provides comprehensive and objective evaluations of adverse events by experts, then broadcasts the lessons learned to the wider cardiology community in a non-punitive environment.

Introduction

The VA Clinical Assessment, Reporting, and Tracking (CART) program is a national clinical quality program that monitors the safety of all cardiac catheterization procedures performed across VA. As part of its mission, the program has developed a novel and unique approach to monitoring and reviewing any major adverse event that occurs during one of these procedures—the CART Coronary Major Adverse Event (COR-MAE) program. On a monthly basis, 11 VA interventional cardiologists from across the US join in a teleconference to discuss safety and quality issues of cardiac catheterization. They discuss individual adverse events that have occurred in catheterization labs to raise precipitating systemic issues that contributed to the events, and identify how to avoid complications in the future. Interventionalists, experts in the field, provide profound and valuable input from their own experience.

Key Information

The CART COR-MAE program has been years in the making. In 2004, leaders from various domains in VA proposed a national clinical quality program, CART, to generate real-time data to assess and monitor quality of cardiac catheterization procedures across VA. The implementation of this novel program uses a clinical software application integrated into the VA EHR. By 2009, OABI installed the software and began recording standardized patient procedural data on all coronary angiographies and Percutaneous Coronary Interventions (PCIs) across VA. This data supports local and national analysis as well as overall quality improvement.

Context

Because of the wealth of data collected in real time from catheterization labs, clinicians expressed a desire and demonstrated the ability to incorporate a national peer review system into these procedures. The CART COR-MAE peer review program began in 2011 as a way to address safety in the 79 VA cardiac catheterization labs. This program, based at the CART coordinating center in Denver, CO, monitors any in-lab major adverse events (defined as death, stroke, emergent percutaneous coronary intervention, or emergent need for bypass intervention) that occur during a diagnostic angiogram or PCI, then generates a real-time alert to the CART coordinating center and the Cor-MAE program so that a peer review can begin. Reviewers from a committee of 11 to 13 VA interventional cardiologists from around the US convene to review each case. Two committee members then review EHRs and images pertinent to the procedure and interview the local medical staff overseeing the case. Using this information, the reviewers assign the event one of three levels: Level 1 (no quality issues identified), Level 2 (potential quality issue identified), or Level 3 (definite quality issue identified). Committee members review cases deemed Level 2 or Level 3 via teleconference. The team shares decisions with the local site's cardiology team and chief of staff. The system's construct protects peer reviews from legal discovery for personnel employment or disciplinary action, fostering a non-punitive environment that can appropriately focus on any systemic issues that may have contributed to adverse events, rather than individual blame. The reviews are robust and thoughtful, and VA's cardiac community holds them in high regard. Many occur in lieu of local site reviews, thus saving practitioners and hospital staff time and effort. Finally, committee members file these events and reviews, and they track and share any patterns or areas of special interest with the broader community of VA cardiac catheterization laboratories.

Practice Description

VA CART COR-MAE Program is a unique national program that has significantly advanced peer review processes and improved the safety of Veterans in all VA catheterization laboratories. Because this program is facilitated by the electronic VA CART application, all major adverse events are detected in "real time," allowing the peer review process to begin immediately. Each year, 40,000 Veterans undergo diagnostic angiogram procedures and 10,000 undergo PCI procedures. Every one of these Veterans is part of and benefits from this safety-monitoring program. Since program inception, the program has reviewed 173 events. Of these, 144 (83 percent) were Level 1. Any events given a Level 2 or 3 designation involved action taken by the local site to prevent similar events in the future. Quality improvement opportunities identified in these reviews then spread to the larger VA Catheterization Lab community.

Replicability

The COR-MAE program and its components of real-time event detection, national peer review by experts, and dissemination of its insights, is scalable to other areas of health care and in a variety of health care settings. For example, this process exists for another cardiac procedure, transcatheter aortic valve replacement, and will monitor safety for these procedures in the same way that the Cor-MAE monitors safety for coronary catheterization. Similar programs are also under development to monitor electrophysiology and peripheral vascular procedures in catheterization laboratories.

Recognition

Candice Gillmann, Tom Maddox, Steve Bradley, John Rumsfeld, Hans Gethoffer, Bob Jesse, Bernadette Speiser, Greg Noonan, Alec Arney, Megan Petrich, Steve Fihn, Yuri Walker

Education to Reduce Unnecessary Myocardial Perfusion Imaging

David Winchester, MD, MS, Staff Cardiologist

North Florida/South Georgia Veterans Health System, Gainesville, FL
david.winchester@va.gov

This simple, effective approach to educating clinical providers significantly reduced unnecessary cardiac stress testing through specialty-specific education.

Introduction

Unnecessary tests result in reduced access to care and wasted spending. They do not benefit patients and, in some cases, cause them direct harm. Efforts to reduce unnecessary testing, however, often do not have a human face. Finding an uplifting anecdote about someone getting an appointment two days earlier or avoiding a dose of unnecessary radiation is a challenge. From a systems perspective, however, initiatives to reduce unnecessary testing can have a dramatic impact.

To reduce potentially harmful unnecessary tests, we created Education to Reduce Unnecessary Myocardial Perfusion Imaging (ERUMPI) in the North Florida/South Georgia Veterans Health System (HCS). This program consisted of didactics and printed materials targeted to specific health care provider types (PC, cardiology, etc.). Content included recommendations about cardiac testing and tips for managing heart disease. We tracked the frequency of unnecessary cardiac testing in our nuclear lab and showed a decrease of unnecessary testing from 5 percent to less than one percent (P<0.001).

Key Information

Dr. David Winchester started the ERUMPI program in FY 2015 in the North Florida/South Georgia Veterans HCS. Team members included a nurse researcher and physicians from Imaging, Nuclear Medicine, and Cardiology. We collaborated with PC and Hospital Medicine in order to deliver our didactics. Medical Media helped by printing posters, which we sent to clinics throughout the HCS. VISN 8 funded the project with an Innovation grant and supported Dr. Winchester and our research nurse. The most resource-intensive part of the process is tracking the appropriateness of testing, which typically takes about ten minutes per patient when conducted retrospectively by someone reading the patient chart.

Context

The North Florida/South Georgia Veterans HCS includes two medical centers and several satellite clinic locations. One facility (Malcom Randall VAMC) reads all nuclear cardiac stress tests, which simplified the analysis of data. A significant challenge, however, is that these tests can be ordered by any physician or provider at any of the facilities within the HCS. Adequately educating all providers is a logistically difficult task.

Practice Description

After establishing the baseline level of unnecessary studies, we created and delivered didactic presentations at a variety of locations. Based on prior data, we were aware that the pattern of unnecessary tests was different based on provider type: PC and cardiology physicians both order unnecessary tests, but for different reasons. As such, we developed the educational materials to be specialty-specific. The lecture aired via intranet to all PC outreach clinics during an established educational seminar series to maximize the reach. We surveyed providers after the lecture; all felt the content was helpful and 78 percent agreed ("strongly agree" or "agree") that they intended to change their practice because of the content.

Replicability

This practice is easily reproducible. Physicians and providers appreciated the content. We specifically attribute success to 1) targeting the content to each specialty, and 2) making the recommendations a collaborative discussion as opposed to a punitive experience. The challenge we have at this stage is to understand whether the process has lasting results. In reports of other efforts to change behavior through education, a regression follows an initial positive response to prior practice. This deserves further study at our facility.

Recognition

VISN 8, Susan Stinson

Integrated Management and Polypharmacy Review of Vulnerable Elders

Anna Mirk, MD, Physician, Geriatrics and Extended Care

Atlanta VA Health Care System, Decatur, GA

anna.mirk@va.gov

The Integrated Management and Polypharmacy Review of Vulnerable Elders (IMPROVE) intervention combines evidence-based best practice with Patient-Centered Care (PCC) to reduce harmful polypharmacy and improve the ability of older Veterans and their caregivers to manage medications safely through a face-to-face structured visit with a clinical pharmacist.

Introduction

The Integrated Management and Polypharmacy Review of Vulnerable Elders program is an integrated medication management program to address polypharmacy in community-dwelling Veterans aged 85 and older at risk for medication-associated problems and loss of independence.

Mr. X is a 93-year-old widowed Veteran diagnosed with lymphoma and early stage dementia. During the 12-month period prior to the IMPROVE intervention, medical records show that Mr. X had a total of 21 outpatient visits and one ED visit. At that time, he was taking 29 different medications and his 30-day supply of medication from VA cost a total of $506.48. Mr. X, his daughter, and his primary caregiver agreed to meet with the geriatric clinical pharmacist in his PC geriatrics clinic as a participant in the IMPROVE program. During the session, the clinical pharmacist, Dr. K, eliminated six medications, which included three that could interact adversely with warfarin. Notably, the month following the IMPROVE intervention, Mr. X's VA medication costs decreased from $506.48 to $273.24 for a 30-day supply. These figures do not reflect several vitamins that Dr. K also eliminated.

At 12 months post-intervention, analysis shows that the number of medications that Mr. X took continued to decrease to 18. His cost for a 30-day supply also decreased to a post-intervention total of $50.34. In addition, Mr. X's outpatient visits decreased to a total of nine, with no Emergency Room (ER) visits. Mr. X's daughter said that Dr. K was "very helpful" and not only helped her father, but also helped her, the caregiver. She said that participating in the session had improved her (and her father's) ability to take medications as prescribed, and indicated that she now "has less stress and less anxiety" about managing her father's medication.

IMPROVE successfully reduced key medication-related risk factors in a sample of 28 Atlanta VAMC Veterans age 85 years and older taking ten or more medications. Specifically, 79 percent had at least one medication discontinued and, on average, 1.7 medications were eliminated from regimens. Clinicians reduced Potentially Inappropriate Medications (PIMs) by 14 percent. Comparing medication costs and utilization (calls and visits) six months prior- to and six months post-IMPROVE, we found that pharmacy costs (saving $64 per Veteran per month) and health care utilization rates were likewise reduced. Patients and caregivers found IMPROVE helpful (93 percent), with 100 percent recommending the clinic to other Veterans. Cost savings were comparable to or greater than those previously reported for similar interventions.

Key Information

Providers designed the IMPROVE clinical demonstration project at the Atlanta VAMC with the following goals in mind: to promote a team-based collaborative approach to medication management in vulnerable elderly Veterans, reduce the adverse consequences associated with multiple medication use, and advance patient and family-centered care. Overarching goals include improving Veterans' health and independence, reducing health care costs, and preventing the need for institutional care.

During FY 2012 and FY 2013, teams at the Atlanta VAMC and Atlanta site of the Birmingham/Atlanta Geriatric Research Education and Clinical Centers (GRECCs)—a geriatric clinical pharmacist, geriatrician, and two gerontologists—worked to develop and pilot a patient-centric program to address medication management in vulnerable elderly Veterans living at home and at high risk for medication-associated problems and loss of independence. This clinical demonstration project integrates evidence-based best practices with the expertise, needs, and values of patients, their caregivers, providers, and pharmacists, to develop a medication management program that targets these priorities in concert with the resources of the PACT.

Context

Multiple medication use is highly prevalent and frequently necessary for managing multiple chronic co-morbidities in older Veterans. However, polypharmacy places Veterans at risk for medication-associated adverse outcomes, including adverse drug reactions, increased ED, hospital and PC utilization, and death. Our team developed an integrated medication management program to address polypharmacy in Veterans aged 85 years and older enrolled in the geriatrics PC Clinic taking ten or more medications. This cohort represented the top 5 percent of medication users enrolled in the clinic. By virtue of VA Geriatrics and Extended Care T-21 funding, an interdisciplinary team of clinical and scientific content experts developed and evaluated the IMPROVE intervention.

Practice Description

The IMPROVE model was designed with input from Veterans, family caregivers, and PACT providers and pharmacists through a series of focus groups and qualitative interviews. Providers also identified potential facilitators and barriers to implementation and uptake. They recruited high-risk Veterans and their caregivers through a letter and a follow-up phone call. Each IMPROVE clinic visit involved a face-to-face clinical pharmacist consultation during which all medications were reviewed with the Veteran and family caregiver(s). Providers evaluated each regimen and, if indicated, adjusted for appropriateness and safety. They also assessed barriers to tailor each Veteran's visit with specific education, strategies, and tools in support of successful medication management.

The program provided pharmacists with several tools to assist in a systematic evaluation of medication management concerns and quality of prescribing. A built-in CPRS template guided the pharmacist visit. The template included medication reconciliation, a systematic review of all medications to verify indication and check for redundancies, drug interactions, Potentially Inappropriate Medications (PIMs), and proper therapeutic monitoring. The template also included assessments for level of medication assistance available, goals of care, health literacy, and barriers to adherence. When necessary, clinicians gave pillboxes, illustrated medication schedules, low vision aids, and other adaptive devices to the Veteran. Communication of recommendations with the

PCP occurred by co-signature on the note, or same-day consultation for urgent concerns. At the discretion of the pharmacist, they conducted a face-to-face follow-up visit or phone call.

Replicability

In 2011, the VHA Geriatrics Pharmacy Taskforce recommended that facilities offer "individualized pharmacy review for high-risk patients on multiple medications." This recommendation was in line with the increasingly integrated role of the clinical pharmacist in the PACT and the recent requirement that Medicare Part D Medication Therapy Management Programs offer this service to select patients with chronic disease. The IMPROVE project provides this service with a focus on the PACT, patient and family-centered care, and use of existing best practice standards for medication management and safe prescribing for older adults.

The engagement of PACT members and a clinical pharmacist who championed the model enhanced the success of our pilot project. The effort involved in recruiting, scheduling, and assessing Veterans who participate in the program requires a local champion and support from the PACT, as well as local leadership, to ensure resources and time are appropriate. Given the success of the pilot, ORH funded the program during FY 2014 and FY 2015 RH to translate the model to target rural older Veterans in CBOCs. Given the lack of geriatric medicine experts in the CBOC setting, they added additional components to the intervention in the form of academic detailing, and provider audit and feedback on prescribing habits. Preliminary results show successful translation and significant improvement in prescribing quality.

Recognition

Anna Mirk, LaWanda Kemp, Katharina Echt, Molly Perkins, Anna Vandenberg, Theodore Johnson II, Christine Jasien, Florence Longchamp, Aaron Bozzorg, Melissa Stevens, Beverly Abrams, Joette Lowe, Atlanta VA, VISN 7

Nurse-Initiated Sepsis Protocol & Nursing Education

Kristin Drager MSN RN CNL CEN

William S. Middleton Memorial Veterans Hospital, Madison, WI
kristin.drager@va.gov

This sepsis program provides nurses the education and tools to recognize sepsis early and use a nurse-driven protocol to initiate diagnostic and treatment interventions in collaboration with the provider, resulting in an improvement in Veteran outcomes and reduction in hospital resource utilization and costs.

Introduction

Sepsis is a serious medical problem. The overall mortality rate from severe sepsis or septic shock ranges from 30 to 60 percent and it is the tenth leading cause of death in the US, with costs nearing $17 billion. Evidence supports marked improvement in patient outcomes if clinicians identify sepsis early and implement an evidence-based protocol at the time of recognition.

Since sepsis programming at the William S. Middleton Memorial VA Hospital began in 2012, providers at the facility have diagnosed more than 700 hospitalized Veterans with sepsis. Among Veterans diagnosed with sepsis and treated with the sepsis protocol in the ED, there has been an 80 percent decrease in the progressive worsening of stages of sepsis once hospitalized, a 60 percent decrease in mortality rate, and an average reduction of five bed-days-of-care per patient, resulting in a 43 percent cost-saving per patient. Because this program focuses on nursing education and the protocol is nurse-initiated, nursing staff can better advocate for Veterans and deliver evidence-based care that results in improved outcomes.

Key Information

In 2012, a Clinical Nurse Leader (CNL) led/collaborated the development and implementation of new sepsis programming. Sepsis programming includes a nursing education program and a nurse-initiated sepsis protocol that clinicians utilize in the ED and Intensive Care Unit (ICU) settings. Medical-surgical, psychiatric, infusion clinic, and Community Living Center (CLC) nurses receive sepsis education and a sepsis guideline to facilitate early recognition of sepsis with corresponding Situation, Background, Assessment, and Recommendation (SBAR) scripting that clinicians utilize when communicating patient concerns to the provider. Inpatients meeting severe sepsis and septic shock criteria move to the ICU setting where the nurse-initiated sepsis protocol begins. With this new programming in place, a significant number of hospitalized Veterans now receive time-sensitive, evidence-based care for sepsis.

Context

The William S. Middleton Memorial VA Hospital in Madison, WI, is a 129-bed medical facility with 85 acute care beds, a 26-bed CLC and an 18-bed residential treatment program. Our facility provides tertiary medical, surgical, neurological, and psychiatric care, and is a national center for heart, lung, and liver transplants. It is also an Epilepsy Center for Excellence. We serve 130,000

Veterans living in 15 counties in south central Wisconsin and in five counties in northwestern Illinois. Because our medical facility provides care for Veterans with complex medical conditions, sepsis is a common problem with serious implications.

Practice Description

Programming includes the development of a new nurse-initiated sepsis protocol for our ED/ICU RNs and nursing sepsis educational programming for all Registered RNs. Physician, nursing, pharmacy, and education staff participates as well.

For ED and ICU nurses: if there are abnormalities in the patient's vital signs and they exhibit specific signs and symptoms of infection, nurses can initiate the sepsis protocol in collaboration with the provider. By allowing nursing staff to initiate the protocol, we found that recognition and diagnosis of sepsis and time-sensitive treatment interventions occurred much sooner.

For inpatient nursing staff: we developed evidence-based sepsis guidelines aimed at helping them recognize sepsis quicker. A scripted communication tool helps them better articulate their concerns to the provider, leading to prompt identification of sepsis and transfer to a higher level of care so the sepsis protocol can begin.

We developed nursing education for ED/ICU and inpatient nursing staff regarding the pathophysiology of sepsis, stages of sepsis, and treatment interventions. We deliver education to existing staff and new staff within the nursing orientation program.

Replicability

Prior to 2012, the William S. Middleton Memorial VA Hospital did not utilize a sepsis protocol. After identifying this gap in care, a CNL formed an interdisciplinary team of vested stakeholders to create a sepsis committee to initially focus programming in the ED. Because we cared for so many septic Veterans, staff was eager for additional sepsis education and a nurse-driven sepsis protocol that delineated evidence-based treatments. After the sepsis programming began in the ED, word spread throughout the hospital. Inpatient nursing staff expressed great interest and programming spread organizationally, with widespread buy-in. We implemented programming systematically and used Kotter's Change Model, which was instrumental in the initial implementation and successful sustainment of this programming.

Any VA site that does not have a sepsis protocol or provide sepsis education to their nursing staff regarding the latest Clinical Practice Guidelines (CPGs) would benefit from this promising practice. The essential components for this programming exist and are replicable at other facilities. Facilities must establish a champion to lead an interdisciplinary sepsis committee of vested stakeholders. Committee members would ideally include representation from nursing, medicine, pharmacy, education, and performance improvement.

Recognition

Becky Kordahl, Elizabeth Fayram, Cindy Phelan, Sue Heidrich, Heather Royer, Interdisciplinary Sepsis Committee Members, nursing staff

Identification of Malnutrition and Nutrition-Focused Physical Exam

Anne Utech PhD, RDN, LD, Deputy National Director, Nutrition and Food Services
VA Central Office, Washington, DC
anne.utech@va.gov

VA Registered Dietitian Nutritionists (RDNs) perform Nutrition-Focused Physical Exams (NFPEs) to assess Veterans for a variety of nutrition diagnoses and for signs and symptoms of malnutrition, improving interdisciplinary care.

Introduction

Approximately 15 to 60 percent of hospitalized patients are malnourished in the US. Malnutrition leads to increased illness, decreased function and quality of life, and increased health care costs. Identification of malnutrition is the first step in correcting the condition and it is important to ensure that VA practitioners are aware of and comfortable using the standardized 2012 American Society Parenteral and Enteral Nutrition (ASPEN) and Academy of Nutrition and Dietetics (AND) guidelines for malnourished patients.

Mr. X came to the Salt Lake City VAMC with cardiac failure and joined a waiting list for a heart transplant in December of 2013. Kim Engelby, Registered Dietitian/Nutritionist (RDN), assessed him with a mildly compromised nutrition status upon admission. He required a biventricular assist device (BI-VAD) due to his poor heart function. Complications led to a decline in his nutrition status and he met criteria for Severe Acute Disease Related Malnutrition. Providers told the Veteran he needed to improve his nutrition status to receive a heart transplant. He focused on improving his intake and worked closely with his nutritionist. During his stay, Mr. X gained motivation and weight. After seven months of medical complications and improvements, he was nourished enough to receive a transplant in July of 2014 and continues to do well.

At the James A. Haley VAMC in Tampa, FL, many RDNs did not feel competent in performing a Nutrition-Focused Physical Exam (NFPE). Team members initiated a weekly conference sharing case examples of implementation of the malnutrition criteria via "Malnutrition/NFPE Rounds." Rounds involved an impromptu call out to staff when an RDN had determined that a patient met at least two characteristics of the malnutrition criteria. Malnutrition Rounds were an effective way to assist RDNs in becoming comfortable and proficient in completing a NFPE.

Key Information

RDNs perform NFPE to assess Veterans for a variety of nutrition diagnoses and for signs and symptoms of malnutrition. Early identification ensures that clinicians implement and communicate appropriate interventions throughout the care team. To improve interdisciplinary care of Veterans with malnutrition, it is imperative to utilize new adult malnutrition criteria and International Classification of Diseases (ICD) 10 coding. The National Nutrition and Food Services (NFS) Program Office, along with the Clinical Nutrition Subcommittee (CNS), implemented this program through NFS Strategic Goals during 2013–2016. This practice exists at all VAMCs.

Context

The CNS leadership utilized the American Society for Parenteral and Enteral Nutrition (ASPEN) consensus statement to form policy and reshape practice among the RDNs, ensuring that all were trained to work at their highest level of practice. In 2014, 1,923 Veterans met adult malnutrition criteria. In 2015, this figure rose to 14,419 and continues to increase. Approximately 67 percent of malnourished patients will experience further decline in their nutritional status during their hospitalization. Identification of malnutrition can potentially prevent complications related to malnutrition. Proper diagnosis of malnutrition also has the potential to promote higher reimbursement rates. The FY 2016 NFS strategic goal for malnutrition is to educate interdisciplinary teams on appropriately identifying malnutrition and documenting it.

Practice Description

CNS decided that identification of malnutrition was a top priority for RDNs. A subgroup of three RDNs from CNS led the strategic plan and created annual goals for VHA RDNs to promote understanding and competent usage of the ASPEN criteria. NFS developed "cheat sheets," training sessions, and templates, and tracked outcomes. Each year, the Strategic Goal has advanced from promoting more RDN identification of malnutrition to passing this knowledge on to other pertinent medical providers.

Replicability

With the help of the VA Employee Education System (EES), NFS developed appropriate training tools to train all RDNs to ensure they had the knowledge to begin implementing NFPE practice at their respective facilities. Beginning in FY 2014, the malnutrition Strategic Goal leaders educated the field on the new criteria for diagnosing malnutrition through conference calls, monthly strategic plan updates, creating and providing sample templates for documentation, and working with Managerial Cost Accounting to create a specific Event Capture Code to capture workload and quarterly articles in the NFS newsletter.

Recognition

Kelli Horton, Gail Schechter, Kristy Becker, Jim Brewer, Sherri Lewis, Julie Kurtz, Sara Perdue, Jamie Leuthold, Ellen Bosley, Anne Utech, VA NFS Field Advisory Committee, CNS

Development of a Prostate-Specific Antigen Tracker for Prostate Cancer

Michael Chang, MD Chief of Radiation Oncology
Hunter Holmes McGuire VAMC, Richmond, VA
michael.chang3@va.gov

This practice enhances the quality of patient care by using the Electronic Medical Record (EMR) to passively monitor patients who are at risk for developing recurrent cancer of the prostate, enabling early intervention.

Introduction

One of my patients, whose Prostate-Specific Antigen (PSA) was rising after definitive radiotherapy five years before, was picked up by the tracker and brought in early for salvage brachytherapy to cure his prostate cancer. Had it not been for the PSA tracker, his disease might have progressed beyond our ability to cure him. We reached out to him and he was so appreciative and relieved that he might still be able to be cured.

Key Information

We proposed expanding the practice of creating a PSA tracker for patients who have been treated with prostatectomy so that as soon as their PSA rose, they could be referred for early intervention with salvage radiotherapy. Early intervention with radiotherapy while the PSA is rising but still low potentially increases survival and prolongs quality of life.

Context

We are a level 1 facility serving 50,000 unique Veterans and are a national referral center for prostate cancer patients. We have been striving to improve the treatment of all cancer patients across VA enterprise. We hope someday that our practice will expand to cover all VA patients through the creation of an early warning PSA failure detection system for patients who have been treated for prostate cancer but continue to be at risk for recurrence of their disease.

Practice Description

Once patients are treated with surgery or radiation, they still have a significant risk of their cancer coming back as reflected by their PSA values rising. By working with Systems Engineers, we created a computer algorithm that interrogates the corporate data warehouse, which holds all VA data to identify patients with prostate cancer whose PSA are rising. The algorithm can be used to create a list of patients who have failed or who have not had their PSA checked recently. That list can then be reviewed to identify who might benefit from early intervention with salvage radiation therapy or brachytherapy. These patients can be salvaged before the PSA rises to a level where they are no longer curable.

Replicability

We adopted this practice because prostate cancer patients live a very long time and their cancer can come back up to ten years or later. During that time, patients may miss appointments, forget to get their PSA checked, and may have their disease progress without them knowing it. This system helps make sure these at-risk patients are getting the care they need. With assistance from VACO, the Veterans Engineering Resource Center (VERC), and the National Program Office of Radiation Oncology, we hope to develop this idea further and expand it to more facilities within VA.

Recognition

Sandra Troeschel, Kristine DeSotto, Paul Taibi, Michael Hagan

PACT Pharmacy in Minneapolis Veterans Affairs Health Care System Opiate Safety Initiative

Elzie Jones, PharmD, CPS

Minneapolis VA Health Care System, Minneapolis, MN
elzie.jones@va.gov

This multi-disciplinary project helped managed patients on high dose opioids for tapers, goal setting, and therapy maximization to significantly reduce daily opioid doses, creating a safer environment for our patients.

Introduction

Mr. X, a patient with chronic low back pain on high dose methadone 40mg every four hours (over 2,000mg morphine equivalents daily), presents to the clinical pharmacist for management of an opioid taper. The patient is very upset that his medications are being decreased and states that he needs them to live. During the interview, he is asked what his one wish or goal would be should his pain be better and his medication lower. He states, "I would like to try to fly again, but that will never happen. You can't have a pilot's license when you are taking methadone, and I will NEVER be off methadone." After one year of working with the pharmacist to taper methadone to 5mg twice daily, the patient states he is ready to be off completely. He still has pain, but it is no worse than before the taper. Now, however, he is able to think clearly and be more functional. He brought his pilot's license application with him, which he plans to complete when his methadone is completely gone.

Key Information

Minneapolis Veterans Affairs Health Care System (HCS) developed a plan for an Opioid Safety Initiative (OSI) in 2011 and implemented it in 2012. Because no program development funding was available, we utilized the resources we had available, namely the PACT CPS. Led by a designated clinical pharmacist pain specialist, the PACT Clinical Pharmacy team managed the majority of patients on high dose opioids (greater than 200mg morphine equivalents daily) for tapers, goal setting, and therapy maximization. Through this focused program, the teams were able to significantly reduce daily opioid doses, creating a safer environment for our patients.

Context

Minneapolis HCS is a large, 1a facility that serves a wide variety of Veteran patients in the upper Midwest. In 2014, we served over 100,000 unique patients. We have services at our main facility and 13 CBOCs. Minneapolis HCS also offers services for Spinal Cord Injury (SCI), one of four polytrauma Centers of Excellence, and, since 2014, a CARF-accredited Pain Rehabilitation Program (Commission on Accreditation of Rehabilitation Facilities). Prior to the CARF-accredited program, no formal pain program was available for our patients, making pain difficult for providers to manage. Minneapolis HCS was consistently an outlier concerning the amount of opioids prescribed. With the implementation of the OSI, patients were given a new resource to help manage and treat their pain in a safer and more effective manner.

Practice Description

Prior to implementation, the PACT CPS group (initially six members, currently 15) met to discuss goals, concerns, and resources needed to ensure the OSI program would be successful. A Pharmacy Pain training and competency program was developed with the help of the entire group. The PACT Pain CPS educated, trained, and signed off on the competency to ensure each CPS had the necessary skills, and that training was consistent across the group. The pain competency is now a core competency of the PACT CPS. All PACT CPSs were also trained in Motivational Interviewing (MI), which was key for communicating effectively with patients.

Veteran cases were discussed with or referred from the PCP for case management and/or tapers. Veterans were observed for approximately six months before being discharged back to PC. Follow-up was generally monthly, more frequently in some cases depending on the patient's response and needs. The tapers were generally 10 to 20 percent decrease per month. Our experience showed that tapering faster generally led to poorer patient acceptance.

Replicability

At the time of program initiation, PCPs were struggling to help patients manage their pain. The PACT CPS group recognized the problem and felt it was a very important project to undertake. A pain champion was identified (Dr. Peter Marshall, MD) to facilitate communication with the medical staff. The Office of Strategic Integration (OSI) formed with support from the medical center leadership (Chief of Staff, Facility and VISN Director) to ensure buy-in from key stakeholders. All medical and pharmacy staff was trained prior to implementation. Pharmacy Informatics (PI) developed a tracking tool for providers to have knowledge of their patients who noted as the highest risk. These lists were distributed to both PACT CPS and PACT teamlets. PACT CPS met with their individual PACT teamlets to develop plans for managing patients.

Each VA facility has the availability of PACT CPS for their teamlets, and the training and competency is easily reproducible and transferable. The tracking tool is now available nationally, eliminating a step needed for implementation of an OSI.

Recognition

Peter Marshall, Anders Westanmo, Kevin Burns, Tessa Kemp, Melissa Atwood, Todd Naidl, Jennifer Bolduc

Overdose Education and Naloxone Distribution

Alan Kershaw, RPh, Inpatient Pharmacy Clinical Specialist

VA Boston Healthcare System, Brockton, MA
alan.kershaw@va.gov

The Overdose Education and Naloxone Distribution (OEND) program provides Veterans with information on opiate overdose and teaches them how to prevent accidental opiate overdose using nasal naloxone.

Introduction

Two years ago, soon after the opiate overdose was declared an epidemic in the state of Massachusetts, the Chief of Pharmacy of Boston VA Healthcare System (HCS) presented me with the task of addressing the problem locally.

We were one of the first VA facilities in the country to develop a nasal naloxone-training program for Veterans with current or previous opioid dependence, enlisting an interdisciplinary team consisting of pharmacists, nurses, psychiatrists, and social workers. The OEND Program is an intervention plan developed with the guidance of the Massachusetts Department of Public Health.

Key Information

OEND trains at-risk Veteran patients on proper nasal naloxone administration in addition to preventing, recognizing, and responding to an opiate overdose. However, educating individual Veterans as they are admitted to the hospital is not enough, because they cannot save themselves in overdose situations. So I ask these patients to take the OEND handbook and teach friends and family members how to reverse an opiate overdose with nasal naloxone, so that we can exponentially create an awareness of the opioid epidemic and reverse the upward trend of overdose deaths that the state of Massachusetts has experienced over the past 15 years.

During the past two years, Boston HCS Pharmacy Department has dispensed over 500 nasal naloxone rescue kits to Veterans. All VA Boston police carry rescue kits on their belts and have training in its proper use, and we have begun to make kits available for emergency use in various residential and clinical areas on campus deemed high risk.

Context

The topic of opiate overdose prevention arose at a Morbidity and Mortality (M&M) meeting, and was escalated to the Pharmacy and Therapeutics Committee (P&T), where Robert Henault, RPh CDE, Chief of Pharmacy for Boston HCS, was responsible for finding a volunteer from his department willing to start an OEND program. We began as a pilot study on a 15-bed detox unit at Brockton VAMC. It began in February 2014, and I saw my first patient the following April. We felt monitoring a smaller and more specific unit would be more manageable to track admissions.

I work as a clinical pharmacist at VA Boston's campus in Brockton, MA, where the hospital serves Veterans with spinal cord injuries; we have transitional care and community residential areas, as well as a building dedicated to acute and long-term mental health. Initially, my primary focus was on Veterans admitted for opiate detox.

Practice Description

I start each workday by screening overnight admissions for Veterans with a history of opiate abuse/dependence that would benefit from OEND training. After I develop a list of eligible patients, I begin to monitor their progress notes daily, and must wait for their detox to get to a point where they are comfortable enough to talk about OEND. Communication with nursing staff is essential. If we approach the Veteran at a time when they are feeling better, they are more likely to accept the offer for OEND training and get the most out of this opportunity. After the education is completed, a note is entered in the CPRS, where I add the PCP as a co-signer, notifying them that their patient successfully completed the training. I prescribe the nasal naloxone rescue kits for the Veterans to be added to their discharge prescription package.

After various committees reviewed the pilot, we agreed to expand the OEND program to include two acute mental health units, 25 beds each, to bring my daily monitoring capacity to 65 beds total.

Over the past two years, I have taught over 310 Veterans resulting in 40 opiate overdose reversals. Those taking credit for these life-saving measures are mostly Veterans and their friends. An additional ten reversals have been recorded, five by other Boston VA facilities, and another five by Boston VA Police department.

Replicability

This practice was implemented at Boston VA HCS with the goal of helping to reverse the upward trend of accidental opiate overdose in our state, and should be adopted by any state in the US where accidental opiate overdoses are on the rise.

Recognition

Vincent Ng, Michael Charness, Robert Henault, Grace Chang, Kathryn Lange, Lisa Rolek

Providing Veterans Safe and Responsible Options for Medication Disposal

Jeanne Tuttle, National Pharmacist Program Manager

Pharmacy Benefits Management Services, VA Central Office, Washington, DC

jeanne.tuttle@va.gov

Prescription drug abuse has now surpassed car accidents and guns as the leading cause of accidental death. To help address this epidemic, this project provided Veterans with safe and responsible options to dispose of their medication. To date, Veterans have returned over 21 tons of medications.

Introduction

Beginning in the fall of 2014, Pharmacy Benefits Management (PBM) Services began outreach and communication to the field about the importance of providing Veterans with responsible medication disposal options. Many in the field expressed concerns about the requirements in law for the onsite receptacle option. Therefore, in early 2015, PBM initiated a pilot at six medical facilities involving both pharmacy and VA Police. Results of the pilot showed overwhelming support for the practice by Veterans and staff and there are now over 70 receptacles in use throughout VA. PBM also worked with a vendor to develop customized signage to engage Veterans in the practice. Providing these options to Veterans:

- Promotes medication safety in the home.
- Reduces the chance of intentional and accidental poisonings.
- Reduces the risk of drug diversion.
- Safeguards the environment.

Key Information

To help address the prescription drug abuse epidemic, in September of 2014 the Drug Enforcement Administration (DEA) published "Disposal of Controlled Substances; Final Rule." This regulation gives patients safe and responsible options for disposing of medication. Based on this rule, PBM instituted a practice to provide Veterans a safe and responsible mechanism to dispose of unneeded medication in alignment with VA's commitment to patient-centered care. To date, Veterans have returned over 21 tons of medications that have been destroyed in an environmentally responsible manner and PBM has received many positive comments from the field:

- Pharmacy Chief and Police Chief: "This is a real customer-friendly, Veteran-friendly, community-positive system."
- Veteran X: "Appreciate the convenience."
- Pharmacy: "A Veteran volunteer at the information desk was very enthusiastic about the receptacle. He has been telling others and even brought his expired meds in."
- Nursing: "Long overdue."

- Mental Health Provider: "Great option to get excess meds out of the hands of patients who may do harm to themselves if allowed to stockpile."
- Pharmacy: "Facility staff are very supportive and happy to spread the word."
- Police Chief: "Patients have commented that they are very thankful that we have the container now which provides them with a safe and legal method to dispose of unwanted medication."

Studies indicate that a majority of patients do not promptly or properly dispose of their unused, unwanted, or expired medications but rather store them in the home, often times unsecured. This increases opportunities for accidental poisoning (especially in children), diversion, and non-medical use. The National Survey of Drug Use and Health data indicates greater than 50 percent of people using pain relievers non-medically obtained them free from friends and family. The National Drug Control Strategy lists proper medication disposal as one of the major areas to reduce prescription drug abuse.

When patients dispose of their unused medications, it is typically in the household garbage or by flushing them down the toilet or sink with pharmaceuticals ending up in a solid waste landfill and in the water supply. There is an estimation that over 250 million pounds of pharmaceuticals are disposed into the sanitary sewer system each year and as a result, an Associated Press investigation found concentrations of over 50 pharmaceuticals in the drinking water of 24 major metropolitan cities having detrimental effects on aquatic species and possibly on human health and development.

Context

PBM is aligned under Patient Care Services (PCS) at VACO and has several programs decentralized throughout the country to provide organizational and clinical leadership to VHA Pharmacies. A survey conducted in VISN 5 prior to implementation of the DEA final rule showed 13 percent of respondents stated they returned medications directly back to the pharmacy or medical center. This poses both health risks to staff and security storage issues, especially at CBOCs that do not have an onsite pharmacy. In addition, returning controlled substances directly back to health care staff is not legal under DEA regulations. The challenge was to find a solution for all Veterans to have a safe method to dispose of medications, which would be in alignment with federal law and would safeguard staff.

Practice Description

The process started with the formation of an inter-professional Subject Matter Expert (SME) workgroup at the national level to discuss and analyze the options DEA was proposing in the draft regulations. Concurrently, an Executive Decision Memo was developed to ensure funds would be available to support the implementation of the practice. Once the regulations were published, outreach at the VISN, facility, and program office level was instrumental in garnering support as well as ensuring VHA staff engaged Veterans in a legal manner. Mail back envelopes and guidance for distribution as well as Veteran marketing materials reached each facility while the onsite receptacle pilots took place. Resources at the national level for standard operating procedures, staff education, Veteran engagement, and forms to gather the required documentation are post edit to a SharePoint site. Feedback on return rates by facility are provided to the field on a monthly basis so that facilities can assess their progress and make any needed changes. An announcement is in place for the My HealtheVet website. Information on disposal was also published on the

PBM MedSafe website with a link on the VA A–Z Health Index: http://www.pbm.va.gov/PBM/vacenterformedicationsafety/vacenterformedicationsafetyprescriptionsafety.asp.

Replicability

Key factors for successful uptake and rollout of this national initiative include:

- Engaging SMEs proactively to help determine Veterans' needs
- National funding to ensure implementation would not be hampered due to the lack of funds at any one facility
- Strong communication plan and outreach on all levels
- Identification and solicitation of peer champions
- Creating the needed tools and resources nationally rather than depending on each facility to develop locally. This conserves resources (developed one time vs. 150+ times) and also ensures standardization
- Ongoing feedback to facilities on their progress

Recognition

Northern California HCS, New Mexico VA HCS, Jesse Brown VAMC, Clement J. Zablocki VAMC, William S. Middleton Memorial Veterans Hospital, VA Maine HCS, Cincinnati VAMC

GeriPACT

Kenneth Shay, DDS, MS, Director, Geriatric Programs
VA Central Office, Washington, DC
kenneth.shay@va.gov

The GeriPACT practice is a specialized PACT practice that employs clinical teams with advanced geriatrics care competencies to provide geriatric-principled care to elderly patients.

Introduction

Geriatric Patient Aligned Care Team (GeriPACT) originated as Geriatric Primary Care (GPC) at several sites in VHA in the late 1990s, in response to the need for clinical teams with advanced geriatrics care competencies to follow frail elderly outpatients who had experienced rehabilitation and functional optimization in Geriatric Evaluation and Management (GEM) inpatient and outpatient programs.

Here is a great example of how that program helped an individual Veteran. Mr. X is a 92-year-old WWII Veteran of the 10th Mountain Division ("the Ski Troops") who received two Purple Hearts and a Bronze Star for his work as a radioman in the Italian Alps. He has lived independently since his wife died when they were both in their early 80s. He began receiving PC from VA, where he also works as a volunteer, after a family member suggested the social atmosphere at VA might be beneficial. He has hypertension, benign prostatic hypertrophy, cataracts and lens implants, and two hearing aids. When he experienced three falls over a six-month period, his PACT consulted GeriPACT.

GeriPACT evaluated his medication regimen and determined that was to blame. They simplified his drugs and he requested his care continue with GeriPACT because he felt he received better care there. When he turned 90, GeriPACT staff noted that he was devoting less attention to his personal appearance. Then, in consultation with an adult daughter who lived nearby, he agreed to receive weekly homemaker support to assist with dressing and bathing. The aide reported signs of cognitive decline and, following the necessary assessment, Mr. X reluctantly agreed to stop driving. GeriPACT arranged for his involvement in an adult day care program where he could receive his medications, have a nutritious lunch, participate in regular activity (including Tai Chi to enhance his balance and 30 minutes daily on an exercise bicycle), and socialize.

Key Information

Through interdisciplinary assessment and development of a comprehensive plan of care, frail elderly Veterans who experience rehabilitation and functional optimization are able to remain living in the community. However, without a geriatrics team to oversee their subsequent health care management, many of these patients' health declined when their PC teams deviated from Geriatric Evaluation and Management (GEM) recommendations due to time pressure and other factors. In the early years of the new millennium, Geriatrics and Extended Care (GEC) recognized the value of officially establishing GPC. By the time PACT was introduced in 2010, there were four to five dozen GPC programs overseeing the care of about 30,000 Veterans. When it was mandated that all PC in VA be termed "PACT" and staffed accordingly, all GPCs were renamed GeriPACT, although many have struggled to receive staffing at the PACT level (i.e., for each provider there should be one RN, one LPN, and one clerical person).

Context

Over 50 percent of the Veterans seen in PACT annually are age 65 or over. Most of these older Veterans experience successful management in the brief appointments they have with PACT two or three times per year. Nevertheless, there is a small subset of Veterans, perhaps 3 to 5 percent, whose needs are unaddressed in the PACT setting. There are numerous reasons for this shortfall, including 1) multiple interacting and unstable clinical conditions; 2) multiple medications requiring monitoring and management; 3) the need to coordinate care and services with non-VA health systems also involved in the Veteran's care; 4) interactions with housing, nutrition, family, and mental health factors; 5) the high prevalence of cognitive impairment due to stroke and dementia; and 6) PACT personnel's limited comfort dealing with the non-medical aspects of patients' care needs. As a result, this subset of patients substantially impedes clinic flow by either requiring much longer clinic time or more frequent visits because only a fraction of their needs can be addressed in one appointment. In some cases, both situations exist. They are high-utilizers of health care resources, both planned and unplanned.

Practice Description

The major differences between PACT and GeriPACT are:

- GeriPACT has a dedicated social worker and a dedicated clinical pharmacist, because psychosocial and medication issues are universally key complications in each GeriPACT patient's care.

- The provider in GeriPACT has a level of advanced training or clinical experience in assessment and management of patients living with the decline, chronic disease, and cognitive compromise that frequently accompany advanced age.

- GeriPACT panels are limited to 2/3 the size of PACT panels, permitting appointment lengths to be slightly longer. Appointments are longer because these patients may need to have instructions repeated. It may take more time for staff to review their extensive medical and pharmaceutical histories. Typically, these patients may ambulate, dress, and undress more slowly. And to meet these patients' needs, it is often necessary to work with one or more family members or caregivers. When a VA system offers GeriPACT, the PACT practices at the site run more efficiently because these patients who need more time and attention are attended to with the GeriPACT, not the PACT, schedule.

The GeriPACT team is available for consultative support to co-located PACT teams whose patients can benefit from the input of clinicians with advanced geriatrics expertise, even as PACT continues to manage their care. These factors enhance PACT patient access and improve PACT and GeriPACT patient and family satisfaction. When frail older patients receive management according to geriatric principles as they are in GeriPACT, they experience less need for use of Emergency Rooms (ERs), visit hospitals and nursing homes less, and, when admitted, have shorter stays. All of these factors work to enhance access for other Veterans, by reducing the overall costs of care and freeing up space and appointment slots.

Replicability

GeriPACT has expanded since 2010 from about 50 programs serving 30,000 Veterans to over 75 programs serving nearly 55,000. Every VISN presently offers the service in at least two sites and, in some networks, in every medical center. GeriPACT is the dominant source for "Comprehensive Geriatric Evaluation," a service mandated (as one of the "Non-institutional Cares") to be available to Veterans by statute. It is an approach to care that has been demonstrated by both VA and non-VA studies to enhance older persons' functional status, reduce medications, and improve quality of life.

In March 2016, a GeriPACT Summit was convened in Albany, NY, that attracted over 120 VA clinicians. Supported by their VISNs (all networks were represented), clinicians shared best practices and identified critical data and policy needs necessary for further expanding the program.

Recognition

Birju Patel, William Kavesh, James Powers, Tom Hornick, Sathya Maheswaran, Carmen Arick, Steve Barczi, Paul Cherniack, Michael Godschalk, Marianne Tanabe, Carrie Pohl

Developing and Expanding Antimicrobial Stewardship to Reduce Inappropriate Antibiotic Use and Consequences of Antibiotic Overuse

Kelly Echevarria, PharmD, Infectious Diseases CPS

South Texas Veterans Health Care System, San Antonio, TX
kelly.echevarria@va.gov

Implementation of an effective Antimicrobial Stewardship Program (ASP) enhances Veteran safety by reducing complications of inappropriate antibiotic therapy, such as adverse drug events, antibiotic resistance, and Clostridium difficile (C.difficile) infection.

Introduction

The CDC estimates over two million people per year are sickened with antibiotic-resistant bacteria resulting in over 23,000 deaths. Another quarter million patients require hospital care for C.difficile diarrhea resulting in 14,000 additional deaths. Antibiotic use is the most important risk factor for both of these outcomes. VHA Directive 1031 requires all VHA facilities to implement an ASP and publish an annual report, but the practices that are most effective in reducing inappropriate antibiotic use are not clear. In addition, one of the major goals of the National Action Plan to Combat Antibiotic Resistance released in March of 2015 is the requirement for ASPs in all acute care hospitals, with specific deliverables regarding reduction of inappropriate antibiotic use by 2020.

There is a personal significance to this goal for me. Early in my career at South Texas VA Health Care System (HCS), I became friends with a disabled Veteran and VA volunteer with whom I worked. Despite a myriad of health problems, he always had a smile and worked tirelessly to make our jobs easier and allow us more time to care for our Veteran patients. Because of an antibiotic he received for a possible urinary tract infection, he developed an episode of severe C.difficile diarrhea and ended up in the intensive care unit (ICU). Although he recovered fully, he went on to suffer numerous relapses, resulting in continued hospitalizations, additional time in intensive care, surgeries, and finally a prolonged stay in the long-term care unit until he passed away as a result of the complications incurred by the hospitalizations. This was all due to a single course of antibiotics, which were potentially unnecessary. I still have the angel he gave me when my daughter was born and it remains in her room 14 years later. His face is the one I see when I think of why we must identify situations where antibiotic use is unnecessary or inappropriate.

Key Information

Development of the ASP at South Texas VA HCS was initially a collaboration between the Infectious Diseases CPS (IDCPS) at South Texas VA HCS and an Infectious Disease (ID) physician, with approval through the Antibiotic subcommittee, Pharmacy and Therapeutics Committee (P&T) and Clinical Executive Board (CEB). Initial efforts were focused on high-risk patients, such as those with bacteremia and patients in the ICU, but expanded to other areas over time. Documentation of positive results provided to hospital committees allowed justification to expand personnel resources. Additional impetus and support for the need for this type of program came from national recommendations from the Infectious Diseases Society of America, the CDC and ultimately from a VA Directive and Presidential Action Plan.

The National VA Antimicrobial Stewardship Task Force provided many useful tools, example policies, educational resources, and collaboration to encourage the development of ASP across VA, but there remained much uncertainty about the logistics of implementation and best practices for ASP.

Context

South Texas VA HCS is a level 1a teaching facility in San Antonio, TX. Besides the usual ICUs, medical and surgical wards, and Community Living Centers (CLCs), we also have a bone marrow transplant unit, inpatient spinal cord injury unit, and inpatient polytrauma unit. These specialty patients are often at increased risk of antibiotic overuse, antibiotic resistance, and C.difficile infection. In addition, as a teaching facility, we have a large number of providers prescribing antibiotics, often rotating in and out of South Texas VA HCS, making education and consistency of practice a challenge.

Practice Description

The beginning of our formal ASP was in 2009, with the development of a policy and physician/pharmacist champion. Over the next several years, we worked to identify the best ways to impact antibiotic use broadly given a relative lack of data tools and staffing (at that time we had two Acute Care CPSs and no dedicated physician time for ASP). We took a systematic approach to implementation, and tools developed by the National Antimicrobial Stewardship Task Force facilitated many of the activities and initiatives.

Positive results of these systematic activities have included:

- Increased encounter tracking for ASP activities and restricted antibiotic consults.
- Cost avoidance related to ASP activities from $125,000–$250,000 annually.
- Many quality improvement projects and medication use evaluations resulting in local and national posters and presentations.
- Improved susceptibility profiles for P.aerugionsa and S.aureus, with stable levels of susceptibility for other common pathogens.
- Reduction in overall inpatient antibiotic use from an average of 349 Days of Therapy (DOTs) per 1,000 days present in 2009 to 291 DOTs per 1,000 days in 2015.

Replicability

Several factors continue to contribute to the success of the South Texas VA HCS ASP. Probably the most important factor is the presence of personnel with dedicated FTE time for ASP activities, and excited and motivated people in those positions who take ownership in the program and its success. The purchase of available third-party software (Theradoc) greatly improved efficiency of ASP activities through specialist reports and alerts. Strong IT support in the form of Pharmacy clinicians with strong knowledge of CPRS and VistA as well as provider viewpoint allows for the development of tools that are helpful in guiding decisions about antibiotic therapy without being overly intrusive. I think it also helped to do things one step at a time. It is possible to replicate what we did by following a systematic process:

1. Develop a policy and appoint a Pharmacy and Physician champion who takes ownership in the ASP with allotted time for ASP activities.

2. Engage providers, nurses and pharmacists, and get their input regarding antibiotic use at the facility in addition to how they feel the ASP Team can help them.

3. Gather data on antibiotic use patterns, antimicrobial resistance patterns, and opportunities for improvement. Good IT support to develop useful and efficient reports can greatly facilitate this process. In addition, students and residents can also be helpful for data collection.

4. Review the Assessment Task Force (ASTF) SharePoint site for examples of initiatives and educational materials.

5. Select one opportunity for antibiotic improvement (such as increasing intravenous to oral conversion). Collect baseline data, implement, and then collect follow-up data.

6. Track and report relevant outcomes (such as workload, interventions, antibiotic use, resistance, and C.diff infections) as initiatives are implemented.

7. Once improvement is documented in an area, select another area for improvement and repeat.

Recognition

Jose Cadena-Zuluaga, Jason Bowling, Kelly Echevarria, Marc Weiner, Courtney Ortiz, Kelly Echevarria, Mark Wong, Makoto Jones, Matt Samore

Anticoagulation Improvement Project

Ellen A. Jones, PharmD, CACP; CPS

VA Central Western Massachusetts Healthcare System, Leeds, MA
ellen.jones@va.gov

This Anticoagulation Improvement Project has resulted in improved care to Veterans using a systems redesign model. Significant improvement in Time in Therapeutic Range (TTR) has resulted in fewer hemorrhages and ischemic strokes among those Veterans on anticoagulation therapy.

Introduction

Patients receiving warfarin for anticoagulation benefit from better control, as they have fewer bleeding and clotting events. Percent TTR is a measure of anticoagulation control. The goal of our project was to improve TTR in VISN 1, using a process improvement approach. From May of 2013 to September of 2014, VISN TTR improved from 64.2 percent to 67.7 percent, compared with a flat trend at 64.5 percent for the rest of VA during the same period. This improvement equates to prevention of approximately 20 major hemorrhages and 12 ischemic strokes within our VISN during that period, resulting in a cost savings of approximately $1.5 million over two years.

One medical center in particular experienced significant improvement in the quality of care provided. At the start of the systems redesign project, this site had a TTR of approximately 52 percent, among the worst in VA. Over 13 percent of patients were lost to follow-up, defined as being on warfarin but not having been tested in over 56 days. Patient satisfaction with warfarin care, at 59 percent highly satisfied, was the lowest in VISN 1 by far. After one year of using the newly created VISN algorithms and Dashboard, as well as improving their processes of care with the help of staff from New England Veterans Engineering Resource Center (VERC), that medical center's TTR increased to approximately 63 percent (average for VA), lost to follow-up came down to less than 1 percent (ideal), and patient satisfaction score increased to 70 percent (on par with the rest of VISN 1).

Many people are apprehensive about change, and in the case of the Anticoagulation Clinic (ACC) project, ACC staff initially had concerns about making changes to clinical practice and work processes. However, staff attitudes changed dramatically during the course of the ACC Improvement project. For example, one staff person remarked that all her initial concerns were "totally disproven" by the project. ACC staff across VISN 1 note that TTR is better, patients experience better outcomes, they have more control over their workload, and they have new and better ways to train incoming pharmacists to deliver ACC care. An ACC staff person remarked, "I think [TTR performance tracking] helps for inspiration. It helps drive people to do better." Furthermore, ACC staff has increasingly embraced the concept of quality improvement. A frequently expressed view point shared among ACC staff regarding TTR is that "…it's not just about a number, it's about improving patient care and saving money…TTR gives you something to reflect on and know that what you're doing actually is having an impact…" Staff feels empowered to make changes and they feel proud of their site level and regional level accomplishments.

Key Information

In 2011, VISN 1 approved an Executive Decision Memorandum (EDM), which initiated a two-year project to unify the outpatient anticoagulation care in the VISN in an effort to improve anticoagulation care. A VISN anticoagulation coordinator was hired and an industrial engineer from the VERC was detailed to initiate a systems redesign of the VISN's ACCs. Each medical center chose a site level coordinator to represent the team. Over the initial two years of the project, significant results were experienced in the areas of improved TTR, decreased rate of lost to follow-up, and improved patient satisfaction. This led to the creation and subsequent approval of a second EDM, which supported continuation of the project to sustain the gains and continue improvement.

Context

It has been estimated that approximately 10,000 Veterans receive long-term anticoagulation from VISN 1. Using cost models, it has been determined that the VISN could save approximately $1 million a year through prevented events in atrial fibrillation patients by improving TTR by 5 percent. The challenge that has been addressed was finding a model of best practice that supports a TTR of 70 percent or greater. It was identified that centralized anticoagulation services is a best practice over decentralized services. This created a challenge to re-structure many of the ACCs within the VISN. Another challenge was decreasing the number of patients who were lost to follow-up. At the start of this project, there was approximately a 20 percent rate of lost to follow-up. After the development of the VISN anticoagulation Dashboard, the rate dropped to less than 5 percent in about one year.

Practice Description

The initiation of the project required hiring a VISN anticoagulation coordinator and an industrial engineer to head the project. Next, medical center coordinators were selected within the VISN. The team was detailed on the goals of the project and provided training on systems redesign and improvement work. Meetings were coordinated both in-person and via teleconferencing. During the meetings, the team looked for waste within the work performed at each site and identified best practices both within and outside of the VISN. Travel was coordinated to visit a VA facility that was identified as a top performing site (this was outside of VISN 1). Visits to the different sites within the VISN allowed for observation and feedback to the local ACCs.

In looking for best practices, the team identified the need for a VISN SharePoint, a VISN Dashboard, and VISN anticoagulation algorithms/policies. These tools were developed by the group and with the help of the VERC and the Data Management Office. Tests of change were performed to determine if the tools created were effective. Problems were identified and improvement continues even as this is being written.

Replicability

This practice was adopted by our VISN due to the identification of a need to improve patient outcomes while also saving money on health care costs. It was a successful project because the support provided was sufficient to produce positive outcomes. The VISN and local leadership allowed the team time to enact the changes, but also provided resources and training needed to make the project successful. Education on systems redesign and Lean and Motivational Interviewing

(MI) was integral to the success of this project. Support for travel was necessary to allow for observation, analysis, and collaboration. These key tools have allowed our team to be successful.

Part of the initial goal of this project was to allow for replicability of our work. Since the outcomes of this project have been proven successful, several tools that were created for our VISN's ACCs are now available on a national level. Many of the algorithms and policies created as part of this project are being adapted as national algorithms and policies. The influence of our work can also be appreciated in the development of the 2015 National Anticoagulation Directive. Additionally, a national anticoagulation Dashboard is being developed with the influence of this project.

Recognition

Angela Park, Ashley Benedict, Timothy Schmoke, William Lukesh, Adam Rose, Megan McCullough, Beth Ann Petrakis, Michael Mayo-Smith, James Schlosser, Sampath Narayana, Allison Marshall, Pamela Sweeney, Dale Cyr, Candida Perez, Ellen Jones, Jennifer Kinney, Patricia Callahan, Carolyn Malikowski, Christine Kearns, Jaime Correia, Margaret Quillin, Meghan Quilter, VISN 1 Anticoagulation Teams

Warfarin to Direct Oral Anticoagulants Conversion Process

Courtney Pawula, CPS

VA Health Care System, Phoenix, AZ
courtney.pawula@va.gov

This innovative practice allows patients to maintain clot and stroke prevention while reducing the burden of warfarin, which in turn helps improve quality of life.

Introduction

The use of warfarin for prevention of clots or stroke can be quite overwhelming for a patient and his/her family. There are many restrictions on diet, medications, and health management, as well as the necessary labs that range from every few days to every few weeks. Additionally, the constant medication dose changes can be difficult to manage, particularly for older Veterans or those who live alone.

The Direct Oral Anticoagulants (DOACs) have the benefit of a regular dosing schedule, fewer medication interactions, limited drug interactions, less impact of acute medical changes, and less frequent monitoring. This improves Veteran quality of life by limiting the amount of interactions as well as the amount of time they have to spend at VA obtaining labs and having appointments. Beyond the basic benefits of these agents, literature has shown similar and, in some instances, superior prevention of clots/stroke as well as similar or better bleed risk compared to warfarin. While the patients themselves may not automatically recognize these benefits, they certainly affect the Veterans' lives.

Key Information

A PACT pharmacist within Phoenix VAMC implemented this practice after learning about it from colleagues at Sierra Nevada VA Healthcare System (HCS). I led this implementation from proposal to conversion. The proposal went through submission and approval by Phoenix VAMC Pharmacy and Therapeutics Committee (P&T) in February 2014; adoption and implementation occurred in fall 2014. This practice improves patient outcomes and quality of life and can decrease health care costs.

Context

Phoenix VA is a 1b tertiary medical hospital that has multiple CBOCs. Within Phoenix VAMA, a centralized Anticoagulation Clinic (ACC) manages all patients on warfarin. Prior to 2015, the ACC was short-staffed and had more patients enrolled per FTE than recommended by VHA guidance. The development of this program helped to identify the patients with the lowest Time in Therapeutic Range (TTR) and pull them out of the ACC. While this was a benefit to the patient (to help improve their outcomes), it also helped to improve the ratio of anticoagulation patients per FTE.

Practice Description

This process started by talking with previous co-workers from Reno about their similar project and obtaining the Structured Query Language (SQL) code that they had written to find their patient lists. Once the SQL code was obtained and processed through our Patient Data Warehouse, I reviewed the percentage of patients with a TTR less than 60 percent, which literature has shown is effective for preventing clots/strokes, to determine the potential impact of the project. From there, a proposal was sent to P&T to get the ok to convert clinically appropriate patients. Once approved, the review process began.

Every 3–4 months, our pharmacoeconomics team provides a list of the patients with TTR less than 60 percent. I work with the pharmacy residents one day per week to review the list, and then determine if patients are appropriate for a switch in therapy. The determination is based on: renal function, current hemoglobin and platelets, bleed risk, history of bleed, history of malignancy, history of non-adherence, or anything else that would be considered an exclusion factor provided by Pharmacy Benefits Management (PBM). If a patient is appropriate for conversion, a CPRS note is entered to their PCP and specialist with recommendations for conversion, including specific drug and dosing recommendations. If the PCPs agree, the patient is contacted by me or the resident to discuss benefits and risks of the new agents compared to warfarin. If the patient agrees to switch, the patient has a face-to-face visit with me or the resident and thorough medication education is provided. At this time, the patient will also complete new labs (International Normalized Ratio, metabolic panel, and blood counts) to ensure it is safe to switch to the new agent. When converted, I contact the patient by phone for the first three months to assess tolerability and adherence; at one month after initiation, repeat labs are completed to ensure the medication remains safe. After the first three months, the patient undergoes tracking by their PACT pharmacist for the next three months and is then discharged back to their PCP for a follow-up every six months. As of December 2015, we reviewed 320 patients with about 45 percent success in converting to the new agent.

Replicability

The most important factor for this program was being allowed to have protected time to review and see these patients for conversions. In terms of replicability for other VAs, I believe they need to have someone interested in completing similar work, buy-in from the providers, buy-in from pharmacy management to provide protected time for reviews and completing education/conversions, and someone able to run the SQL software through the Patient Data Warehouse for their facility.

Recognition

Michael Harvey, Arthur Allen, Todd Rowland

Swallow Strengthening Oropharyngeal Clinical Program

Nicole Rogus-Pulia, PhD, CCC-SLP, Advanced Geriatrics Fellow
William S. Middleton Memorial Veterans Hospital, Madison, WI
nicole.pulia@va.gov

Swallow STRONG is a patient-centered multi-disciplinary clinical program for Veterans with dysphagia that provides therapy to restore and maintain safe and effective swallow function.

Introduction

Mr. X enrolled in the Swallow "Strengthening Oropharyngeal" (STRONG) Clinic in December 2014 with initial complaints of food and pills stuck in his throat and choking events with saliva at night. Eating was becoming less enjoyable for him. His baseline Videofluoroscopic Swallow Study (VFSS) confirmed aspiration with thin liquids as well as mild pharyngeal residue. The cause of his dysphagia (swallowing disorder) was unclear (no specific underlying associated medical diagnosis). Mr. X was highly motivated to improve as he felt that dinner with his wife was not enjoyable anymore. He was not able to converse with her while eating, as he had to concentrate on his swallowing. He enrolled in the Swallow STRONG Clinic and can be described as the model patient. Despite a technical error with the device at one point, as well as a trip to Florida during his enrollment, he followed the therapy schedule as outlined and kept all his appointments.

By the end of treatment, his swallow improved to within normal limits for his age. He was no longer aspirating and only had mild pharyngeal residue. He reported being able to talk to his wife during a meal because he does not have to concentrate as much on swallowing. Mr. X felt that his swallow improved substantially and the results of his VFSS confirmed his reports.

Key Information

Swallow STRONG is a patient-centered multi-disciplinary clinical program for Veterans with dysphagia that was developed at the William S. Middleton VA Hospital in Madison, WI. This program has been funded by a Geriatrics and Extended Care (GEC) T21 grant from FY 2013 through FY 2016. Additionally, in FY 2015, three VA expansion sites were added in New Jersey VA Healthcare System (HCS), Chicago (Hines) VA Hospital, and St. Louis (John Cochran) VAMC. In FY 2016, a fourth expansion site, the Cincinnati VAMC, was added. The main goal of Swallow STRONG is to improve swallowing/eating-related transitional care for Veterans with dysphagia. The intervention provides therapy to restore and maintain safe and effective swallow function resulting in more independence and improved health status, thereby reducing hospital admissions, length of stay, and long-term institutionalizations. Multidisciplinary support for patients provided as part of each in-person visit allows for the ability to address various swallowing-related concerns using an integrated approach to dysphagia management. Patient-centered outcomes, in addition to physiologic and health-related outcomes, ensure a focus on quality of life in addition to improved health status. We also utilize telehealth for follow-up visits with patients at their CBOCs, providing optional home visits when needed.

Context

The William S. Middleton VA Hospital in Madison, WI, is an 85-bed acute care hospital, with an additional 26 beds for sub-acute care (transitional care/rehabilitation/and hospice), as well as 18 beds in the hospital's residential rehabilitation treatment center. More than 270,000 Veterans with dysphagia account for 350,000 visits and admissions to VA facilities annually. It has been estimated that up to 22 percent of adults above the age of 50 years and upwards of 40 percent of those within institutional settings suffer from dysphagia. Swallowing pressure reserve, the relationship between isometric (maximal) tongue pressures and tongue pressures during swallowing (submaximal), is lower with advancing age, which places older adults at higher risk for dysphagia. A number of medical conditions also frequently lead to dysphagia, including stroke, head and neck cancer, or respiratory conditions. The major complications of dysphagia include malnutrition, dehydration, and aspiration pneumonia. Pneumonia is the fifth leading cause of infectious death in those 65 and older and the third leading cause in those beyond 85 of age. A recent study found dysphagia to be an independent predictor of aspiration and non-aspiration pneumonia in patients 70 years of age or older discharged from an acute geriatric hospital unit. Standard of care treatment for dysphagia currently consists of compensatory approaches that do not affect underlying physiology of the swallow and recommend the use with every swallow. These may negatively affect quality of life and thereby result in low patient adherence. Rehabilitative exercises are ready for use that affect underlying swallow physiology, but they are not progressive in nature nor tailored to the patient's baseline level. Additionally, online feedback regarding performance is not frequently available and the intensity as well as frequency of these exercises often varies.

Practice Description

The Swallow STRONG program employs an intensive, eight-week systematic, multi-disciplinary approach to dysphagia treatment. Each patient matches with a dedicated Speech-Language Pathologist (SLP) who follows him or her throughout the entire eight weeks of treatment. The therapy approach utilized is Isometric Progressive Resistance Oropharyngeal (I-PRO) therapy facilitated by the Swallow STRONG® device. This is a quantitative approach to oropharyngeal strengthening, based in the core principles of exercise physiology derived from the sports medicine literature. The device includes a custom-molded mouthpiece with embedded pressure sensors.

There are two required in-person clinic visits during which Veterans see the SLP, a nurse or respiratory therapist, and a dietician. The patient's respiratory status is monitored by the nurse or respiratory therapist allowing for quick identification of any associated illness. The dietitian assesses nutritional status and makes dietary adjustments and recommendations to maximize nutritional intake while effectively managing dysphagia. This unique combination of providers allows us to treat dysphagia more comprehensively.

Tracking a variety of outcomes occurs over the course of treatment. Functional swallowing changes are quantified using videofluoroscopic swallow evaluations at baseline and at final (eight week) appointments. Penetration-aspiration scale scores representing airway invasion and oropharyngeal residue (material left in the mouth/throat after the swallow) ratings are measured for each swallow. A dietary intake questionnaire is administered and Functional Oral Intake Scale (FOIS) scores are derived to quantify level of oral intake. Patients also complete a dysphagia-specific Swallowing

Quality of Life survey (SWAL-QOL) and rate items related to swallowing symptoms and effort related to swallowing using a visual-analog scale.

Replicability

Specific factors that contributed to successful implementation of the Swallow STRONG program in Madison VAMC and our four expansion sites include dedicated clinicians, support from hospital leadership, referrals from primary providers, and dissemination of clinic outcomes to other VAs and hospital providers. A high number of severe and chronically dysphagic patients are treated by speech pathologists across VAs and private sector hospitals. Not all of these patients respond positively to standard of care dysphagia treatment. To replicate this program in other facilities, there would need to continue to be adequate staffing. Two of our expansion sites were able to implement and sustain this program with low staffing needs. Without continued tracking of outcomes, this program can be easily implemented by existing staff with the only necessary costs being the purchasing of devices and mouthpieces. To continue the multi-disciplinary approach to dysphagia management while minimizing time dedicated to the program, bimonthly team meetings could be set up in place of all clinicians being present at each in-person visit for patients enrolled.

Considering improved patient outcomes and substantial projected cost savings provided by this program, the costs to its further dissemination throughout VA system are quite low. In addition, Swallow Solutions, LLC administrators would consider a price reduction for bulk orders, which would provide additional cost savings. The expansion of this program to three additional sites over three years (with the Cincinnati VA site added in FY 2016) supports that this program can be successfully disseminated to additional sites, thereby demonstrating cost-effective replication.

Recognition

Megan Light, David Crawford, Suzanne Roscher, Kathy Groves, Jill Zielinski, JoAnne Robbins, Ken Shay, Karen Massey, Susan Kloss

Impact of a Pharmacist-Managed Heart Failure Post-Discharge (Bridge) Clinic for Veterans

Michael Brenner, Pharm.D. BCPS-AQ Cardiology, CPS

VA Ann Arbor Healthcare System, Ann Arbor, MI
michael.brenner@va.gov

The Heart Failure (HF) post-discharge clinic is a pharmacist-run clinic that was implemented to reduce readmission rates for HF. Patients admitted for HF exacerbation, as a primary or secondary diagnosis, or a new diagnosis during the recent hospitalization, are seen in the clinic within 7–10 days after discharge.

Introduction

A Veteran was seen in the Heart Failure Post-Discharge Clinic six days after a recent hospital admission for HF exacerbation. He presented to clinic with no change in symptoms due to fluid retention since his recent hospitalization. His ability to perform daily activities was limited due to shortness of breath. He had fluid retention in his abdomen and from his lower extremities up to his thighs. He was frustrated because he attempted to improve his symptoms by making lifestyle modifications. It appeared that perhaps he was released too soon from the clinic and was at high risk for readmission. In clinic, his diuretic was changed to a different agent in the same class when it was discovered he had a suboptimal diuretic response. When he followed up several weeks later, his symptoms significantly improved and he felt back at his baseline after losing 15 pounds of fluid. He no longer experienced shortness of breath unless he walked at a brisk pace. He was able to increase his physical activity and perform daily activities. His ability to become more independent and less reliant on his sister significantly increased.

Implementing the HF post-discharge clinic has made a significant impact to Veterans and caregivers. In this clinic, Veterans are given close follow-up to ensure they receive optimal care and extensive education to understand the importance of reducing hospitalizations and improving survival. The clinic has captured patients who are on the path toward a HF readmission within a short timeframe after hospital discharge as well as patients who were perhaps released too early.

Key Information

Beginning in 2010, the HF cardiologist and I came up with the idea to implement a HF post-discharge clinic to address the higher than average rate of HF readmissions at our facility. We both met with the chief of cardiology, chief of ambulatory care, and chief of internal medicine. Once the support was received, data on a subset of patients was collected as a pilot before we officially went forward. A consult was created and implemented into CPRS. Meetings took place with different internal medicine physicians and care coordinators for each medicine team so that when this patient population was identified in the hospital, the consult could be generated during the hospital admission. Promotion of the clinic included face-to-face and emailed detailing, presentations at morning report with the internal medicine teams, and meetings with cardiology fellows, chief residents, and nurse care coordinators. The clinic was officially implemented at the beginning of 2011. Frequent HF hospitalizations diminish quality of life and increase reliance on family members and financial burden to families, and can lead to mortality. In addition to the impact to the patient, HF also increases health care costs, hospital readmission rates, and average length of stay, and decreases hospital bed availability. This clinic sought to be a solution to those problems at VA Ann Arbor Healthcare System (HCS).

Context

VA Ann Arbor HCS is a level 1A tertiary care facility located in Ann Arbor, MI, and a part of the newly consolidated VISN 10. It is a teaching hospital with close ties to the University of Michigan Medical Center located just down the street. The cardiology section at VA Ann Arbor Healthcare System provides specialty care for Veterans who receive PC in Ann Arbor as well as other VA hospitals throughout the state of Michigan and northwest Ohio. Subspecialty clinics are limited at other VA facilities in Michigan, especially for HF. Since many patients come to the HF clinic from other VA hospitals, it was becoming increasingly difficult to accommodate patients in the existing HF clinics within a short timeframe after a hospital admission. An increase in the time to follow up has been shown to increase the risk for hospital readmission. Developing the HF post-discharge clinic has allowed the patients to receive attention in a shorter period and reduced hospital readmission rates within 30 days.

Practice Description

The HF post-discharge clinic is a pharmacist-run clinic that was implemented at VA Ann Arbor HCS to reduce readmission rates for HF. Patients admitted for HF exacerbation, as a primary or secondary diagnosis, or a new diagnosis of HF during the recent hospitalization, are seen in the clinic within seven to ten days after discharge. Clinic occurs one-half day per week and visits are 60 minutes per patient. The pharmacist interviews each patient to address the reason for the recent hospital admission, assess current symptoms and lifestyle, and provide medication reconciliation. Once all the information is collected, these patients are discussed with our HF attending to confirm the assessment and plan. The HF cardiologist answers any patient questions. The pharmacist then makes medication adjustments and recommends appropriate monitoring parameters when indicated. Patients are followed by the pharmacist via face-to-face or telephone until patients are established or seen in the HF or general cardiology clinic.

The HF post-discharge clinic has been successful based on a reduction of 30-day readmission rates and death compared to usual care. Usual care was defined as a patient who received follow-up in the pre-existing HF clinics or by a PCP. Time to follow-up was significantly shorter in patients who attended the post-discharge clinic (11 ± 6 vs. 20 ± 23 days, p<0.0001), and time to first all-cause readmission trended longer in the post-discharge clinic group (41 ± 19 vs. 34 ± 25 days, p=0.11). There was no difference in 90-day death and all-cause readmission between groups (p=0.12). However, risk-adjusted 30-day death and all-cause readmission was significantly lower in patients who attended post-discharge clinic after discharge (10 vs. 22 events, adjusted HR 0.40, 95 percent CI 0.19-0.86, p=0.02). The most common pharmacist interventions made in the post-discharge clinic were adding medications (42 percent) and stopping medications (39 percent); possible adverse drug effects were identified in 28 percent of post-discharge clinic patients.

Replicability

This clinic was established to attempt to lower readmission rates for Veterans with HF and improve access to care, thus supporting our mission of Veteran-centered care. The success of this clinic was due to the support of our HF cardiologist, the chief of cardiology, HF providers, chief of ambulatory care, and chief of internal medicine and due to the buy-in from key players on the inpatient side of the house. The clinic was successful in recruiting patients as the inpatient providers saw the ease of placing a consult to the service and ensuring that care was available post-discharge. The consults could often be scheduled prior to the patient even leaving the hospital, which increased patient satisfaction and comfort at the time of discharge.

Gathering support from administration and colleagues based on hospital data are vital to implementing a pharmacist-run post-discharge clinic. In addition, close communication with different sections within the hospital has been a key component to the success of the clinic and ensuring that everyone is on the same page. In order for this to be replicated in other facilities, clinic space, availability to see patients in a short timeframe, available support staff, a cardiologist, and a clinical pharmacist with advanced knowledge in HF would need to be in place.

Recognition

Scott Hummel

Pharmacy Pain eConsult

Abigail Brooks, PharmD, BCPS, CPS in Pain Management; Christine Vartan, PharmD, BCPS, CPS in Pain Management

West Palm Beach VAMC, West Palm Beach, FL
abigail.brooks@va.gov

The Pharmacy Pain electronic consult (eConsult) service allows PCPs to consult a Pain CPS for assistance with various chronic pain management requests. The Pharmacy Pain eConsult service has increased timely access to pain management specialists.

Introduction

The Pharmacy Pain electronic consult (eConsult) service allows PCPs to consult a Pain CPS for assistance with various chronic pain management requests. The eConsult service has grown over the years and the workload has provided justification for a second Pain CPS. A Pharmacy Residency project completed in 2013 found that there were 288 Pain eConsults placed during the period of July through December 2013; this number has increased more than trifold with 1,122 Pain eConsults placed from July through December 2015. Additionally, in 2013, a majority (74 percent) of PCPs surveyed indicated overall satisfaction with the Pain eConsult with time and access cited as the most important factors for determining their overall satisfaction. The Pharmacy Pain eConsult service has continued to be a very efficient practice for the West Palm Beach VAMC and the Veterans served by the facility. Increasing access to pain management specialists in a timely manner continues to be the driving force behind the success of the Pain eConsult service.

Key Information

The West Palm Beach VAMC's Pharmacy Pain eConsult service started in 2013 in response to the overwhelming need for pain management guidance from PCPs. Prior to implementation, PCPs were consulting with Pain CPSs via curbside consult or telephone calls. Stakeholders in the development of the eConsult service included the Pharmacy Service, specifically the CPS in pain management, the Physical Medicine and Rehabilitation service (which includes the Chronic Pain Clinic), and the PC service.

Context

The West Palm Beach VAMC serves Veterans from a seven county area in southeastern Florida, with 64,467 Veterans served in FY 2014. In addition to the main medical center in West Palm Beach, a number of services are offered to patients in six CBOCs. The West Palm Beach VAMC also has 149 acute inpatient beds as well as a 120-bed Community Living Center and 15-bed Blind Rehabilitation Center. A large number (31 percent) of Veterans served by the West Palm Beach VAMC are between the ages of 65–74 years old and served in Vietnam (35 percent), with Veterans from WWII and other conflict eras served as well. The Pharmacy Pain eConsult service was developed to streamline requests from PCPs for pain management assistance and provide recommendations directly in the patient's chart.

Practice Description

The service was set up for the pain management CPS to facilitate specific provider needs for chronic pain patients, including 1) querying the Florida Prescription Drug Monitoring Program (PDMP), 2) opioid dosing conversions, 3) opioid tapering, 4) drug screen interpretation, 5) non-opioid pharmacotherapy recommendations, and 6) opioid pharmacotherapy recommendations.

A full and extensive chart review is completed for both non-opioid and opioid pharmacotherapy recommendations, including past medical history, previous medication trials, previous chronic pain non-pharmacotherapy treatments, social history, mental health treatment history, and potential drug interactions. The most complicated patients are typically discussed with a physician in either the Pain Clinic or Physical Medicine and Rehabilitation service. Opioid Safety Initiative (OSI) parameters are referenced frequently in the consult assessment and recommendations, which reinforces the most important clinical rationale to providers who are not specialists in chronic pain. Ideally, this information is then disseminated and explained to the patient on a more basic level by the provider. Pending the outcome of the chart review, recommendations may go beyond just medications but also may include recommendations for physical therapy, chiropractor or acupuncture evaluation, pain psychology, or other necessary services. Occasionally, patients will be referred to the Pain Clinic for a full evaluation and then followed by the pain management CPS.

Replicability

The Pharmacy Pain eConsult service was developed based on frequently asked questions by PCPs who requested assistance with pain management. With this service, the consult is implemented directly into CPRS. A similar consult can, and has been, implemented at other VA facilities using consult categories appropriate for the needs of the facility.

Recognition

Mitchell Nazario, Ramon Cuevas-Trisán, John Meléndez-Benabe, Nick Beckey, Hiroko Forbes

Modified Early Warning Scores and White Blood Cells

Dawn Harris, MSN, RN-BC, CNL, VHA LHC YB, VHA-CM
North Florida/South Georgia Veterans Health System, Gainesville, FL
dawn.harris@va.gov

The Modified Early Warning Score (MEWS) and White Blood Cells (WBC) is a tool implemented at the Malcom Randall and Lake City VAMCs to recognize early signs of clinical deterioration and sepsis in patients.

Introduction

MEWS is a tool used by hospitals to recognize early signs of clinical deterioration in patients. In addition, the tool is used to initiate early interventions and management by increasing nursing attention, informing the provider, and activating a rapid response call and/or code blue team. The MEWS tool involves assigning a numeric value to several physiologic parameters, such as the blood pressure, heart rate, temperature, respiratory rate, and level of consciousness also known as the Alert, Voice, Pain, and Unresponsive (AVPU) scale. In addition, adding WBC to the MEWS was identified as another parameter to recognize early signs of sepsis in patients. These parameters help to derive a composite score that is used to identify patients at risk for clinical decline.

A positive MEWS score greater than three has been associated with poor patient outcomes. The purpose of integrating MEWS + WBC with CRPS/VistA is to provide staff with a report and clinical reminders to assist with timely management of patients and increase nursing awareness and knowledge of recognizing early signs of clinical deterioration.

Key Information

The MEWS and WBC promising practice was led by Dawn Harris, MSN, RN, Clinical Nurse Leader, by implementing a MEWS Committee to develop an action plan utilizing evidence-based practice to improve the current practice. Russell Jacobitz, BSN, RN, Clinical Applications Coordinator, played an integral part in the technical development of the VistA MEWS database to build a report and clinical reminders in CPRS.

MEWS was initially implemented and piloted for two months from May to July 2014 on 3 West, a 30-bed medical-surgical telemetry unit. A MEWS report was established by Clinical Informatics that automatically calculated the MEWS score of three or greater for patients identified as positive. The report was printed by the charge nurse after vitals are taken. Nurses then assessed the patient and notified the provider for interventions, as needed. In August 2014, MEWS was initiated in the Malcolm Randall VAMC and Lake City VAMC medical-surgical units. Processes were developed on how, when, and who would print the MEWS report which have been sustained. Additional processes included adding clinical reminders to the patient's chart to serve as another visual aid for nursing staff, creating a MEWS template to document interventions and monitor progress, and staff education. In January 2015, MEWS + WBC were implemented to identify early recognition of sepsis in patients.

Context

MEWS was initiated at the Malcom Randall and Lake City VAMCs due to various clinical practice problems. There was a lack of recognition from staff to identify early signs of clinical deterioration in patients regarding physiological parameters, such as changes in vital signs, level of consciousness, and sepsis. This has been an ongoing issue due to poor communication, lack of follow-up among clinical staff, and poor assessment skills regarding trends in parameters. Although nurses are ultimately responsible for reviewing vitals, many times they become overwhelmed due to the acuity of patients and overlook trends that may indicate a possible decline in a patient's condition. As a result, many patients were being transferred to a higher level of care for issues that could have been addressed if early signs of changes were identified and treated in a timely manner.

Replicability

Replication of this practice for others would need to include strong collaboration with Clinical Informatics, Nursing/Physician leadership, and ongoing communication.

Recognition

Russell Jacobitz, Michael Ross, Andreas Zori, Sheneka Mortley, Julie Whitney, Stephanie Beckham, Ileana Koerner, Amy Manna, Michelle Williams, Carrol Graves

Fall Prevention Practice and Protocol Gap: Identifying Improvement Areas in Acute Care

Anastasia Rose, MEd, MSN/MHA, RN, CCRN-K
VA Portland Health Care System, Portland, OR
anastasia.rose@va.gov

This clinical project examined how fall prevention protocol recommendations were applied to Veteran inpatient practices, identifying areas to improve.

Introduction

Patient falls are the most common adverse event reported in hospitals and can lead to undesired outcomes, including, but not limited, to hospital-acquired injuries, prolonged hospital stays, medical complications, increase in health care cost, litigation, loss of confidence of mobility, disabilities, and increased mortality for elderly patients. Most falls are preventable and nurses play a critical role in identifying patients at risk for falling. Multi-component programs have shown to be effective in reducing falls. Some of the successful multi-factorial interventions include post fall review, patient education, staff education, footwear advice, and toileting.

The purpose of this quality improvement project was to understand current fall prevention practices on two acute care units at VA Portland Health Care System (HCS), to detect gaps between the hospital fall prevention protocol and actual work practices, and to identify areas for improvement.

Key Information

Two trained graduate-level RN VA Nursing Academic Partnerships (VANAP) faculty led this project. Information was collected from February to April 2015 on two medical-surgical units. The hospital fall prevention protocol issued in 2011 included the following initiatives: definition of a fall, interventions reflecting fall prevention standards of care for all patients, interventions for identified high fall-risk patients based on Morse Fall Scale score, patient education key points and materials, documentation standards, and post fall care. In 2015, the Fall Prevention Workgroup led by a medical-surgical Clinical Nurse Specialist (CNS) restructured fall prevention goals to integrate an individualized and interdisciplinary approach to fall prevention.

Context

VA Portland HCS is a 277-bed facility providing inpatient critical, acute, psychiatric, long-term, skilled, and hospice care on two campuses. VA Portland HCS annually serves approximately 85,000 Veterans in Oregon and southwest Washington. Veterans are a predominantly aging population. The risk for falls increases significantly with age and older adults are more likely to be injured from a fall. Veterans have a 25 percent greater chance of falling compared to the civilian sector. VA Portland HCS has historically underperformed when compared to national benchmarks for like facilities on falls with injury per 1,000 days of care. Preventing falls decreases hospital expenses by reducing length of stay and costs associated with the treatment of adverse effects.

Practice Description

Unit staff helped identify patients who were high risk for falls. Patients assigned bed alarms, safety attendants, or those assessed as being medically inappropriate did not participate in interviews. Project RNs conducted semi-structured patient interviews to obtain patients' understanding and perception toward fall prevention activities. As part of the interview, project RNs provided fall prevention education using the VA Portland HCS fall education brochure. Patients' room environments were also observed at the time of interview. The project RNs evaluated if Universal Fall Precautions were implemented and if any additional interventions were utilized for patients assessed to be at high risk for falling. Subsequent chart reviews examined the following factors: patient age, sex, admitting diagnosis, secondary diagnosis, recent Morse Fall Scale score, mental status, and documentation that patient education was completed by nurses. Environmental assessments were conducted for items noted in the fall prevention protocol.

Information was obtained from 37 Veterans: 20 patients from a medical-surgical unit and 17 patients from a vascular unit. The environmental assessment revealed variation in adherence to the fall prevention nursing protocol. For example, some recommendations had high adherence: more than 90 percent of patients had skid-free footwear and call-light within reach. Other recommendations had lower adherence: 60 percent of patients had urinals at bedside and 50 percent had a fall-risk sign posted outside of the room. The results indicate the largest areas for improvement were improving patient fall prevention education, patient environment of care, and nurse adherence to fall prevention protocol recommendations. Providing patient education that promotes patient engagement and informing nurses about gaps in fall prevention practices may be effective in strengthening the fall prevention program.

Replicability

We believe that the project findings will be informative to anyone who may be struggling with reduction of patient falls in an institutional setting. Our multi-method examination (observation, patient interview, chart review) of fall prevention practices can be used by nurses who want to identify practice gaps and improve fall rates in acute care settings.

Recognition

Hiroko Kiyoshi-Teo, Nicole Carter, United States Department of Veteran Affairs Office of Academic Affiliations, Office of Nursing Services VANAP Program

Redesigning Educational and Competency Requirements for Environmental Management Service

Karen DiDomenico, BSN, RN, Veteran Health Education Coordinator

VA Connecticut Healthcare System, West Haven, CT

karen.didomenico@va.gov

This educational program was developed to standardize training, ensure and maintain competency, and define the role of Environmental Management Service (EMS) Technician as an integral part of the patient-centered care team.

Introduction

The Operating Room (OR), Environmental Services, Emergency Medical Services, and Veteran Health Administration of Connecticut (VHACT) Leadership identified several challenges in standardizing the OR cleaning processes. The cleanliness of any OR is imperative for healthy patient outcomes and seamless management of OR patient flow. These departments in conjunction with the Hospital Education Department addressed the challenges utilizing evidence-based information and practices from VHA facilities across the nation. Utilizing the VHA VEIN (VA Educators Integrated Network), the VHA national education email group and the wonderful consul of an EMS education specialist from St. Louis, a plan was organized.

The core work group consisted of the OR Nurse Manager, EMS leadership, the Hospital Education team, and the generous efforts of the consultant. A total system/department review revealed the need for standard operating procedures (SOPs), reinstituting cleaning checklists, and incremental EMS staff. Nursing and Hospital Education took the lead role in seeing this project to fruition. A new position, the EMS Clinical Educator, was created and filled by a RN. The EMS Clinical Educator included the Infection Control Department to round out the necessary expert knowledge needed to accomplish the task. The group utilized the practices from similar hospitals, and the Association of perioperative Registered Nurses set standards to write SOPs, develop EMS staff competencies, and create a certification program, which all EMS employees must "graduate." As the program evolved, the procedures, education, and SOPs were generalized to departments besides the OR, such as Interventional Radiology, Endoscopy, and the Catheterization Lab. The process became known as the Environmental Management Service University. Over the past two years, 70 staff have profited from the University program.

Cleanliness outcomes were measured via a patient satisfaction survey (Survey of Health Care Experience with Patients (SHEP) scores) and OR cleanliness monitoring by the nurse manager and nursing supervisors. The baseline SHEP score was 54 percent which was below the national average. Post educational intervention the SHEP score has improved to 79 percent which is above the national Veteran satisfaction average.

Key Information

EMS University came to fruition on day four and five of New Employee Orientation week by the EMS educator in response to an insufficient orientation for EMS staff. EMS University originated at VA Connecticut Healthcare System (HCS) and included all new EMS staff from both West Haven and Newington campuses. The EMS educator collaborates with Nursing Service, Safety Office, EMS leadership, and Infection Prevention. The development of these programs help support the reduction in hospital-acquired infections, provide staff with an improved perspective of the workplace, and increase employee engagement from EMS staff.

Context

VA Connecticut HCS is a level 1a medical center that provides both inpatient and outpatient care to Veterans and their families. VA Connecticut HCS has seven OR suites, Post-Anesthesia Care, Ambulatory Procedures, Endoscopy, Cardiac Catheterization, Interventional Radiology, Mental Health Services, Medical Emergency Room (ER), Psychiatric Emergency Room (ER), Rehabilitative services, Blind Rehabilitation Program, Community Living Center, Cancer Center, PC, Specialty Care, and Recreational and Integrative approaches to health care. The challenge of providing a healthy environment of care in all of these arenas is addressed in EMS University. The practices directly improved the environment of care and infection control practices. EMS University and the OR certification and competency program contribute to the overarching goal of zero hospital-acquired infections created by cleaning deficiencies.

Practice Description

The initial step in the process was to bring the content expert from the St. Louis VAMC to VA Connecticut HCS to validate the competency of the EMS clinical instructor. Together they were able to perform the initial competency validation of supervisors, including the Acting Chief of EMS, and EMS staff who were assigned to the OR. A competency schedule was identified in order to maintain competency of EMS staff assigned to the OR. All EMS OR staff, including supervisors, is competency validated initially and at the following intervals: one month, three months, and then annually while assigned to the OR. This process is completed in collaboration with the OR leadership to identify rooms available for cleaning and reviewing the results after a cleaning has been completed.

EMS University entailed the development of a comprehensive curriculum, to include all learning, tasks, and skills necessary to perform the duties assigned. The EMS instructor obtained the necessary equipment, including a housekeeping cart. Ultimately, EMS University has succeeded due to the dedication, support, and collaboration of all involved in meeting the common goal of improving environmental services.

Replicability

Both EMS University and the OR certification process were adopted, because of an Office of Inspector General (OIG) inspection and citations. Overall, the organization was determined to improve cleaning and infection prevention outcomes. The EMS service line was under-resourced and lacked SOPs and competencies. Given these factors, the organization's leadership was motivated to improve environmental cleaning. VA Connecticut HCS now maintains procedures, policies, and checklists that can be made available to any other VA facility. In addition, staffing requirements, to assure sufficient human resources are available to achieve these outcomes, can be shared. At this time, VA Connecticut HCS has been visited by both the Boston and Providence EMS representatives, who have met with the local EMS educator to share the program elements and outcomes. VA Boston HCS has adopted the EMS clinical instructor role (one FTE).

Recognition

Randolph Torralba, Karen Didomenico, Suzanne Teixeira

Improving Moderate Sedation Practice: Real-Time Documentation, Electronic Forms and Simulation Learning Technique

Candace Nowlin, MSN, Nurse Educator

Ralph H. Johnson Medical Center, Charleston, SC
candace.nowlin@va.gov

Our interdisciplinary team applied lean and VA system engineering methodologies to transform our current moderate sedation documentation process in the ED, defining our workflow from the bottom up. We provided training using high-fidelity simulation resulting in improved organizational and Veteran outcomes.

Introduction

A 35-year-old OEF/OIF Veteran arrives via ambulance to the ED having sustained a dislocated shoulder from falling from a five-foot ladder. This is a common scenario, whereby physicians and nurses need high levels of knowledge, training, and competence in Moderate Sedation Procedures (MSPs); this both assists the patient back to his/her baseline functional status and alleviates pain in a safe manner. Moderate Sedation is a method in which a team of health care professionals uses sedating agents to diagnose or treat patients effectively; in the majority of cases, the patient is able to go home a couple of hours after the procedure. Through an analysis and comparison of our current practice and evidence-based/best practices in MSPs, our leadership team sought an opportunity to improve our practice utilizing the most recent standards of care related to MSPs. Moderate Sedation is considered a high-risk procedure requiring constant patient surveillance by the health care team. Moderate Sedation also offers a more humane approach than pain medication alone in many instances. It is also an alternate for general anesthesia in some instances, especially if general anesthesia is too risky. The ED leadership team and education faculty had rising concerns in regard to previous issues in Moderate Sedation use related to the following: 1) a very small area on forms for documenting pertinent patient information; 2) an inability to track paper documents retrospectively; and 3) documents that were missing crucial elements of Moderate Sedation according to Joint Commission (JC), American Society of Anesthesiologists and VHA Directives 1039 & 1073.

New electronic templates in CRPS, the core electronic record in the broader VistA platform, allow for hard-stops, which are user-friendly. CPRS templates designed by the team contain up-to-date components of MSP standards of care with critical components for pre-procedure, intra-procedural, and post-procedural assessments. Future outcomes related to patient satisfaction, improved pain control, ease of documentation for staff, and decreased length of stay in the ED are intended to exceed previous outcomes for Veterans receiving MSPs.

Key Information

MSPs occur frequently at Ralph H. Johnson VAMC and require highly trained and competent staff, proper equipment, and guidelines for safe practice. Examples of procedures that may utilize MSPs are cardiac catheterizations, reduction of dislocations, foreign body removals, or endoscopic exams.

The facility continues to be a Five-Star facility in the southeast US, and continuously drives to use research and innovative approaches to improve care for its patients. A Team Systems Coach assisted core team members using TeamSTEPPS® to improve processes for Moderate Sedation from January 2016 to March 2016. Nineteen rapid experiments were performed by the Simulation expert and Nurse Educator to include real-time charting and use of high-fidelity manikins. Pre-assessments, intra-procedural and post-procedural assessments were documented containing all the critical elements included on the new electronic forms in CPRS. Training of ED staff occurred over a three-week period, which included one-hour sessions of completing the electronic documentation records, simulation of MSPs, other didactic training modules, and some one-to-one training if needed. Our "Go Live" date for changes in MSP in the ED was announced and documentation thus far has been captured at 100 percent in the electronic records with all the necessary components to promote safe patient care related to Moderate Sedation. The ED goal is to be in 100 percent compliance with documentation that is now electronic versus paper forms that can be lost, and/or difficult to read.

Context

The Ralph H. Johnson VAMC serves Veterans residing in the southeast corridor, coastal South Carolina, and portions of coastal Georgia. The ED was the piloted area for the new practice guidelines, including electronic, real-time charting, and all the JC criteria for charting.

The Ralph H. Johnson VAMC is a 145-bed primary, secondary, and tertiary care medical center that provides acute medical, surgical, and psychiatric inpatient care, and both primary and specialized outpatient services in southeastern South Carolina and Chatham County, GA. The VAMC supports the Vet Centers in North Charleston, SC, and Savannah, GA, and operates the outpatient clinics in Savannah, GA, and Myrtle Beach, SC. Currently, the medical center is operating 98 beds and a 20-bed nursing home.

The medical center is closely affiliated with the Medical University of South Carolina (MUSC) and supports 84 resident FTEs in medical and dental specialties, as well students from nursing, pharmacy, social work, and allied health disciplines. Charleston VAMC is a partnership site for VA Nursing Academy in collaboration with the MUSC School of Nursing. The Research Service has more than 100 research investigators involved in more than 300 research projects. The ED tends to approximately 25,000 patients annually, operates 24 hours/day, seven days a week, and accepts ambulances from three surrounding counties adjacent to Charleston Harbor.

Practice Description

Collaboration began among team members using True Lean form. Current practices, paper forms, equipment, policies, and protocols were examined and compared to best practices and research related to MSPs. The team leaders involved in the implementation plan consisted of a nurse educator, simulation coordinator, and clinical applications coordinator. A gap analysis was performed utilizing JC standards, American Society of Anesthesiologists standards and VHA Directives related to Moderate Sedation. It was realized that our practice needed to be more precise and documentation should be in real time and contain all the elements required for Moderate Sedation. Medications used for MSPs could be lethal, may cause respiratory arrest, or may lead to circulatory collapse if meticulous surveillance, documentation, and training were not in place in the future. The implementation plan to executive leadership included all areas of the hospital that used Moderate Sedation. Nurse educators, ED physicians, ED clinical nurse leader, ED nursing management, and nursing staff participated in meetings, emails, training sessions, and equipment review. All emergency staff participated in simulation learning that successfully demonstrated patient assessments and critical elements for documentation of MSPs. The ED at Ralph H. Johnson took a lead in best practices for MSP, using EHRs and updating best practices.

Replicability

Updates in Moderate Sedation have improved our documentation and procedures to an elevated standard of care. A team approach, including leadership, education, and staff made it possible to execute the implementation plan. The management team was committed to improving care in this aspect of documentation and is progressive with utilizing sophisticated health technology. Other clinical areas of the facility or other VA facilities could easily adopt the electronic forms with critical elements of evidence-based practices in MSP. Embracing change is often difficult in any organization but is much easier with stakeholder buy-in. Leadership, teamwork, thinking outside of the box, and daring to be creative produced success for the ED team with the help of education, leadership, an informatics nurse, and a systems redesign coach.

Recognition

ED staff

Antibiotic Follow-Up Telephone Calls

Gloriann Watson, PharmD, Chief, Pharmacy Service

VA Pacific Islands Healthcare System, Honolulu, HI
gloriann.watson@va.gov

VA Pacific Islands Healthcare System (VAPIHCS) instituted a new practice of reaching out via telephone to Veterans receiving antibiotic prescriptions in a manner that allows direct patient contact, notwithstanding the vast, thousands-of-square-mile expanse of the geographic region we serve.

Introduction

In FY 2015, VAPIHCS instituted a new practice of reaching out via telephone to Veterans receiving antibiotic prescriptions. The practice has allowed us to enhance access particularly for Veterans with limited resources who live in rural areas, including those in Guam and American Samoa.

Of the Veterans we contacted through this practice, 12 percent identified an issue or concern with their medication. Pharmacy Service staff have been able to assist these Veterans with their concerns, which otherwise may have gone unaddressed, in a timely way. Of the Veterans called, 95 percent acknowledged their appreciation of the follow-up call. Interestingly, of the 5 percent who did not, 12 percent reported having an issue with the medication they received, which our staff was then able to address. While utilized for those receiving antibiotics, our practice is not uniquely suited to antibiotics. Subject to resource allocation, a similar practice can be implemented across any range of drugs or services with equal success.

Key Information

We adopted the practice of telephonically contacting each antibiotic recipient in FY 2015 and have continued the practice into FY 2016. Although there were initially some reservations from Pharmacy Staff because of the added responsibilities and doubts regarding efficacy, the feedback from the clinical pharmacists more than a year into the practice has been uniformly positive. Staff has been amazed at the impact the follow-up calls have made. We also incentivized the practice by rewarding the clinical pharmacists who made the most calls with a 59-minute time off award, which created a healthy competition for all. Moreover, Veterans have directly expressed their appreciation for the concerns expressed by staff and for the opportunity to learn more about the drugs they are taking. While usually efficacious, antibiotics are not without risks, including Clostridium difficile (C.difficile) infection, allergic reactions, and the development of tendinitis and/or resistance. It is our responsibility as Pharmacists to ensure our Veterans are taking their medications correctly and responsibly.

Context

VAPIHCS provides outpatient medical and mental health care through its Ambulatory Care Clinic on Oahu (Honolulu) and through seven CBOCs, including West Oahu, Hawaii (Hilo and Kona), Maui, Kauai, American Samoa, Guam, and Saipan. Long-term care, inpatient mental health care and residential PTSD services are also provided. The expanse of care coverage across the Pacific exceeds the size of the contiguous 48 states and crosses three time zones. The facility and the Pharmacy Service, in particular, are committed to providing high-quality care to Veterans throughout our region of responsibility, including even the far-reaching rural areas.

Practice Description

When a Veteran receives an antibiotic from the outpatient pharmacy, the clinical pharmacist, pharmacy resident, or pharmacy student provides on-the-spot medication consultation at the front window. Within three days, a follow-up telephone call is made to reconnect with the Veteran, to ensure that the antibiotic is being administered and stored correctly, to inquire regarding any adverse effects, and to confirm that the Veteran is aware of the available pharmacy and emergency resources should the need arise. We also remind the Veteran of the importance of finishing the antibiotic course, even if relief (or even resolution) has already been experienced. Before concluding the call, we invite questions and address any Veteran concerns.

Replicability

We adopted this practice because Pharmacists are partners in drug safety. Medications improve quality of life for many Veterans, but also pose serious risks. Although we provide medication consultation at the time of dispensation, patients may be overwhelmed by the amount of information provided at once and in a public place, which may lead to an incomplete understanding. Providing a follow-up telephone call a few days later, after the Veteran has had an opportunity to begin administering the antibiotic, and while the Veteran is in the comfort and privacy of his/her home, can lead to a better understanding of the importance of their medication and improve adherence.

This practice also gives pharmacists, pharmacy residents, and pharmacy students in the outpatient pharmacy some time away from their prescription verification and checking responsibilities to use their extensive education and experience to teach our Veterans about their medications, to address any concerns, and to build confidence and relationships for the future.

Recognition

VAPIHCS

Zoster Immunization Transport to the Veteran's Home: A New Standard of Practice for Veteran-Centered Care

Ruby Wood, RN-BC, MSN, MBA, CHPN, Nurse Manager HBPC

VA Eastern Kansas Health Care System, Leavenworth, KS

ruby.wood@va.gov

This Veteran-centered practice addresses safe transport of zoster vaccine to the homes of rural Veterans to reduce the incidence of shingles. We purchased a vaccine transport system, developed policies, trained nurses, and implemented this progressive, preventive program in FY 2016.

Introduction

Home Based Primary Care (HBPC) nurses provide all types of immunizations, but prior to this project, homebound Veterans in rural remote areas did not have access to zoster immunization for the prevention of shingles unless they traveled to the nearest VAMC, which could take an hour. The current guidelines also posed a barrier to care due to the 30-minute stability window after the vaccine is reconstituted, after which time it loses potency.

In evaluating this challenge, a team of nurses and pharmacists researched information about possible ways to improve this situation. The team learned that the experts at Merck Manufacturing recommend reconstituting the zoster vaccine upon removal from the freezer. We also learned that the zoster vaccine could be stored and/or transported at refrigerator temperature (between 36°F and 46°F) up to 72 hours prior to reconstitution. The team identified a special vaccine transport carrier that maintains the stable recommended temperature for 12 hours, and is supported by scientific evidence.

The HBPC team implemented the zoster vaccine project in January 2016 and has provided zoster immunizations to Veterans in five service areas with no adverse effects. Our Veterans benefitted from reduced risk for contracting shingles. We continue to collect data to monitor for future cases of shingles in Veterans who were immunized following the implementation of the new standard of practice. Veterans benefitted because more clinic time opened up for those in need of service. The zoster vaccine project could also decrease the pharmacy cost by decreasing the waste of unused reconstituted vaccine.

Key Information

This standard of practice was shared with other HBPC programs, along with policies, immunization standard of practice, safe transport container guidelines, competencies for immunizations, EpiPen Auto-Injectors®, and nursing education guidelines. My team implemented the project at the Eastern Kansas Health Care System (EKHCS) VA Leavenworth and Topeka campuses beginning in January 2016. I led the project, collaborating with staff nurses from HBPC and pharmacists. This project is making a difference in the quality of life for all Veterans that can avoid a shingles eruption, which causes uncomfortable disabling symptoms that wax and wane for months after a breakout.

Context

EKHCS VA is a Midwest facility with two campuses an hour apart. We serve approximately 37,000 Veterans in urban and rural areas. Some of the Veterans on our panel have a history of homelessness, low income, and are underserved. In the HBPC program, we serve 310 geriatric Veterans with many chronic illnesses, and some have barriers to accessing care, such as undependable transportation, being homebound due to illness, and addiction issues, including drugs or alcohol. Several of the Veterans on the HBPC panel have been on service for several years, due to the stability provided by the HBPC interdisciplinary team. They come to rely on the team for most of the care provided to improve their health, including immunizations.

Practice Description

The practice is about safely transporting zoster immunization directly to the home of the Veteran to reduce the incidence of shingles. The team gathered facts about immunizations from the Centers for Disease Control and Prevention website and research articles, and via interviews with Merck Manufacturing and McKesson Transport Company. The group met weekly and compiled resources to write policies and protocols, and put together a proposal to discuss with the Pharmacy and Therapeutics Committee (P&T) and our medical staff providers. Both groups accepted and approved the project and encourage our team to move forward. We selected nursing team leaders as immunization champions, and they assisted with completing nursing competencies and setting up Microsoft Excel spreadsheets for data gathering.

Replicability

This project was successful due to the persistence of our nurses and the pharmacists working many hours to ensure a great outcome. This project had great support from the beginning from physicians who understand the importance of immunizations and the barriers that Veterans face accessing care. We will share this project with all HBPC programs nationally after more data is gathered. It should be very easy to replicate at any VA facility, and the team will share all resources and experiences encountered with the project.

Recognition

Jennifer Thomas, Roselle Schanker, Tracy Jo McCombs, Kathy Overmyer, Kelli Christy, Barbara Burklund, David Elcock, Susan Parks

Personal Health Planning Process

Elizabeth Recupero, DO, PC Physician

VA Boston Healthcare System, Jamaica Plain, MA
elizabeth.recupero@va.gov

The Personal Health Planning (PHP) Process is a patient-centered approach to PC that incorporates Veterans' goals and values while at the same time addressing their health and well-being.

Introduction

A 30-year-old OEF/OIF Veteran presented to my clinic for his annual exam. He reported feeling depressed and angry at his life since his discharge from the US Army. He had gained a significant amount of weight (70 pounds), and was feeling like a failure in life. He told me, "Everyone sees me as a fat guy and not a war hero." I used the Whole Health Review of Systems (WHROS) to assess the areas of his self-care, as well as his values and beliefs. I discovered that he was a husband and father of three young children. He was attending college as a full-time student and delivering pizza at night to support his family. Interestingly, this Veteran told me that he and his family "lived on pizza" as it was a free and easy meal.

Using the organizing principles of the PHP Process, I worked with this Veteran to create shared goals, which we then transformed into a personal health goal. This Veteran was able to say to me, "I will not eat pizza." This was the starting point of his Specific, Measurable, Achievable, Relevant, Time-Bound (SMART) goal. I arranged for monthly follow-up appointments with our clinic LPN for a weigh-in as well as health coaching around weight loss.

Each month, our LPN would report that this Veteran was making significant progress and that I would be impressed with how well he was succeeding. When he came to the clinic four months later, I was astonished with his success. He had lost 30 pounds, and not only was he "not eating pizza," he was eating healthy snacks and meals, exercising daily, and most impressive to me he had included his children in his lifestyle changes. His "daddy-time" was spent cooking healthy meals and doing exercise and sports with his children. He told me that I changed his life. I told him that he did that all on his own; I had merely asked him if he could give up pizza.

Key Information

The PHP Process, which encompasses all of Whole Health and Patient-Centered Care, is used during new and follow-up PC visits. Early patient feedback has demonstrated a high level of satisfaction among Veterans who experience this process. There is also a high level of provider satisfaction.

Context

We serve an urban Veteran population that includes both men and women across multiple PC practices. Our goal was to increase patient engagement to improve health outcomes. We were focusing on "changing the conversation" to adequately address the health and well-being of our Veterans with a focus on disease prevention by engaging Veterans in their own self-care.

Practice Description

This practice utilizes the entire team of providers and support staff within PC. Through patient-centered language, shared goal and agenda setting, Whole Health assessment, and health coaching, the entire PC Team works to engage Veterans in their health and well-care by activating them to become more involved in their own areas of self-care. The PHP Process is a simple model that involves four organizing principles: 1) Whole Health assessment; 2) shared goals; 3) personal health plan; and 4) skill building and support. For success, all members of the PC Team need to be involved in this model.

Replicability

Two years ago, three PC teams (provider, RN, LPN or health technician, and Medical Support Assistant (MSA)) were selected within VA Boston Healthcare System for a pilot in collaboration with the Office of Patient-Centered Care and Cultural Transformation. During the pilot, we developed a process that started with the exploration of patient values centered on health, assessing health behaviors across eight components of health, and culminating in setting personal health goals. This PHP process incorporated patient-centered communication to stimulate discussion on status of chronic conditions and health risks, and shared agenda setting and health goals (as defined by provider/team and patient) that aligned with their attitudes, beliefs, and values. We created new tools to facilitate this process: an introductory Whole Health patient brochure, a WHROS (combination of traditional and WHROS), and a personalized health plan summarizing health risks, shared goals, and personal health goal(s). Since January 2016, we have doubled the PACT teams involved and we are currently in the midst of spreading our work throughout all Boston VAMC PC clinics.

Commitment from executive and PC leadership is the most essential factor to the success that we had in spreading the PHP Process throughout VA Boston. Furthermore, PHP requires a team approach to patient care. Individual clinician coaching and observation with feedback to promote competency at goal setting is also required. This process also expands on the foundation that clinicians learn in training.

Recognition

The Office of Patient-Centered Care and Cultural Transformation, Mary Gallagher-Seaman, Whole Health Workgroup, Michael Charness, Jacqueline Spencer

Designated Women's Health Providers

Sally Haskell, MD, Deputy Chief Consultant, Women's Health Services

VACO, Washington, DC

sally.haskell@va.gov

Assignment of women Veterans to Designated Women's Health PC Providers has increased quality and satisfaction with VA care for women Veterans.

Introduction

PC for women Veterans is provided by a specially trained Designated Women's Health Provider (DWHP). DWHPs receive training to provide general PC and gender-specific care to women Veterans. To ensure that every woman Veteran has the opportunity to choose a DWHP, Women's Health Services (WHS) provides education and training in the unique health care needs of women Veterans (including post-deployment issues) through a Women's Health Mini-Residency program. Research has shown that quality of care and satisfaction increase when women receive care from a DWHP.

VA's External Peer Review Program (EPRP) is part of VA's quality performance process in which reviewers select monthly random samples of Veteran's health records to review for appropriate and timely preventive and chronic disease care. Using data from EPRP, Women's Health Researcher Dr. Bevanne Bean-Mayberry discovered an interesting and promising trend. Although all women Veterans had very high rates of receiving appropriate preventive care overall, Dr. Bean-Mayberry found that women assigned to a DWHP were even more likely to receive age-appropriate cervical cancer screening (94.4 percent vs. 91.9 percent) and breast cancer screening (86 percent vs. 83.3 percent) than women not assigned to a DWHP. Of note, women Veterans were more likely to receive breast and cervical cancer screenings than women who have Medicaid, Medicare, and commercial insurance.

Dr. Lori Bastian, another Women's Health Researcher, questioned whether an assignment to DWHPs changed women Veteran satisfaction with care. Dr. Bastian used data from VA Survey of Health Care Experience with Patients (SHEP), using the Consumer Assessment of Healthcare Providers and Systems (CAHPS) Patient-Centered Medical Home survey. The results found that women assigned to a DWHP had higher overall experiences with care compared to women assigned to other PCPs and, in addition, women assigned to DWHPs were more satisfied on six composite scores, including access, communication, shared decision making, self-management support, comprehensiveness, and office staff.

Key Information

To provide the highest quality of care, VA implemented a policy in 2010 that women Veterans be assigned to a DWHP who has either documented extensive experience or has continuing medical education credits in women's health. These physicians or advanced practice nurses are able to provide both routine PC and gender-specific care, in the context of a longitudinal provider-patient relationship.

VA now has DWHPs in every medical center and most CBOCs. Each health care system has a Women Veterans Program Manager (WVPM) and a Women's Health Medical Director/Champion responsible for overseeing the delivery of services to women Veterans. Additionally, each VISN has a WVPM VISN Lead responsible for coordinating women's health programs across the VISN. This system of care has improved quality and satisfaction among women Veterans.

Context

The population of women Veterans using VA health care has doubled in the last decade with over 600,000 women Veterans enrolled for VA health care in 2015. As a health care system that has historically provided care to a mostly male population, several years ago VHA found that some PCPs were not up-to-date in women's health, and there were gaps in women's care when they were referred from their PCPs to other providers for routine gender-specific care, such as Pap smears, contraceptive care, and menopausal management.

Practice Description

WHS has trained over 2,500 providers in women's health and is in the process of training additional providers to ensure that every woman Veteran has the opportunity to receive her PC from a DWHP. Approximately 70 percent of women Veterans are currently assigned to a DWHP.

Replicability

Since implementing policy for assigning women to DWHPs in 2010, VA has advanced quality of care and satisfaction for women Veterans and developed a model of care that may potentially be exported to improve quality of care for women in other health care settings.

Recognition

DWHP, WVPM

Improving Gender Disparities in the Department of Veterans Affairs

Nancy Maher, PhD, Program Analyst
VACO, Washington, DC
nancy.maher@va.gov

Since 2008, VA has reduced gender disparities in most Healthcare Effectiveness Data and Information Set (HEDIS) performance measures through a five-year system-wide redesign plan to ensure that women Veterans receive high-quality comprehensive care, clinical quality measures are reported to leadership, and feedback is given to providers.

Introduction

There are currently over 1.8 million women Veterans in the US, and approximately 440,000 of them used VA health care in 2015. In 1988, women represented 4.4 percent of the total Veteran population. This rose to 10 percent in 2014 and is projected to be 11 percent in 2020. It is a major goal of Women's Health Services (WHS) and VA that women Veterans receive the highest quality care, equitable to that of their male counterparts throughout the VA health care system. To that end, VA began reporting health care quality measures by gender starting in 2007. These measures included gender—neutral indicators of health care quality in mental health and cancer screening, preventive care, and chronic disease management among others. Although VA typically outperformed the private sector in these quality measures, significant gender disparities were noted within VA, with higher percentages of male Veterans being screened for mental health conditions and cancer as well as receiving vaccinations than female Veterans.

In 2008, a strategic plan focusing on improving women's health care was implemented throughout the VA health care system. During this time, quality measure disparities between men and women Veterans were reported to VA leadership, and provider specific data were released in 2010. In 2011, gender disparity improvement was included as a performance measure in VA leadership annual performance plans and VISNs were required to work toward reducing gender disparities through local quality improvement initiatives. To assess the impact of these activities, WHS conducted a 2013 retrospective study analyzing gender-neutral clinical quality measures, most of which demonstrated a decreasing trend in gender inequities over the five-year span from 2008 to 2013. For instance, national gender disparities significantly narrowed or disappeared in depression screening rates (from 6 percent to no difference); PTSD screening (from 5.8 percent to no difference); percentage of ischemic heart disease patients with low-density lipoprotein (LDL)>100 mg/dl (from 18 to 9.4 percent); and in percentage of diabetic patients with LDL >100 mg/dl (from 14 to 6 percent).

Key Information

In 2008, WHS launched a five-year VA health care system-wide redesign plan to ensure that women Veterans receive comprehensive care from providers proficient in women's health care, that clinical quality measures are reported to leadership by gender, and feedback is given to providers. In 2011, gender disparity improvement was included as a performance measure in the Healthcare Leadership

Annual Performance plan, resulting in increased attention to this issue. Each VISN was required to choose a performance measure with a gender disparity and develop local quality improvement initiatives targeted toward reducing disparities. Best practices implemented by VISNs included education, support and involvement of leadership, collaboration between programs and systems redesign, standardization of processes and electronic reminders, and significant patient engagement. Success of gender disparity mitigation was found to be dependent on multi-dimensional interventions aimed at patients, providers, and systems of care. The issue of equitable care is of paramount importance to VA as more and more women become patients of VA health care system. Examining disparities allows a health care system to better understand and address how different patient populations experience care (e.g., provider bias, access to care, care fragmentation, cultural barriers) as well as improve care delivery so that all patients benefit.

Context

The patient population served by this promising practice is enrolled women Veterans who are actively using the VA health care system. Currently, over 650,000 women Veterans are enrolled in VA health care. This number will likely continue to increase as more and more women are serving in the military; in fact, VA estimates that by 2040, women will make up 18 percent of the total Veteran population. Historically, VA health care systems served primarily male Veterans, thus it has had to make significant structural, organizational, provider, and cultural adaptations to provide equitable care for women and to become a health care system that women Veterans prefer to use. Tracking gender disparities in clinical quality measures has assisted leadership in identifying and addressing local issues that may contribute to these disparities in health care delivery to women.

Practice Description

WHS continues to monitor gender data for clinical measures nationally, by VISN, and by individual VA health care systems. These measures are reported quarterly in the Gender Report produced by the Office of Analytics and Business Intelligence (OABI). The data are gathered by VA's External Review Program, which randomly samples medical records of Veterans receiving VA care. Based on previous methodology, differences of 5 percent or more are considered clinically significant. In 2015, most gender differences have dropped below the clinically significant range, but small disparities remain in measures of pneumococcal and influenza vaccination rates and diabetes care at the VISN level and cholesterol management in high-risk patients nationally.

Replicability

The specific factors leading to the success of the practice are continued involvement, leadership, and oversight provided by the WHS program to mitigate gender disparities in health care quality within the entire VA health care system. Additionally, the continuous gathering of data by the OABI on clinical quality measures by gender and the nationwide availability of the EHR provide the tools necessary for replication in every VA site in the country. Other local factors contributing to the reproducibility of this practice include the presence of providers and other health care professionals dedicated to women's health and preventive care in every VA health care system, including women Veteran program managers, health promotion disease prevention coordinators, and women's health providers and staff.

Recognition

Patty Hayes, Sally Haskell, Alison Whitehead, Joe Francis, Steven Wright

Health System Approach to Enhancing Reproductive Health Care Delivery

Laurie Zephyrin, MD, Director

VACO, Washington, DC

laurie.zephyrin@va.gov

Many Veterans of reproductive age (18–45 years old) have health conditions that require treatment with medications that pose a risk to a developing fetus or breastfeeding newborn. VA launched an initiative that includes tools that leverage VA's national EHR. These tools enable VA providers to initiate conversations regarding preconception care, disease management, and contraception to ensure that women Veterans and their babies have the best possible outcomes.

Introduction

Reproductive health care is an integral component of comprehensive health care for women Veterans. Optimal reproductive health is not simply the absence of reproductive disease but a state of complete physical, mental, and social well-being. As a reproductive health care provider for women Veterans, I recognized that there were a number of opportunities for initiatives to improve the reproductive health care offered by VA for women Veterans. Several of my patients were women Veterans with mental health conditions that required medication. When some of them became pregnant, they had to weigh the risks and benefits of staying on the medication. VA needs tools to initiate these discussions with women before they became pregnant and other providers echoed this need across the health care system. There was a recognized need for innovations addressing safe prescribing and preconception care.

To address these needs, the Teratogenic Drugs (TDrugs) Initiative was initiated to provide alerts for high-risk medications through VA's electronic medical record system. Given their complex medical histories, many women Veterans who use VA health care have medical or mental health conditions that require medications that may pose a risk to a fetus or breast-fed infant. TDrugs enhances the ability of VA providers to counsel women on the risks and benefits of monitoring versus discontinuing the use of potentially harmful medications before or during pregnancy and while breastfeeding.

These innovations are critical tools for VA health care providers since they will make important reproductive health information readily available to them and to their patients. TDrugs is an enhancement of CPRS/VistA that notifies clinicians of potentially unsafe medication use in reproductive aged women. In doing so, it gives providers an important tool to initiate conversations around preconception care, contraception and disease management, and medications and lactation.

Key Information

Many Veterans of reproductive age (18–45 years old) have health conditions that require treatment with medications that pose a risk to a developing fetus or breastfeeding newborn. Research indicates that one in two women Veterans of reproductive age who filled prescriptions at VA pharmacies received at least one such medication, but only 20 percent had documented use of contraception. To enhance awareness of the reproductive safety of medications, VA launched a specific order check in the EHR to notify providers when prescribing a high-risk medication to a woman of reproductive age. Additional enhancements have been developed to include a computerized system of notifications, alerts, and reminders to facilitate risk/benefit decision making when prescribing these medications and to prompt review of contraception use. This enhanced electronic record functionality will advance patient safety in women of reproductive age. Collectively this set of enhancements makes up TDrugs.

Context

Currently women Veterans of reproductive age (18–45 years) make up 42 percent of the total women Veterans who use VA health care. Reproductive health care is one of the top five health care needs among women Veterans in this age group. However, many of these women Veterans also have multiple and complex medical and mental health conditions that may affect the delivery of reproductive health care and management of reproductive health conditions. For example, one in two women Veterans in this age group fills a prescription at VA pharmacy that is potentially teratogenic. Without ensuring proper counseling and contraception, these women Veterans are at increased risk of miscarriage or delivering a baby with a congenital malformation. Therefore, to provide the highest quality reproductive health care for women Veterans an integrated, multi-disciplinary approach is needed that engages key stakeholders across the entire health care system.

Practice Description

TDrugs leverages VA's national EHR. These tools enable VA providers to initiate conversations regarding preconception care, disease management, and contraception to ensure that women Veterans and their babies have the best possible outcomes. Currently, TDrugs is implemented at several test sites and will begin rolling out nationally in late 2016.

Replicability

TDrugs required support from local IT offices and various national program offices to be implemented successfully. This included VA Office of Women's Health Services, the Office of IT, and Pharmacy Benefits Management. Additionally, we engaged medical and research experts in the field. Our efforts were further supported by the growing body of peer-reviewed research on women Veterans' reproductive health that highlighted the need for programs around safe prescribing. At each test or pilot site, we engaged the women's health leadership and the broader medical center leadership. Support of the medical center leadership ensured dedicated IT, which was crucial for the implementation. In advance of the national rollout of this innovation, our team has already planned a series of informational cyber seminars and trainings. Our expectations of success are also based on feedback from VA women Veterans program managers, maternity care coordinators, and women's health care providers regarding the ongoing need for tools, such as TDrugs.

Recognition

Patricia Hayes, Sally Haskell, Deanna Rolstead, Karen Feibus, Laurie Zephyrin, Anthony Puelo, Robert Ruff, Kenny Condie, Dan Petit, National CPRS Clinical Workgroup, Rob Silverman, Lisa Longo, Chasitie Levesque, Lydia Safko, Deneen Askew, LuAnne Barron, Mara Catalano, Yolunda

Coleman-Jenkins, Fran Cunningham, Caitlin Cusack, E. Bimla Schwarz, Stacy Garrett-Ray, Chester Good, Niharika Goyal, Glenn Graham, Margaret Heimann, Jim Hewins, Jason Hunt, Kristian Johnson, Seun Joseph-Adebo, Don Lees, Elizabeth LeMonds, Chasitie Levesque, Bruce Levine, Lisa Longo, Janet Markle, Melissa McNeil, Don Michalak, James Sanders, Lynn Sanders, Roberto Santos, Todd Schippers, Elizabeth Schwarz, Jeanie Scott, Robert Silverman, Pradnya Warnekar, and Laurie Zephyrin

Taking Action on Survey Data at All Levels of the Organization to Improve Patient Care

Dee Ramsel, PhD, MBA, Executive Director
VACO, Washington, DC
dee.ramsel@va.gov

Taking action on survey data at all levels of the organization improves employee engagement, which ultimately improves Veteran care.

Introduction

Seth Moulton is a freshman Democrat Congressman from Massachusetts. He is also a Veteran, and completed four tours of duty in Iraq. Before he became a US Congressman, he went to VA for health care. He shared his story with National Public Radio in 2015 and described how despite good experiences with clinicians, he was discouraged by long waits for appointments, being trapped in circular referrals, being given incomplete information, scheduling and IT issues, and even incorrectly being given Advil® after surgery rather than Percocet®.

Vietnam Veteran Mr. X went to his local VA hospital for a heart catheterization and stent. He was nervous about the procedure, but reassured by the attentiveness, efficiency, and professionalism of the staff and clinicians. He was warmly greeted as soon as he arrived, and was shown to the waiting room. Mr. X did not wait long for the procedure to begin, it proceeded smoothly without incident, and he received his medication, information, and instructions before leaving. Staff members were more attentive after recent efforts to recognize good performance, increase morale, and improve leadership visibility.

How do we have a positive experience every time?

These are but a few actual improvements that have been made in VA sites nationwide as a result of using survey data to increase organizational health and provide the quality care Veterans deserve. Healthy organizations work together and go the extra mile to prevent Veterans, like Seth, from falling between the cracks, and ensure more Veterans have an experience similar to Mr. X. Healthy organizations are places employees are proud to work, and places where Veterans are confident they will get the care they deserve.

A Veteran's experience is the sum of hundreds of interactions, relationships, and attitudes that often occur behind the scenes, out of his/her view. How long a Veteran waits to be seen depends partly on how well staff communicate with each other. Whether a Veteran feels respected by his/her clinician is shaped by the clinician's own feelings of respect, satisfaction, and engagement. How quickly a mistake is caught and corrected depends on whether the culture is focused on learning or on blame. We know that healthy organizations—where staff are engaged, valued, and supported—tend to be more effective, efficient, and enjoyable places to work and receive care.

Healthy organizations encourage everyone to contribute to improvement, from the most junior employee to the most senior executive. VA includes everyone's contribution through an annual census survey that is the top diagnostic tool to understand employee engagement, VA All Employee Survey (AES). This gives all employees a voice and forum to help improve the system. Issues raised in the 2014 and 2015 AES led to impactful improvements in the care Veterans receive in facilities nationwide.

Key Information

Improvements from using AES data include: one pharmacy was able to fill prescriptions three minutes faster. A facility saw their patient satisfaction scores increase (SHEP; Survey of Healthcare of Experiences of Patients). Another facility found ways to expand telehealth services, increase appointment slots, and improve opiate safety. One service line was able to reduce patient complaints from 47 the previous year, to nine. Others reported $300,000 in savings that could be reallocated to other needs. Improved communication between clinicians led to quicker adoption of changes in therapy. Equipment was repaired and reinstated faster. Employee morale increased because of better relationships and more trust in leadership. These and many similar improvements made real, tangible differences in the care Veterans received and the day-to-day lives of employees.

These, and similar improvements, were made in many sites nationwide, and were championed by dozens of supervisors, service chiefs, and executive leadership teams. NCOD manages the AES, and collected information about improvements that resulted from using the survey data in 2014 and 2015 (reports are available to all VA employees). These improvements made real, concrete differences in the lives of Veterans and employees. In many cases, these improvements came at little or no cost, such as increasing leadership visibility and openness to questions or feedback. The practice of using survey data to affect change also addresses a multitude of specific concerns in specific groups that would be difficult to discover and resolve any other way.

Context

Using survey data to inform change helps ensure communication occurs between leaders who make decisions and staff who work face-to-face with Veterans. Sometimes in large organizations, this communication can break down. Having regular focused conversations, and setting goals for improving climate that are grounded in data, can prevent this breakdown and can actually strengthen the organization. These improvements benefit everyone in VA regardless of status—Veteran, employee, leader, or labor partner.

Practice Description

Successful leaders at all levels, and from many different facilities across VA, encouraged discussion about ways to address concerns raised in the survey data and ways to maintain strengths. Although each group faced unique challenges, collaboration was a consistent and unifying theme across sites that reported improvement. Successful leaders actively involved staff and other stakeholders in discussions about change, and made those discussions as transparent as possible. Typically, the Medical Center Directors (MCD) set general priorities for the facility and tasked service chiefs with specific issues in the data from their areas. In turn, the service chiefs often empowered frontline supervisors to present and discuss the data from their workgroups through meetings, focus groups, or listening sessions. Roseburg VAMC illustrates the value in this process; they saw significant increases on many indices of organizational health from 2014 to 2015, which the MCD directly attributed to considering workgroup-level AES data and empowering everyone to address concerns at the lowest and most specific levels possible.

The first step in using AES data is to review the facility AES reports produced by NCOD. These reports provide statistical comparisons to benchmark groups across years for several levels of organizational data. This allows local leadership to prioritize areas for discussion and account for statistical concerns associated with measuring attitudes. More specific data about occupations or service lines are usually accessed via Pyramid data cubes that are then used to drive specific discussions at the lowest possible level. Results and recommendations from these discussions are generally communicated back up the organizational hierarchy where they are prioritized and implemented. Utilizing employee-led workgroups to plan the implementation is considered a strong practice.

Replicability

One of the most promising aspects of this practice is its generalizability. Using survey data to inform action and improve care can be done at any site. All VA sites have access to organizational health survey data (from multiple time points throughout the year), and at workgroup or service levels in the case of the AES. Another promising aspect is that discussion only costs time—there are no fees associated with presenting, discussing, and planning around survey data. Groups that make changes based on AES data tend to see substantial improvements in efficiency and service as previously mentioned.

Leadership support and trust are important prerequisites for these improvements. Leaders who welcome feedback and collaboration encourage the open, frank discussions necessary to improve care. To spread this practice, leaders should create environments that encourage communication, asking questions, and group learning.

Recognition

Organizational Assessment Subcommittee, VHA NCOD

SPECIAL POPULATIONS

Paws of Freedom

Michael Cortright, Acting Director, VHA Innovation Program
VACO, Washington, DC
michael.cortright@va.gov

Paws of Freedom seeks to improve Veterans' mental health by pairing them with companion dogs. The program links Veterans with trained companion dogs and any handler training required. VA also provides Veterans with medical care for their companion dogs.

Introduction

The number of suicides, family abuse, and PTSD occurrences affecting Veterans who are returning to civilian life after military duty continues to rise. Veterans often face unemployment, broken relationships, addiction, and depression during this transition. A bond between animals and Veterans, particularly dogs, has shown noted improvements in anxiety levels, sleep duration, and exercise, as well as decreased hypervigilance, and decreased feelings of isolation. Everyone needs a loyal friend, and that concept is not lost on Veteran organizations and animal shelters working to pair Veterans with companion dogs.

Paws of Freedom creates and leverages partnerships between VHA and programs that train companion dogs. The program links Veterans with trained companion dogs, as well as any handler training that is required. VA also provides Veterans with medical care for their companion dogs.

Paws of Freedom has an immediate impact on Veteran lives. In 2014, records of Veterans who adopted dogs through the program showed Veterans were thrilled with their adoptions. By January 2016, the program expanded, pairing 68 dogs with Veteran owners. Presently, 100 percent of Veterans in the program are reporting they are happy with the impact of their new companion. Program highlights showing "the human face" of the project (and the canine face) live on the Paws of Freedom page of the VHA Innovation Whole Health and Wellness Resource Bundle, a VA intranet site.

- "He's a good cuddle buddy, always paying attention to me and he does his job. When I get angry, he gets my attention. He jumps up or puts his paw on me to distract me, and it helps remind me that I'm no longer in the military."
- "Having a companion dog has made me a lot happier."
- "It will give you someone to keep you feeling good about. Dogs can make you see a reason to keep going on."
- "I feel he is a companion who unconditionally loves me."
- "My dog makes me less anxious, and I feel safer at home."
- "His presence definitely makes me feel safer at home."
- "He has made us very happy. He has also put us on a schedule. We cannot imagine our life without him."
- "He takes our minds off whatever is wrong. He is really smart and loving."

Key Information

VA pairs rescue dogs with Veterans, particularly those with PTSD or other emotional health issues. The program is unique because the dogs receive their training from prison inmates from another program called Prison Pups N Pals. Dogs in the program originate from the Humane Society and receive 14 weeks of obedience training at the Tomoka Correctional Institution with oversight by West Volusia Kennel Club.

- The Humane Society sterilizes microchips and vaccinates the dogs prior to placement at the prison, and all dogs adopted have passed the American Kennel Club (AKC) Canine Good Citizen Test.

- American Society for the Prevention of Cruelty to Animals' (ASPCA) uses Meet Your Match Canine-ality to identify a personality and lifestyle match between dogs and Veterans.

- Veterans participating in Paws of Freedom attend informal training sessions at Tomoka Work Camp, where they communicate with the dog's handlers, practice basic obedience commands, and bond with the dog.

- Following dog placement, Veterans have additional resources available, including access to an animal behaviorist, additional obedience classes, and grant money for veterinary care.

- Veterans are encouraged to talk with their dog and establish a caring relationship with the effect of improving the severity and persistence of the mental health symptoms they face.

Context

Veterans who suffer from conditions, such as emotional detachment, loneliness, and avoidance, and with co-occurring diagnoses, such as anxiety and depression, are good candidates for the program. Most Veterans participating in the current program are enrolled in the Orlando VAMC system (or a VAMC within a reasonable distance), referred by a mental health provider, have a mental health diagnosis (in the pilot, 100 percent of participants have PTSD diagnosis with some co-occurring conditions), and are from varying war eras. Veterans are pre-screened for the program with two areas of focus: 1) Patient-Centered Care (PCC; i.e., identifying what the Veteran is seeking and helping the Veteran determine if their "wants" are a good match with their "needs") and 2) exclusionary factors (i.e., already owning a dog, housing issues, active substance abuse, active psychotic symptoms, recent history of violence).

Practice Description

On the VHA Innovation Whole Health and Resource Bundle, the original innovator, Jennifer Muni-Sathoff, outlined best practices for starting a similar program:

- Collaborate with a successful prison dog-training program in your community that is working with an established humane society with a staff veterinarian. Not all dogs sent to the training program will be good matches for Veterans. Implement the ASPCA "Meet Your Match Program" through the partnering humane society. This is a great tool for pairing the right dog with the Veteran.

- This is a mental health recovery oriented program. All participants should complete a comprehensive plan of care and recovery (mental health treatment plan).

- Utilize the PCC Model. Complete the Initial Eligibility Assessment Screening (IEAS) and review the medical record to determine whether a companion-house dog will be a good match for a Veteran's expressed wants and needs. Veterans should have a realistic view of the dog they will receive. This is not a service dog. This is a house pet who is most likely recovering from its own trauma of loss or abuse.

- Veterans should visit the training facility to bond with the dog, learn the dog's trained obedience commands, and determine any specific training commands. Facility permitting, Veterans may work with the inmate trainers during scheduled sessions, along with a VA social worker who is present for all visits. Clinicians should document all visits in the medical record.

- Dog-Training Process: 14 weeks (two cycles of basic obedience training with some individualized tasks depending on the Veteran's request and dog's capacity to learn). Inmate trainers maintain a daily journal of the dog's progress, which is provided to the Veteran at graduation. Dogs are sterilized, microchipped, and current with vaccinations prior to placement in the prison.

Replicability

Given the number of Veterans suffering from emotional and mental health issues throughout VA, the demand for similar programs is high. The program is highly replicable in other geographical areas with a strong and supportive team. The team and extra effort needed for the coordination between the animal shelter, dog trainers, and Veterans is crucial to success. The program continues to be successful on its own in Orlando.

Recognition

Jennifer Muni-Sathoff

Novel Approach for Controlling Photophobia in Combat Veterans with Traumatic Brain Injury: Artificial Pupil Contact Lenses

Mary Jackowski, PhD, OD, Rehabilitative Optometrist

Syracuse VAMC, Syracuse, NY

mary.jackowski@va.gov

The use of Artificial Pupil Contact Lenses (APCLs) as a reliable treatment of severe photophobia in combat Veterans with Traumatic Brain Injury (TBI) has become a standard treatment option of our Vision Rehabilitative Service (VRS).

Introduction

Over 20 years ago, as a low vision specialist in an ophthalmology department, I encountered a new population of patients with severe light sensitivity. A local physiatrist was working with patients with mild Traumatic Brain Injury (or concussion) who complained of a new, post-traumatic intolerance to normal amounts of ambient lighting, outdoor lighting, and indoor lighting. This persistent photophobia accompanied ocular discomfort and/or a disabling headache. At the time, these patients had received a full visual exam with normal results, and received no resulting treatment. The symptomatic patients had taken to wearing dark sunglasses and reported analgesic overuse. At the time, low vision specialists had available colored lenses to treat disabling glare in patients with ocular disease. Initially, we reported acceptance of these lenses by patients with symptoms following a head injury. Specifically, we reported increases in their visual performance (e.g., improved reading rate, contrast sensitivity). However, these lenses were not particularly helpful to patients with profound light sensitivity. They created color distortion, allowed the transmission of more light overall, and provided no real value. Patients preferred wearing dark sun wear or employing avoidance techniques.

More recently, young combat Veterans returning from deployment provided us with another population of highly photophobic subjects. Sixty to seventy percent (60 to 70 percent) of Veterans with a history of mild head injury complain of a more persistent photophobia than is usually seen in the private sector. These Veterans perceive light as a noxious stimulus often associated with headache/ocular discomfort that is separate from other pre- or post-traumatic headache profiles. Symptoms may appear during active duty, but often go unnoticed until post-deployment periods. These are young people returning from war, re-entering busy civilian lives, sometimes reluctant to complain about disability. Clinicians had assured many patients of a normal ocular health status, and many presented with symptoms that were not successfully treated. As with private sector patients, they self-treated with any available manner of light stimulus reduction. However, these maneuvers had a cost. For example, the fiancé of a newly engaged couple complained about the emotional effects that sun wear use and minimal eye contact had on their relationship and family life. Another symptomatic Veteran used avoidance body behaviors (crouching, head down, chin-to-chest loss of eye contact). Others complained of missing workdays because of exposure to commercial work light, with employers unaccepting of accommodations. Veterans returning to school reported being unable to tolerate the florescent glare in classrooms, creating reduced visual performance and discomfort, even to the point of discontinuing their education. A female Veteran reported her inability to walk into her child's school building without using sunglasses.

Context

Examination of Veterans' ocular health revealed normal structure and physiology. Standard brain imaging did not identify causes. Current treatments included avoidance behaviors, environmental modifications, and light-filtering lenses. These treatments offered some alleviation, but were difficult to implement in challenging situations. Headache/pain medications provided variable amounts of relief, but carried with them undesired side effects. Symptomatic Veterans had to modify the effects of noxious lighting by refraining from participation in daily activities. Photophobia also had a negative impact on mood, personal relationships, and perceived enjoyment of life. Many Veterans acclimated to chronic use of dark, wrap-style sun wear worn indoors and outside. This maladaptive practice introduced additional problems, including loss of central visual acuity and image contrast, potential increases in light sensitivity, and loss of all-important eye contact in social/work situations. Throughout our network, Veteran case managers refer Veterans with significant photophobia to our clinic. We have developed a detailed intake questionnaire, heavily weighted with questions addressing light levels and effects on visual performance. Given the steady flow of Veterans aged 20–45 years with persistent post-injury photophobia, and of the general ineffectiveness of current treatment options, we found it necessary to identify other strategies for reducing the amount of light entering the eye.

Practice Description

Within the last three years, we have been successful in using Artificial Pupil Contact Lenses (APCLs). Currently, the APCL in use is a standard 14-millimeter opaque contact lens with a fixed 4.5-millimeter clear, optically correctable center. Medical suppliers offer these commercially available lenses in a variety of pupillary diameters and iris colorations. These APCLs make a prosthetic repair of iris defects resulting from congenital, traumatic, or surgical events that cause glare and light sensitivity. The contact lens provides an opaque covering of the cornea and limbus. The APCL reduces light entering the eye, but unlike sunglasses, it selectively reduces peripheral light levels leaving central vision unobstructed. Subjectively, when normal subjects wear the APCL in standard room lighting, there is an immediate reduction in perceived brightness and a clear edge to the peripheral field at about 70 degrees of eccentricity.

After Veterans receive a detailed intake questionnaire, those reporting significant light sensitivity also receive a ten-point questionnaire modeled after the Brief Pain Inventory (BPI) (Cleeland, 2009). The questionnaire evaluates the effectiveness of different therapies in achieving clinical outcomes. The questionnaire uses a zero to ten rating scale, providing estimates of "worst," "least," and "average" intensity of symptoms, both before and with APCLs. Importantly, this questionnaire helps quantify the effects of APCLs on life activities, in work/social interactions, and perceived mood. After a complete ocular health assessment, including optical correction, dilated fundus, anterior segment exam, and visual perimetry, patients go to a local contact lens specialist for fitting. After a month of successful wear time, Veterans return for a follow-up questionnaire and visual field assessment. In all cases, a Humphrey Visual Field Analyzer (HVAA) without corrective lenses assessed Veterans' visual fields. Clinicians documented small temporal visual field restrictions;

however, for patients with no pre-APCL field losses, the 140-degree horizontal binocular visual field, often used as a requirement for daylight driving, remained intact.

Overall, light reduction reaching the retina is a product of the interaction of the static contact lens aperture and the active biological pupil. Our estimate of light reduction using the 4.5-millimeter pupil contact lens is between 25 and 30 percent. To date, over 40 combat Veterans have claimed relief of symptoms with more than 50 percent improvement across all parameters, including a reduction in headaches. These patients report eliminating the use of sun wear indoors and under cloudy outdoor lighting. Direct bright sunlight still requires the use of additional sun wear. Patients and their families report restoration of normal social interactions. Approximately half of this current group has worn their contact lenses for greater than one year, with replacement lenses provided later. The use of APCLs as a safe and reliable treatment of photophobia has become a standard treatment option of our VRS.

Recognition

Brad Motter, Moriam Abiolu-Osuro, Andrew Taddeo

COVER to COVER: Connecting Older Veterans (Especially Rural) to Community or Veteran Eligible Resources

Jennifer Morgan, Utah Aging and Disability Resource Centers Program Director

VA Salt Lake City Health Care System, Salt Lake City, UT

jen.morgan@utah.edu

Most Veterans are not aware they are eligible for VA benefits. Likewise, trusted community service providers who work in rural areas across the country may not understand how to navigate VA. COVER to COVER bridges that divide, encouraging collaboration between community and VA service providers to ensure Veterans are able to access the resources they need and deserve.

Introduction

In September 2014, the Utah Salvation Army reached out to the local Aging and Disability Resource Center (ADRC) regarding a Vietnam Veteran who was chronically homeless for more than 28 years. The Veteran wanted to get sober and secure housing, but did not have income. Jennifer Morgan, program manager at the state resource center, met with the Veteran and helped him to apply for VA health care and benefits. She educated the Veteran about his eligibility for benefits, and worked with him to apply for VA's Supportive Services for Veteran Families (SSVF) to arrange housing. He also began receiving physical and mental health services from VA, as well as additional assistance from state and federal programs. He now lives in a new apartment, and works for Easter Seals doing outreach with other chronically homeless Veterans.

In roughly the first two years of data collection (April 1, 2013, to September 30, 2015), this collaborative project served more than 1,200 unique Veterans in Utah alone. We created more than 600 referrals to assist Veterans not previously enrolled in VA health care.

Key Information

VA employees train community service providers in Veteran benefits, eligibility, and the application and claims process. They then use that knowledge to increase their referrals to VA while also decreasing processing times from incomplete applications. This is essential, as many rural community agencies have little formal outreach and yet they provide new access points for Veterans and their families to be connected to VA services. Over time, the program has added more formal partners and deepened relationships between community services and their VA counterparts. Additionally, Veteran trust in VA increases when their trusted community connections refer them to VA resources.

Context

Often, older Veterans are unaware they are eligible for VA benefits. Likewise, trusted community service providers in rural areas across the country often are not well versed in navigating VA system. This model bridges that divide, connecting and encouraging collaboration between community and

VA service providers to ensure Veterans are able to access the resources they need. The collaboration allows community providers to identify and educate Veterans about their benefits, often through in-home consultations. VA cannot offer this invaluable process on its own.

Practice Description

This model of collaboration recommends that community resource organizers connect with VA administrators, and then take part in detailed training about military culture, benefits, and claims. All Area Agencies on Aging are able to participate in this project to improve service to Veteran clients. All branches of local VA facilities seeking to build partnerships with community agencies can benefit from this strategy. People in the following roles may find this strategy particularly useful:

- Geriatric and PACT social workers
- State VAs
- VBA and VHA officials in local facilities and medical centers
- All VA outreach points
- Area Agencies on Aging and ADRCs

The decision to participate in this program requires willing partners from local VA facilities, specialists in health care and/or benefits, and from the community aging agencies. A champion is required from each organization, and the champion's supervisors must be willing to allow them dedicated time. This model assumes the concept of a "no wrong door" approach that helps Veterans understand the full range of resources available to them. Rural Veterans now have a new, direct access point to learn about Veteran benefits. They will also get assistance through the application process. VA must maintain open lines of communications between them and community agency administrators to ensure both remain up to date about the holistic picture of resources available.

Replicability

To earn the designation of Rural Promising Practice from the ORH, this program demonstrated:

- Improvement in access to care
- Evidence of improved direct program impact or clinical results for Veterans
- Patient, provider and/or caregiver satisfaction
- Return on investment via reduced costs of care, but not at the expense of quality
- Operational feasibility and replicability at other facilities or service sites
- Strong partnerships or working relationships that maximize efficiency or effectiveness

The program reinforces work that should already be occurring, and creates synergies to allow this work to occur more efficiently. In this sense, no one is implementing a "new program," and therefore the program is easily replicable across the country with the collaboration of the right partners. The partnership involves existing infrastructures that are widely available in rural areas, and as such, it might be possible to sustain the program with existing funding streams.

Recognition

Dedicated administrators, practitioners, and partners

338

Wheelchair Lacrosse: Promoting Adaptive Sports for Veterans and Building Partnerships in the Community

Tiffany Villamin, RN, Clinical Nurse Manager, Spinal Cord Injury; Kenneth Lee, MD, Chief, Spinal Cord Injury Service

Edward Hines Jr. VA Hospital, Hines, IL
tiffany.villamin@va.gov

This approach encourages Veteran participation in adaptive sports through wheelchair lacrosse. The collaboration among several VAs, the Paralyzed Veterans of America (PVA), and community partners is the foundation of several teams forming in the Midwest.

Introduction

When Veterans experience a Spinal Cord Injury (SCI), it has repercussions on their lifespan. Families and caregivers also struggle to manage their care due to complex co-morbidities. The specialty SCI care that VA provides addresses their unique needs and individualizes their care. The quality of life for a SCI patient relates to their relationships with others, as well as reintegration into the community. The SCI service at the Milwaukee VAMC, Hines VAMC, and the local Paralyzed Veterans of America chapters are committed to promoting adaptive sports as a way to support Veterans coping with their disability.

The positive impact on Veterans and their families is the sense of pride, accomplishment, and camaraderie that occurs during team sport activities. They are a prime example of how SCI individuals overcome their injuries and live healthy lifestyles. The Milwaukee Eagles Wheelchair Lacrosse Team and Chicago Cougars Wheelchair Lacrosse Team are composed of Veterans, civilians, and both disabled and able-bodied individuals. This structure allows Veterans and civilians to collaborate and find common ground while participating in adaptive sports.

Over 80 people attended the Chicago Cougars Wheelchair Lacrosse Clinic in March 2016 (two-day event). The goal of the clinic was to raise awareness for the new sport, and ultimately form a team. The Chicago Cougars team is comprised of seven Veterans and five civilians. The Milwaukee Eagles team has 12 Veterans and nine civilians. As the sport of wheelchair lacrosse grows, VA SCI centers and PVA will ensure that Veterans actively participate in the sport.

Key Information

The wheelchair lacrosse clinic was implemented in Chicago (March 2016) and was led by Dr. Kenneth Lee and Tiffany Villamin, RN. Two other clinics occurred in St. Louis (April 2016) and Minneapolis (May 2016). VA facilities supported respective clinics in those areas along with the local PVA chapters. This promising practice enriches the quality of life for disabled Veterans. Promoting wheelchair lacrosse supports VA's initiative to engage more disabled Veterans in adaptive sports. It promotes a healthy lifestyle, as well as improves their overall physical and emotional well-being. This best practice reflects the Integrity, Commitment, Advocacy, Respect, and Excellence (I-CARE) values that VA demonstrates on a daily basis.

Context

The Milwaukee and Hines VAMC SCI centers are collaborating to promote wheelchair lacrosse for Veterans. Although the Veteran population is in the SCI service, they are inclusive of all Veterans. This practice addresses the challenge of engaging disabled Veterans in adaptive sports and facilitates partnerships with the community. Another unique element is the inclusion of civilians, which allows Veterans and civilians to form personal relationships and collaborate.

Practice Description

To create a wheelchair lacrosse team, the first step is to host a clinic to get Veterans engaged in the new sport. The second step is to build a partnership with community resources for space, coaching, and equipment. The Vaughan Chapter PVA, Concordia University of Chicago, and the Rehabilitation Institute of Chicago (RIC) partnered with Hines VA Hospital to successfully implement the clinic. Concordia University of Chicago donated their gymnasium, lacrosse coaching staff, and lacrosse athletes. RIC supported the endeavor by providing athletes and equipment. The Milwaukee Eagles team traveled to Chicago, and also donated equipment to the team.

Concordia lacrosse coaching staff and athletes directed the clinic. They led the wheelchair athletes in lacrosse drills and taught them the rules of the game. At the end of the clinic, the Milwaukee Eagles Team and Concordia athletes simulated a wheelchair lacrosse game. The response and interest in forming a Chicago team generated quickly. Our community partners want to serve the Veteran population, and engaging them in this type of activity advanced the coalition.

Replicability

The practice was successful because of our partnership with community resources, and through the support of the Milwaukee Eagles team. To replicate this endeavor, another SCI center and local PVA chapter would partner with a local collegiate lacrosse team or adaptive sports group. After this relationship forms, a wheelchair lacrosse clinic would be coordinated to engage Veterans and form a team.

The joint effort between several VA facilities and sharing best practices is an important element of our success. VA facilities in VISN 12 (Milwaukee and Hines) stand together in this endeavor and are building coalitions with VISN 15 (St. Louis) and VISN 23 (Minneapolis). The best practice created at Hines VAMC SCI Center is the standard model to follow to form a wheelchair lacrosse team successfully. The goal is to form a Midwest Division (Milwaukee, Chicago, St. Louis, and Minneapolis) and host regional competitions. As the sport grows, it has the potential to join the National Veterans Wheelchair Games as a new sport.

Recognition

Kenneth Lee, MD, The Milwaukee Eagles Wheelchair Lacrosse Team, Vaughan Chapter PVA (Robert Arciola, Maria Hernandez), Wisconsin PVA chapter (Paul Lehman), National PVA (Ernest Butler), Concordia University of Chicago (Gerald Pinotti, Drew Stevenson, Brian Patterson), RIC (Derek Daniels)

STAR-VA: A Veteran-Centered, Interdisciplinary Approach for Managing Challenging Behaviors Among Community Living Center Residents with Dementia

Michele Karel, PhD, ABPP, Psychogeriatrics Coordinator

VACO, Washington, DC

michele.karel@va.gov

STAR-VA is a behavioral team approach for managing dementia-related behaviors among Veterans in Community Living Centers (CLCs). Through Veteran-centered behavioral assessment and care planning, the team helps increase Veteran engagement in pleasant events and decrease symptoms of anxiety, depression, and agitation.

Introduction

Individuals with dementia almost universally experience behavioral symptoms, such as agitation or aggression at some point during their illnesses, reflecting a brain disease interacting with medical, interpersonal, or environmental influences. These behaviors are distressing to the people with dementia, their caregivers, and others in the care environment. National initiatives promote the use of non-pharmacological, psychosocial approaches to help caregivers manage these distressing behaviors. VHA plays a leading role in training, implementing, and sustaining such an approach in our Community Living Centers: STAR-VA. The program originates from Dr. Linda Teri's evidence-based Staff Training in Assisted Living Residences (STAR) program. The program has demonstrated consistent reductions in the frequency and severity of target behaviors, as well as decreased symptoms of depression, anxiety, and agitation among participating Veterans. The large majority of local CLC team members, including all levels of nursing staff, report that STAR-VA provided them new skills to help Veterans, and that the program prepared them to better respond when Veterans with dementia display a difficult behavior.

CLC Associate Chief Nurses whose sites participated in STAR-VA training gave feedback on the program's impact and sustainability. Here are selected quotes from Nurse leaders:

- "We have developed an extensive team of nursing staff mentors. We have trained the medical staff in the Star-VA program and have incorporated recreational staff to implement the Get Active Plans."

- "The direct caregivers have benefited from the program as it recognizes the challenges they face. It helps them feel empowered as they bring concerns to the team members. They have a voice in the treatment plan for those Veterans with dementia."

- "We are pleased with the program's ability to help staff gauge their interactions and identify opportunities to have individualized therapeutic moments."

- "They have seen the results especially with one Veteran who was constantly yelling for his wife. The interventions did have a positive effect for this Veteran and the CLC."

- "STAR-VA education and application can be tailored or adapted to have a positive impact in regards to multiple behavior scenarios."
- "STAR-VA is incorporated in the weekly behavior meetings."

Key Information

Mental health services in VACO, in collaboration with the Office of Mental Health Operations (OMHO), Geriatrics and Extended Care (GEC), and the Office of Nursing Services (ONS) initiated the STAR-VA pilot program and have overseen its expansion over the past five years. VA implemented STAR-VA for two major reasons: 1) national recognition that antipsychotic medications, the mainstay for treating behavioral symptoms of dementia, were not particularly effective and potentially dangerous for people with dementia; and 2) psychologists weaved nationally into VHA CLCs starting in 2008. One of their primary responsibilities was to support CLC teams in behavioral management of symptoms associated with dementia. These professionals needed training to support their teams. The STAR-VA training model evolved to train both a CLC mental health professional (i.e., psychologist or psychiatric provider) and a RN to train the entire CLC team in a structured, Veteran-centered, behavioral care approach ("ABC model"). This approach matters to optimize quality of life and comfort for Veterans with dementia, as well as to empower and engage staff in making a difference in caring for Veterans with complex needs.

Context

Sixty-eight CLCs have participated in the national STAR-VA training program since 2010, representing all VISNs. Eleven new CLCs and staff from 14 previously trained CLCs will participate in the 2016 training program, where the latter will address the challenge of staff turnover of previously trained STAR-VA Mental Health or Nurse leaders. The Veterans served are those with a diagnosis of dementia, who reside in a CLC, and who have repeatedly displayed a distressing behavior of concern to the family or team (e.g., verbal or physical aggression, repeated vocalization, problematic wandering, care refusal, isolative behavior). Due to their neurocognitive disorder, these Veterans have difficulty communicating their needs, (e.g., physical discomfort, boredom, overstimulation, fear, loneliness, etc.), and it is up to their VA caregivers to understand what concerns underlie a "challenging" behavior and address them.

Practice Description

The STAR-VA intervention has three core components:

1. ABCs: Identifying and changing intrapersonal, interpersonal, or environmental activators to and consequences that reinforce or exacerbate the challenging behaviors

2. Pleasant Events: Identifying and increasing, through a structured and individualized process, personally-relevant and meaningful pleasant events consistent with the individual's abilities

3. Realistic Expectations and Communication Skills: Promoting realistic expectations of residents with dementia and increasing effective verbal and non-verbal communication strategies with these residents, including the Listen with Respect, Comfort, and Redirect (LRCR) approach

The STAR-VA training program entails training a CLC psychologist or psychiatric provider to serve as a STAR-VA "behavioral coordinator" and a CLC RN to serve as a STAR-VA "nurse champion." Together, this dyad trains the CLC team, including all levels of nursing staff (especially, our certified nursing assistants). The behavioral coordinator and nurse champion attend a three-day workshop (initially face-to-face, now conducted virtually), followed by six months of consultation (via regular conference calls) with STAR-VA training consultants as they work to implement the approach with Veterans in their CLC. Program resources include an intervention manual, handouts for staff training, a DVD for staff training, and sharing of resources developed by local sites. Attendees participate in program evaluation activities and are encouraged to develop local STAR-VA sustainability plans.

Replicability

Specialists developed the national STAR-VA training program to promote replicability across sites through development of an intervention manual and structured training and consultation process. We are working on additional resources to support program sustainability over time (e.g., additional virtual training resources). We have frequent requests for training from clinicians in other care settings, especially inpatient medicine and inpatient mental health. The training needs to be adapted for use in acute care settings but, given the resources and structure of the approach, it should be a feasible pilot. To date, 68 CLCs have participated in STAR-VA training across all VISNs, with a variability in number of participating sites. In 2016, 25 CLCs will participate: 11 sites for the first time and 14 will re-train a psychologist or nurse leader due to staff turnover.

Recognition

VA Employee Education System (EES) Staff: Brad Karlin, Linda Teri, Eleanor McConnell, Kerri Wilhoite, Elizabeth Czekanski, Lorraine Galkowski, Kim Curyto, multiple CLC psychologist Training Consultants, Jeremy Johnson, Debra Lilly, Katherine Luci, Kathleen Matthews, Caryanne Pope, Brea Salib, Veronica Shead, Bridget Tribout, Connie Eddy, LeShea Nixon

Gerofit

Miriam Morey, PhD, GRECC Associate Director of Research

Durham VAMC, Durham, NC

miriam.morey@va.gov

Gerofit is a group-based exercise program for Veterans ages 65 and older. It offers supervised exercise tailored to functional impairments and patient-directed goals. Program participants experience a significant reversal of declining functional trajectory, high patient satisfaction, and reduced risk of mortality.

Introduction

Each Veteran has a story to tell. A few common themes emerge from the diverse Veterans participating in Gerofit programs across the country. They are all proud to be Veterans, proud to have served their country, and delighted to have found Gerofit.

- One Veteran from Canandaigua, NY, explained, "I started Gerofit one year ago and I've lost 100 pounds. My A1C went from 9.8 to 5.6, my blood pressure is normalized, and my cholesterol went from 200 to 126. I feel 30 years younger. I used to isolate myself and now I have friends and am more outgoing."

- A Vietnam Veteran from Durham, NC, said, "It's much more than the physical. It helps your mind and body, everything; it makes you feel whole again."

- The 96-year-old wife of a World War II Veteran noted, "If it weren't for this program, I don't think we would be walking."

- An 87-year-old Veteran from Los Angeles suffering from pulmonary fibrosis, sciatica, Parkinson's disease, and anxiety feels that Gerofit "saved [his] life. [He has] made amazing progress this year and lots of friends. They should have this at every VA. It decreases costs and increases happy people."

- In Baltimore, two Veterans who are next-door neighbors stopped paying for lawn care and started mowing their own lawns after several months of Gerofit exercise.

- A 70-year-old Veteran from Miami who volunteered with Miami VA Geriatric Research Education Clinical Center (GRECC) exercise programs joined the Miami Gerofit staff as a trainer. Exercise had maintained his health and significantly increased his cardiorespiratory fitness and functional reserve. He recently underwent heart surgery for aortic stenosis, and in less than two weeks, was back leading Gerofit exercise groups six times per week.

Key Information

Gerofit is a group-based exercise and health promotion program for older adults. It offers supervised exercise tailored to functional impairments and patient-directed goals to Veterans ages 65 and above. Gerofit is a model clinical demonstration program originally established in the Durham VA in 1986. The demonstration published a five-year reversal of declining functional trajectory and 25 percent lower mortality rate over ten years among Veterans adherent to the program. Over 1,900 Veterans have participated in the Durham Gerofit program.

In 2014, Gerofit began expanding to other sites across the country with support from the VHA Office of Geriatrics and Extended Care (GEC) and ORH. Program administrators carefully selected partner locations and site directors for their experience and expertise of exercise programs and interventions for older Veterans.

Gerofit can occur in both urban and rural locations, including at VA CBOCs. Gerofit fills a gap in that there are few programs offering personally tailored exercises for older, vulnerable Veterans, a population often excluded from wellness opportunities. Gerofit is very cost effective. The approximate annual cost, per site, is roughly equivalent to the one-year cost of one-to-two institutionalized Veterans.

Context

The Gerofit program focuses on improving the function, health, and well-being of older Veterans. The objective of the program is to maximize years of healthy living and reduce risk for institutionalization. Program findings indicate that older Veteran participants are, on average, functionally 15 years older than their chronological age. Long-term participants have experienced a "compression of morbidity" in that aspects of physical function are improved and then maintained for five years following enrollment. Participation in Gerofit has also shown significant improvements in cardiorespiratory fitness, strength, BMI, cholesterol, and survival (Morey et al., JAGS 1989, 2002). The program aligns with VA Blueprint for Excellence, which seeks to transition from health care to well care.

Practice Description

The Gerofit program is a unique exercise and health promotion program for older Veterans. It is distinct from other programs in that it is not rehabilitation or restorative care. It serves as a lifelong wellness model for health for aging Veterans. A multi-disciplinary team of experts in geriatrics and exercise science developed the supported the program. Gerofit offers multiple types of opportunities for exercise by delivering directly supervised exercise, distance-based counseling, promotion, and education. Monitoring of aging Veterans can occur at local facilities, adult day care centers, and through real-time Clinic Video Telehealth (CVT). In addition, our teams conduct "train-the-trainer" outreach and have developed several geriatric "exercise" clinical rotations that instruct medical trainees, health care providers, and volunteers in the delivery of exercise interventions.

To date, the implementation process has involved a site visit to the Durham VAMC Gerofit program for initial training and interaction with program participants. New program partners gain access to a shared website with numerous training materials and templates. A reverse site visit occurs shortly after patient enrollment begins to assure program fidelity along with regular telephone meetings. The entire group has formed a Learning Collaborative to problem solve and share experiences and findings. Recently, the GEC Mentored Partnership Program has supported emerging sites with short-term funding.

Replicability

There is strong interest in increasing opportunities for health and wellness for our aging Veterans. There are approximately 3.6 million older Veterans not meeting recommended physical activity guidelines suggesting a significant unmet need. The dissemination of this highly successful practice is possible from funding from national offices. Sustainment varies by local environment, and is highly dependent upon leadership support. Replication is highly feasible in VAMCs with strength in geriatrics, a space to accommodate a fitness center, personnel with exercise expertise, and leadership commitment to health promotion. Interest is high from the field to continue dissemination of the program. With appropriate funding this program could roll out nationally.

Recognition

Cathy Lee, Steve Castle, Willy Valencia, Nakole Coleman, Leslie Katzel, Jamie Giffuni, Teresa Kopp, Heather Cammarata, Krisann Oursler, Timothy Oursler, Michelle McDonald, Chuck Ibarra, Karen Massey, Kenneth Shay, Richard Alman, Veteran participants

Mobile Applications to Support Provision of Evidence-Based Psychotherapies

Julia Hoffman, PsyD, National Director, Mobile Health
VACO, Washington, DC
julia.hoffman@va.gov

Mobile applications can supplement face-to-face evidence-based mental health care. They ensure fidelity of gold-standard treatments, decrease the stigma of therapy, support the completion of treatment, and enhance the generalization of skills for Veterans into their real lives.

Introduction

For some, the realities of deployment and military service can result in lifelong mental health challenges if left untreated. In spite of widespread availability of demonstrated psychosocial treatment and services, many Veterans are reluctant consumers. They fail to engage for a variety of reasons ranging from stigma to logistical issues. The rigor of treatments can be intimidating; for example, Prolonged Exposure Therapy (PE) for PTSD requires a detailed retelling of emotionally charged and traumatic events during the therapy session.

Without changing any aspect of the face-to-face elements of treatment, free and anonymous mobile applications, crafted by VHA's Office of Mental Health Services, allow Veterans to use their own devices to record sessions, play them back, complete therapy assignments, and receive homework reminders. Mobile applications provide maximum flexibility and discretion, and allow the Veteran to engage in treatment and following through with it until symptoms have resolved.

Key Information

Experts in our Mobile Behavior Design Lab, located within the National Center for PTSD (NCPTSD) Dissemination & Training Division, developed a suite of mobile applications supporting evidence-based psychotherapies. The NCPTSD provided organization and oversight for the national dissemination efforts of various evidence-based psychotherapies. Thus, the expert clinicians in the field provided input frequently throughout the development process. The DoD's National Center for Telehealth & Technology was a key partner providing valuable insight. The apps support PE, Cognitive Processing Therapy, Acceptance and Commitment Therapy, Cognitive Behavioral Therapy (CBT) for insomnia, alcohol moderation, smoking cessation, and behavioral activation. The first app entered the public app store in 2011. Since then, the mental health apps have achieved broad distribution and uptake. Users have downloaded the apps over 400,000 times. In addition, a survey of clinicians indicated that the Prolonged Exposure (PE) Coach application is used in over 50 percent of encounters within this treatment paradigm. We developed supplementary materials, including clinician's guides, to aid in the successful integration of these tools into clinical practice.

Context

Located in VA Palo Alto Health Care System, the Mobile Behavior Design Lab aims to leverage widely available mobile technology to eliminate barriers in access to high-quality mental health care. Since 2010, our team has convened groups of Veterans with mental health challenges, world-renowned experts, psychotherapy researchers, user experience experts, and frontline clinicians to alleviate challenges of traditional psychotherapy. Any Veteran participating in an active mental health treatment can take advantage of the free apps. In fact, many community providers use the apps with both Veteran and civilian patients. We believe the availability of the apps ensure that high-quality care is available regardless of where a Veteran seeks mental health treatment.

Practice Description

The mobile apps team sought input from 80 Veterans in mental health treatment, world-renowned experts, psychotherapy researchers, user experience experts, and frontline clinicians to alleviate the challenges of traditional psychotherapy. Expert clinicians tested early versions, and we obtained feedback through various public and private channels. Psychologists Eric Kuhn, PhD and Jason Owen, PhD led evaluation and research of the mobile app, in collaboration with researchers and health care providers around the nation.

Replicability

Designing and building mobile applications for VA settings can be challenging. However, when built, leveraging these products in various settings is relatively straightforward. All Mental Health Services apps are free of cost and available in VA and public app stores. Clinician guides help those who are interested bring these apps into care. Providing feedback to the core development team is critical for continued improvement as well as maintaining alignment with emerging best clinical practices. All sites can participate in the ongoing improvement of the tools.

Recognition

Julia Hoffman, VA's National Center for PTSD, DoD's National Center for Telehealth & Technology, VACO offices (Mental Health Services, the Office of Connected Care), Mobile Behavior Design team (Eric Kuhn, Jason Owen, Beth Jaworski, Kelly Ramsey)

Snoezelen Therapy: The Use of Multisensory Stimulation to Advance Geriatric Psychiatry Standards of Care

Georgina Delos Reyes, MSN, RN, Nurse Manager; Joseph De Veyra, MSN, RN, Clinical Nurse Leader, Staff Nurse

VA Long Beach Healthcare System, Long Beach, CA
gina.delosreyes@va.gov

The Snoezelen Therapy employed by VA Long Beach Healthcare System (VALBHS) is a novel, evidence-based therapy that currently produces positive outcomes for patients and staff. This therapy empowers Veterans and staff in an environment that encourages creativity and innovation.

Introduction

The mission of the M1 Inpatient Geropsychiatry unit is to elevate the standard of mental health care. Historically, the unit had a high rate of restraint utilization, and in the past, some described the unit as a "jail-like environment" by some Veterans. Leadership made a decision to utilize non-pharmacological interventions as an alternative to medication and restraints. The unit implemented Snoezelen Therapy, a patient-centered intervention that utilizes multi-sensory stimulation that can reduce neuropsychological symptoms, such as anxiety, depression, and agitation. The intervention uses a variety of sensory equipment that helps patients adapt their responses to sensory stimulation. The word "Snoezelen" is a Dutch word, meaning "to sniff and doze." M1 nurses provide Snoezelen Therapy in the Serenity Room, which includes a sofa, home-like decorations, a bubble water lamp, an assortment of music and meditation audio discs, aromatherapy equipment, squeeze balls, wall projector with various sceneries (e.g., ocean, space, forest, etc.), and soft lighting equipment. Licensed vocation nurse Danee Pisarchuk's experience demonstrates the impact of the innovative intervention on patients and their families:

"One afternoon, I was providing care for a Veteran with dementia and a history of assaultive behavior. While assisting him with Activities of Daily Living, he got extremely agitated and started yelling. I, along with his wife and my manager, accompanied him to the Serenity Room. While conversing with his wife, I discovered he was a huge Elvis Presley fan. I decided to use Snoezelen Therapy and started playing Elvis songs. His demeanor changed as he started to sing along, and within a few minutes, he grabbed his wife's hand and started to cry. He said, 'Thank you so much for loving me.'"

Out of the 60 patients who recently participated in Snoezelen Therapy, 95 percent reported that it was therapeutically effective. There was also a reduction in depression (44 percent) and anxiety (42 percent) after the intervention. Furthermore, the unit successfully provided a restraint-free environment in 2011 and 2014. The intervention has also contributed to above average All Employee Survey (AES) results. From 2013 to 2014, unit innovation (3.9) and overall satisfaction (3.9) were higher than average VHA and VALBHS ratings.

Key Information

In 2010, VALBHS leadership procured Snoezelen equipment. During that year, the Geropsychiatry unit was in the process of transforming from a "jail-like" atmosphere to a home-like environment. Various services, including executive management, MH leadership, volunteers, engineering, infection control, and patient/hospital safety leadership helped create the Snoezelen room. In 2014, the Geropsychiatry unit achieved a grant from VACI, which provided additional equipment, such as mega-pod interactive touch screen, mega-light, sound panel, optic lights, large bubble tube pump, and portable and solar projectors. The unit's shared governance chairs, clinical nurse leader, and nurse manager headed the project. Snoezelen Therapy protocol coincides with the Veteran's treatment plan. The goal of this concurrent treatment option is to optimize recovery by providing an innovative and non-pharmacological intervention.

Context

The VALBHS M1 Geropsychiatry unit is a patient-centered, recovery-based inpatient program. As a division of the MH Health Care Group, it provides acute care and stabilization in preparation for other less intensive outpatient programs. The Geriatric Psychiatry Unit is designed to care for Veterans 55 years or older who require a structured therapeutic and recovery-based environment. The program involves active evidence-based psychopharmacological and psychotherapeutic interventions, education, therapeutic groups, teaching, and research. The primary diagnoses include neurocognitive disorders, such as Alzheimer's, and/or psychiatric diagnosis, such as mood, thought, trauma-related, and substance abuse disorders. The development of the Snoezelen Therapy intervention provides a more patient-centered approach than the typical pharmacological or physical intervention for this complex population.

Practice Description

The unit utilized the Plan, Do, Check, and Act (PDCA) model for quality improvement to implement Snoezelen Therapy. The "Plan" phase involved:

- M1's commitment to implementing evidenced-based, innovative therapies for geriatric psychiatric patients
- Conducting literature review on Snoezelen Therapy
- Accomplishing needs assessment with patients and staff
- Developing timeline and goals
- Providing patient and staff education
- Coordinating with VALBHS executive management, MH leadership, patient safety officer, infection control, volunteer services and engineering departments on equipment and room setup

The "Do" phase involved patient therapy sessions conducted with several patients. The "Check phase" involved assessing patients pre- and post-therapy, monitoring frequency of therapy sessions, and continuously gathering feedback and evaluation. The "Act" phase involved acting on feedback obtained from patients, families, and employees.

Replicability

The practice is successful because of the unit's culture of innovation, the staff's dedication to improving outcomes, and the support of VALBHS leadership. It is possible to replicate the intervention because the staff champions have supported the dissemination of the project, and established a sound implementation process, which they are able to share. The staff and mental health leadership presented a research poster at the American Psychiatric Nursing Association Conference in October 2011, where it received first place in the nursing practice category. In 2013 and 2015, the Office of Mental Health Operations (OMHO) recognized MI's Snoezelen Therapy as a National Strong Practice Project. The Geropsychiatry unit also published the project in an international scholarly journal. Moreover, unit staff provided in-service training about Snoezelen Therapy implementation. Unit champions have also collaborated with other areas to expand the use of Snoezelen Therapy outside of MH, such as the Community Living Center (CLC).

The Snoezelen Therapy employed at VALBHS is a novel evidence-based therapy that produces positive outcomes for patients and staff. This therapy empowers Veterans and staff in an environment that encourages creativity and innovation. The establishment of the M1 Snoezelen Therapy/Serenity Room has cultivated valuable and growing relationships among patients, family members, staff, and hospital administration. Because of this partnership, the impact of this complementary nursing intervention has been positive. It has also promoted safety and fostered patient and staff satisfaction. Thus, the Snoezelen Therapy team improved Veterans' outcomes not because they believed in themselves, but rather the team succeeded because they believed in each other.

Recognition

VISN 22 leadership, VALBHS leadership, Mental Health leadership, Larry Albers, Jessie D' Agostino, Josephine Villanueva, John Tryboski, Pete Hauser, Isabel Duff, Clifford Widmark, Nima Fahimian, Berge Bakamjian, Lynette Fox, Tom Hendon, Rick Banfield, Olivia Parducho, Susan Somes, Mira Castaneda, Janet DeBerry, Sonia Sabado, Joseph Ott, Patterson Jackson, Kris Palazzi, M1 Geropsychiatry staff, interdisciplinary team, M1 Shared Governance Council, Kara Kelly, Melanie Tallakson, Larry Sumait, Crystal Woods, Frencis Barbic, Michelle Gieng, Dorianne Tillano, Edwin Sinson, Loni Caldwell, Debra Martin, Kira Santa Anna, Mark Demesa, Danee Pisarchuk, Nancy Jaboni

Hepatitis C Medication Management Clinic

Audrey Broyer, PharmD, CPS

Manchester VAMC, Manchester, NH
audrey.broyer@va.gov

A multi-disciplinary team of providers and nurses was created to improve Hepatitis C treatment. As part of that improvement, the Hepatitis C Medication Management Clinic (HCMMC) was created to improve access to Hepatitis C medications.

Introduction

The Hepatitis C Medication Management Clinic was developed in response to an increasing demand for Hepatitis C Virus (HCV) treatment upon the approval of new, interferon-free, HCV treatment regimens. The Gastrointestinal (GI) clinic at the facility was understaffed and not able to keep pace as Food and Drug Administration (FDA) approvals of new HCV medications were determined. To provide timely appointments, the HCMMC was started. This clinic has allowed Veterans to be seen within one week of consult and get started on HCV treatment the same day as their visit. Patients are evaluated and cleared for treatment by the GI clinic providers instead of waiting for another appointment with these providers to discuss medication options.

The clinic has allowed our facility to be more flexible, and to treat patients quickly when money is available to fund HCV treatment. For example, Mr. X was sent to obtain HCV treatment through the Veteran's Choice program, as no funding was available at VA at the time. For reasons that remain unclear, the Veteran was referred to a sports medicine physician who was unable to provide the treatment. The Veteran notified the VA GI clinic and was understandably frustrated. On July 31, 2015, Congress approved emergency funding for the treatment of Hepatitis C patients and Mr. X was seen in the HCMMC for the duration of his 12-week treatment. He has since been cured and was very grateful to have received his treatment quickly.

Key Information

The HCMMC was initiated in April 2015. The clinic operates at the Manchester VAMC. The implementation was led by the pharmacy practice, with the assistance of other CPSs, and the GI clinic. The implementation occurred a few months after the interferon-free HCV treatments became available at VA. The HCMMC was not requested or required by supervisors, managers, or facility leaders. Rather, it was initiated based on patient need and the increasing workload facing the GI clinic providers.

Before the initiation of HCMMC in April 2015, the GI clinic at the facility was responsible for 99 percent of HCV treatment. After interferon-free regimens with superior sustained viral response rates were available, GI providers were unable to keep up with the treatment requests of patients. It was determined that a pharmacy-run Hepatitis C medication clinic would allow for an increased number of patients to be treated with HCV medications. Since the inception of this clinic, 44 patients have been seen for medication management solely by the CPS in this clinic, and six patients have been co-managed by the CPS and the GI clinic NP.

Context

The Manchester VAMC is located in Manchester, NH. It is the only VAMC without a full-service hospital. Many Veterans travel to Boston for specialty care, with many traveling long distances. The facility serves Veterans from both urban and rural areas since private sector specialty care can be limited in rural areas of NH. The practice addressed the increase in demand for HCV treatment when the interferon-free treatment regimens were approved by the FDA. These regimens had fewer side effects and improved cure rates when compared to previous treatment regimens. Because of this, many Veterans who were previously not interested in treatment, or who failed previous treatments were presenting to VA requesting treatment for HCV. Without a dedicated clinic for liver diseases, the GI clinic was not staffed to treat the increased number of Veterans requesting HCV treatment. The HCMMC was created to increase access for HCV patients wanting treatment, and for GI patients experiencing increased wait time in the GI clinic because of the increase in HCV treatment.

Practice Description

The HCMMC is a clinic solely for the management of HCV treatment medications. Veterans are seen in the GI clinic for evaluation. If they are screened for treatment, they are then sent to the HCMMC via consult. They can be scheduled quickly, and within one or two weeks of the consult, even the same day (if needed for patients with travel difficulties). During the visit in the HCMMC, the HCV treatment medication and drug interactions are discussed in detail. Since the appointments are face-to-face, the information is tailored based on the Veteran's needs. The Veteran is given the provider's contact information for additional questions or concerns. The patient visit is followed up with lab work and visits every 2–4 weeks until treatment is completed. The HCMMC has 12 patient slots per week.

Replicability

This practice was adopted to improve patient access to HCV treatment. It was successful because of the close working relationship between pharmacy and the GI clinic. This has allowed the two groups to share the workload and avoid duplication.

Other sites could adopt this practice and will do so out of need. It would be important to have the support of the service line managers, as starting a new clinic requires taking time away from existing clinical duties. This practice would not have been possible without the support of pharmacy supervisors and co-workers that agreed to take on extra work so time could be devoted to treating HCV patients.

Recognition

Linda DeOrio, Neil Wesner, Angelo Horatagis, Chrstaline Beem, Patricia Opuni, Kristyn Anderson, Karen Doherty, Van Vu, Jennifer Kinney, Pat Callahan, Mark Connelly, Claire Estes, Kathy Soucy, Robin McInnis

Home Based Primary Care Special Population Patient Aligned Care Team

Darlene Davis, MHA, NHA, RD, National Program Manager, GEC Operations (10NC4)
VHACO Geriatrics and Extended Care, Washington, DC
darlene.davis7@va.gov

Home Based Primary Care (HBPC) PACT provides high-quality, cost-effective, comprehensive, interdisciplinary, PC in the homes of Veterans with serious medical, social, and behavioral conditions. Services include PC, palliative care, rehabilitation, disease management, and coordination of care services.

Introduction

Home Based Primary Care Special Population PACT is a VA home care program that provides comprehensive, interdisciplinary, PC in the homes of Veterans with serious medical, social, and behavioral conditions for which routine clinic-based care is not effective. The best way to describe how the program impacts our Veterans' lives is a real example.

Mr. X is a 77-year-old Air Force Vietnam-era Veteran whose medical history includes; diabetes, heart disease, hypertension, stroke, hypothyroidism, suprapubic catheter for neurogenic bladder, aortic aneurysm, anemia, and peripheral vascular disease with recurrent leg ulcers.

He also had six hospitalizations and extended nursing home stays due to dehydration, acute renal failure, urinary tract infections, and severe Peripheral Vascular Disease (PVD) with non-healing leg ulcers. At the time of admission, he was refusing treatment ("labeled non-compliant"), had little contact with his family, and reported poor quality of life. He was facing long-term placement in a nursing home.

After being enrolled in HBPC, the team took the following action:

- HBPC provider: Worked with the Veteran and caregiver to identify the Veteran's goals and values to drive the plan of care. The provider initiated a medical follow-up plan that provided interventions, communication, and proactively met care needs.

- HBPC pharmacist: Worked with the Veteran, caregiver, and provider to decrease the number of medications. Also established schedules that aligned with the Veteran's goals and priorities.

- Social Worker (SW): Increased the Veteran's disability rating for Agent Orange to 100 percent. Obtained Veteran-directed care to allow the Veteran's granddaughter to be his full-time caregiver.

- HBPC RN care manager: Ended community-purchased care services by teaching the Veteran's granddaughter how to manage wounds and dressings. Routinely monitored the wounds until they healed. Assisted with medication management and ongoing case management support services.

- HBPC dietitian: Provided nutritional support and patient/caregiver education for chronic conditions. The goal was to achieve maximum nutritional benefit for disease management and wound healing.

- HBPC rehabilitation therapist: Conducted functional and home safety assessments, provided for Durable Medical Equipment (DME) needs, and supplied education on fall prevention, home exercise, oxygen safety, fire safety, and disaster preparedness.

Substantial person-centered outcomes were achieved:

- Veteran's family started visiting frequently
- Veteran reported significant improvement in his quality of life
- After HBPC was initiated, the Veteran was no longer hospitalized, nor did he require nursing home placement
- VA, HBPC program not only saved his life but also allowed him to remain safely in his home. It significantly improved his quality of life (financial, social, and medical). The Veteran is no longer considered "non-compliant."

Key Information

HBPC is a Geriatrics and Extended Care (GEC) Special Population PACT and provides personalized, proactive, patient-driven care. The unit of care is both the patient and caregiver. Their combined needs and preferences guide the goals and plan of care. HBPC targets longitudinal-care patients with chronic and serious medical, social, and behavioral conditions, particularly those at high risk for hospitalization, nursing home, or recurrent emergency care. It also targets patients who require palliative care for a serious disease that is life limiting, or refractory to disease-modifying treatment.

Context

HBPC began as a pilot project at six facilities in 1970 and became an established program in 1972. It was designed to serve the chronically ill in the months and years before death, providing needed comprehensive PC services in the home. HBPC began as a unique model of home care, and different from home care available under federal and state programs, such as Medicare and Medicaid. The HBPC model targets persons with complex chronic diseases that worsen over time and provides interdisciplinary care that is longitudinal and comprehensive rather than episodic.

Practice Description

The HBPC program promotes and maintains the Veteran's optimal health, independence, and well-being by providing in-home comprehensive longitudinal care through an interdisciplinary team (physician, nurse, social worker, dietitian, rehabilitation therapist, pharmacist, and mental health provider). HBPC increases access, improves quality, and lowers total cost of care. This is achieved through longitudinal care that includes close monitoring, early intervention, and promotion of a safe, therapeutic home environment. HBPC enhances the Veteran's quality of life, through end of life, by respecting the needs and preferences of the Veteran and caregiver. It addresses symptom management, supports the option of palliative care at home, and supports the caregiver through the grieving process.

Replicability

HBPC was implemented in VHA's largest teaching facilities. The program has successfully expanded to over 330 VAMCs, health care centers, CBOCs, and Reservations. HBPC has grown from serving 7,000 to over 36,000 Veterans daily, and yet population analyses indicate there are approximately 30,000 Veterans with serious chronic disabling diseases, who would also benefit from HBPC. HBPC is not only a proven high-quality, cost-effective program in VA, but it has also been embraced in private sector health care through a successful Medicare demonstration called Independence At Home (IAH). The Medicare IAH demonstration was based largely on the experience, design, and clinical and economic outcomes of VA HBPC model of care.

Recognition

Nationwide VA facilities, which serve Veterans through HBPC services

Medical Foster Home: Where Heroes Meet Angels

Dan Goedken, National Program Manager, Medical Foster Home, Dayna Cooper, National Director H&CBS GEC Operations, Kim Kelley, National Director, H&CBS, GEC Policy
VACO, Washington, DC
daniel.goedken@va.gov

A Medical Foster Home (MFH) serves Veterans who have multiple, complex medical problems, allowing Veterans the choice to receive nursing home level care in a less restrictive, home environment. MFH assists in meeting the increasing demand for Long-Term Services and Support (LTSS) through care in a family setting, while improving quality of life.

Introduction

Mr. X fought in Vietnam. When he returned home he was suffering from PTSD, schizophrenia, and substance abuse. Most of his adult life was spent on the street or in jail. He suffered multiple arrests for burglary and petty theft while trying to secure money. He was malnourished, isolated, and afraid. During his last trip to the county jail he met with a VA Justice Outreach Social Worker who provided him with a chance for a new life.

Mr. X was placed in the Medical Foster Home program. The Veteran's medical team helped him receive VA benefits and his pension, and then followed his medical condition. The team ensured that he ate home-cooked meals, was provided daily medications, socialized with other Veterans, and was treated with dignity and compassion. As a result, Mr. X never went back to jail. He gained 40 pounds and smiled every day. As he neared the end of his life, he chose to die under hospice care in his MFH.

Since the MFH caregiver must reside in the home, the Veteran becomes part of the family. Many Veterans go on outings, family gatherings, and trips and vacations with their MFH families. Ethel Gordon is one such caregiver. Originally from Trinidad, she grew up with a family who provided care to the homeless in her own country. After a career in Mental and Behavioral Health and raising her children, she looked for a way to contribute to the community. She considered fostering children, and in the process learned about VA MFH program. Ethel now includes three Veterans as part of her family, two men and one woman. Each Veteran has their individual story which includes some mental health history.

"We all went to Florida together for vacation," Ethel told me. "We go to church every Sunday. I was able to give them stability. There is always something going on." Her family is also involved, with her college-age children coming home on breaks and bringing home friends. "The Veterans all feel like they are back in college again," Ethel shared. She says the joy it brings to her is much more than what she ever expected.

Key Information

MFH is a VA-approved personal home chosen by both non-service-connected and service-connected Veterans with serious chronic disabling conditions that meet nursing home level of care need. The Veterans entering the program are no longer able to live independently, lack a strong family caregiver, and require daily personal assistance for their long-term care. The MFH meets these criteria of care in a non-institutional setting and at a lower cost than a nursing home. The program began in 1999 by two social workers at the Little Rock, Arkansas VAMC as an alternative to Community Residential Care (CRC). Veterans enrolled in Home Based Primary Care (HBPC) were unfit to live alone safely and did not want to move to a nursing home. Pilots began in 2004 in Tampa, FL, and San Juan, Puerto Rico VA Hospitals.

Context

A MFH serves Veterans who have multiple, complex medical problems. MFH offers Veterans the choice to receive nursing home level care in a less restrictive, home environment. MFH assists in meeting the increasing demand for Long-Term Services and Support (LTSS) through care in a non-institutional setting. It gives Veterans the option to be in a family setting and improves quality of life. More than 3,600 Veterans have now been served in MFH, with an average length of stay of 402 days. The Program is most effective at reducing hospitalizations and Emergency Room (ER) visits. The Program is self-sustaining through cost avoidance of Community Nursing Home and Community Living Center (CLC) costs. MFH provides an alternative to nursing home, in a personal home, at half the cost.

Practice Description

The MFH helps Veterans who have serious chronic disease, disabling conditions, need daily personal assistance, and can no longer safely remain at home because they lack a family caregiver. The MFH program brings together VA support with a person who is willing to open their home and serve in the role of a strong family caregiver. VA MFH Coordinator manages the program, and a VA interdisciplinary home care team provides care in the MFH to the Veteran and training to the MFH caregiver. The MFH is matched with the Veteran's physical, social, and emotional needs, including supervision and protection.

Replicability

Through startup funds provided since 2009, MFH operates in 122 VA facilities in 45 states and territories. The plan is to establish MFH in every VA facility. Caregiver and Veteran satisfaction has received consistently high satisfaction levels. Veterans greatly prefer MFH over facility- based nursing home care with lower overall costs.

Recognition

Little Rock, AR VAMC

Mass Interviewing for Homeless Veteran Outreach

Justin Gallaher, Community Employment Coordinator

Columbus Clinic, Columbus, GA

justin.gallaher@va.gov

Mass Interviewing is a collaborative effort between VA and any employer for the purposes of filling multiple positions with a streamlined interviewing and hiring process.

Introduction

Justin Gallaher is the Community Employment Coordinator (CEC) at Columbus, OH, VA Outpatient Clinic. He is one of over 150 CECs recently employed by VA Homeless Veterans Community Employment Services (HVCES) as part of a national initiative to expand the role of employment in ending Veteran homelessness. As a member of the homeless program team, the CEC leads efforts to establish a local employment collective. The CEC collaborates with VA and non-VA partners to identify local gaps in current employment services, and develops opportunities to engage with local employers committed to helping combat homelessness among Veterans.

Gallaher recently established the mass interviewing program, which exposes Veterans to various employer engagement opportunities, and interviewing processes. For Veterans seeking employment, the program provides a space to receive immediate feedback from interviewers. Interviewers help the Veteran understand what went well and what they can improve on. This type of real-life interview feedback boosts their chances for success in securing employment, even if they don't get hired for that particular job. According to Carl Landry, a Community Outreach Coordinator in Columbus, OH said, "This is still a very new model for us, but we've developed strong practices and we learn something new from each event."

The Columbus VA homeless program staff made a shift from individualized mock interviewing to this mass interviewing strategy, and yielded significant results. To date, 28 Veterans have been hired after mass interviews. Overall, 91 percent of participants received a second interview, and 80 percent were employed through the event. Since mass interviewing started, the employment rates for Columbus' Grant and Per Diem Program (GPD), as well as the Department of Housing and Urban Development and Veterans Affairs Supportive Housing (HUD-VASH) programs have seen significant increases of approximately 53 and 50 percent. The Columbus VAMC's overall homeless program employment rates have more than doubled, from 22 to 45 percent during the same period.

The homeless program team in Columbus, OH, also began hosting job fairs and hiring events at the Columbus VAMC. During those events, employers can disseminate information and interview Veterans. Gallaher and his team have used these opportunities to strengthen relationships with employers, and discuss the concept of mass interviewing with them. To date, five events have brought more than 17 companies to the Columbus VA. More than 100 Veterans have attended, and several received on-the-spot job offers.

Key Information

Mass Interviewing is a "caravan" model developed and implemented by Justin Gallaher at the Columbus VA Outpatient Clinic. While looking at how his housing-focused counterparts used a similar model to introduce several Veterans to multiple landlords in one day, Gallaher wondered if it could work for employment. He adjusted the model to bring together Veterans interested in working in the same industries with multiple employers. He found that conducting mass interviews could introduce several homeless Veterans to multiple employers in the same day. The official kickoff event of the Columbus OPC Mass Interviewing Program was held at the Boar's Head distribution center in Groveport, OH, on October 26, 2015. Additional mass interviewing events continue to be organized.

Context

Employment is critical to helping Veterans exit homelessness. Being homeless makes it challenging for Veterans to search for a job, secure a sit down with an employer, and practice interviewing VHA's Homeless Program addressed the challenge of ending Veteran homelessness in a number of different ways, including the implementation of the CEC across the country. This position focuses on connecting Veterans to internal and community-based resources to address their employment needs and preferences. In search of more effective ways to connect Veterans to prospective employers, Gallaher identified how mass interviewing could vastly improve each Veteran's chances of being employed.

Practice Description

The mass interviewing program, implemented at the Columbus, OH, VA Outpatient Clinic, assigned Veterans to groups by skillset and job category. To be successful, program staff needed to build strong relationships with employers with the right types of job openings in accessible locations. The team began developing employer partnerships by cold-calling potential employers, attending networking events, scouring social media for possible openings, soliciting referrals from recruiters, and working with local military organizations to identify employers and gain their buy-in. Program staff outreached to Veteran groups and assisted them with employment applications as well as improving their interviewing skills.

During the event, Veterans were exposed to various interview processes, as employer styles were somewhat dissimilar. Regardless of the format, Veterans received immediate face-to-face feedback from employers. After the event, the CEC reached out to individual Veterans and the group to review the process, and to adjust the planning of future events. Recognizing that lack of transportation is an employment barrier, the team coordinated transportation to the interview for the entire group. Ultimately, mass interviewing is effective because it eliminates many of the barriers connecting Veterans with employers. It centralizes many of the components of the process. Service providers play a large role in preparing Veterans for the event. Partnering with local VA homeless programs and community service providers maximizes the supports that increase opportunities for Veterans, and assists the CEC in building trusting relationships with employers.

Replicability

The mass interviewing program was successful in Columbus, OH, because it aligned the role and work of the CEC with community opportunities. CECs work every day to connect Veterans to the most appropriate VA and community-based employment services by creating a cohesive community-large platform of resources. The success of the mass interviewing practice is based upon: 1) building employer relationships; 2) engaging and preparing Veterans; and 3) convincing everyone that mass interviewing works toward an endpoint. Although largely dependent on the role of the CEC, establishing partners to support the integration of mass interviewing is key to making the program possible. Other factors influencing the program include logistical support for event organization, and creativity to overcome potential barriers, such as transportation.

Recognition

Columbus Homeless Program team

25 City Coordination to House Homeless Veterans

Keith Harris, National Director of Clinical Operations, VA Homeless Programs and VA Project Manager for 25 Cities

VACO, Washington, DC

keith.harris@va.gov

25 Cities is a collaborative effort with the US Department of Housing and Urban Development (HUD) and the US Interagency Council on Homelessness (USICH) supporting coordinated entry system development and local innovation to prioritize and house homeless Veterans. It involves increasing housing through locally engineered tools. Providing resources in concert with other government and non-profit efforts as part of the national Ending Veteran Homelessness (EVH) campaign.

Key Information

The 25 Cities effort is a key federal strategy that provided technical assistance to 25 communities to mobilize local planning efforts and partnerships to end homelessness. Each community developed effective systems that aligned housing and service interventions. Led by VA, and in partnership with the US Department of Housing and Urban Development and the US Interagency Council on Homelessness, the effort ran from October 2013 through September 2016. The three-year effort brought federal and community partners together to collaborate to address Veteran and Chronic homelessness in the following cities: Atlanta, Baltimore, Boston, Chicago, Denver, Detroit, Fresno, Honolulu, Houston, Las Vegas, Miami, New Orleans, New York City, Orlando, Philadelphia, Phoenix, Portland, Riverside, San Diego, San Francisco, Seattle, Tampa, Tucson, and Washington, DC.

Context

As VA moves closer to its goal of Ending Veteran Homelessness, it is clear that homeless Veterans and their families benefit from the improved collaboration of federal, state, and community-based agencies. It is from this platform that VA, the National Center on Homelessness among Veterans, HUD, and USICH focused on the needs of the cities with the highest per capita homeless Veteran populations through an intensive, data-driven, and community-focused strategy. Through the technical assistance efforts of the 25 Cities Initiative, 19,849 Veterans were housed in 2015. As of March 2016, four communities were acknowledged for ending Veteran homelessness (as per the Federal EVH Criteria and Benchmarks). Those communities included Houston, New Orleans, Las Vegas, and Philadelphia. Two communities, Boston and New York City, ended chronic homelessness among Veterans, and the results of four additional communities, including Miami, Orlando, Portland (Oregon), and Tampa, are currently under review.

Practice Description

The 25 Cities Initiative assembled an integrated team of national experts to work with homeless Veterans programs at the local, state, and federal levels. The team also monitored efforts to end Veteran and chronic homelessness within the identified cities. Effective coordination was a key factor for success, and at the start of the Initiative, communities were encouraged to build local teams responsible for leading aspects of a coordinated housing system. Each city established a leadership team consisting of representatives from VA, local homeless programs, Community-Based Organizations (CBOs), and the Continuum of Care, as well as design, data, outreach and navigation, and landlord teams to spearhead efforts. The organization and role of the team were community-specific in order to address unique local needs.

Collaboration within and between teams was supported by an expert community coach who facilitated goal and strategy alignment. The team of experts and staff supported local coordination efforts by 1) assisting communities in developing and maintaining coordinated entry systems; 2) assisting communities in accelerating housing placement rates through more efficient coordination of VA and community resources and information; 3) helping communities coordinate, create, and maintain a functional list that calculated inflow and tracked housing placements; 4) facilitating and coordinating community partnerships to ensure key players were at the table; 5) promoting and coordinating effective landlord outreach and partnerships to increase available and affordable housing stock for homeless Veterans; and 6) ensuring that communities have sustainable systems in place.

In partnership with VA, HUD, and USICH, the 25 Cities team ensured communities had access to helpful tools and trainings, including national guidance and messaging, interagency policy and memoranda, webinars, community success stories, and promising practices, and sample outreach toolkits and materials. The team not only supported local communication strategies, but also maintained a communication matrix that guided how information moved from the field to the federal level and across various agencies. Information provided to communities was shared via an online interactive platform that provided numerous resources to help communities reach their goals. Additionally, communities experienced quarterly site visits, regular phone and email communications, and customized technical assistance through their community coach. Each community provided weekly, monthly, and annual progress reports. The reports outlined the achievement of goals, the barriers that were addressed, and included recommendations for how to strengthen community teams and systems. All communities received opportunities to communicate directly with representatives from VA, HUD, and USICH national offices through regular check-ins. During each event, the cities were invited to collectively share ideas and successful best practices, challenges, and to request federal assistance. The Initiative demonstrated the impact of partnerships between VA and the community in addressing the unique needs of ending Veteran homelessness across the country.

Replicability

The 25 Cities Initiative attributes its success to the efforts and support by local VA and community partners as well as federal VA support. The partnership allowed each city to produce and institutionalize customizable approaches within the coordinated housing effort. The technical assistance provided through this effort also helped to establish standard yet adaptable strategies for coordinated entry systems, outreach, landlord engagement, and data tracking systems.

The Initiative helped each community develop the practices previously described, and assisted in building sustainable systems that can be replicated and applied to other communities and other homeless populations. The network of partners, program infrastructure, and repository of national resources and guidelines, in addition to the lessons learned and practices developed, will make it easier for communities to adopt similar approaches in the eradication of chronic homelessness for youth, families, and other populations. Many of the distinct practices developed through this effort have been documented and reworked for effective replicability in communities across the country.

Recognition

Local VA staff, community partners, federal partners at VA, HUD, and USICH

Homeless Mobile Medical/Mental Veteran Intervention

Dina Hooshyar, MD MPH, Medical Director
Dallas VAMC, Dallas, TX
dina.hooshyar@va.gov

The Homeless Mobile Medical/Mental Veteran (HMMM-V) Intervention team actively searches the community for Veterans experiencing homelessness and provides them social, medical, and mental health services at point of contact. Their approach is to provide care that is based on Veterans' self-identified goals rather than traditional illness-based treatment.

Introduction

The Comprehensive Homeless Center Program (CHCP) has a long-standing tradition of offering homeless outreach services since 1990, when CHCP became the first VA Comprehensive Homeless Center. Social Workers offer the majority of these services mainly in community, non-VA hospital-based settings. These services consist primarily of meeting the Veterans' basic needs, and generally do not foster opportunities for Veterans to reflect on other important aspects of their lives. Although referrals are made, Veterans do not typically seek medical attention for their medical conditions.

Key Information

Homeless Mobile Medical/Mental Veteran Intervention allows for provision of medical care at point of contact, and provides the opportunity for Veterans to reflect on more than their basic needs. VA Office of Patient Centered Care and Cultural Transformation (OPCC&CT) created the Patient-Centered Care Personal Health Inventory. This inventory facilitates Veteran-clinician dialogue about Whole Health Concepts, i.e., the various elements of wellness. HMMM-V team utilizes this approach as they offer services at homeless encampments, various places not meant for human habitation, and scheduled locations. They have had 185 Veteran encounters. Through actively searching for Veterans experiencing homelessness, HMMM-V clinicians are providing holistic social, medical, and mental health services to Veterans who might not have otherwise received such care.

A critical element in ending Veteran homelessness is bringing services to the Veteran. These Veterans are more likely to engage in care if the Clinician-Veteran interactions are based on Veterans' self-identified goals, rather than traditional illness-based treatment focusing on identified disease(s). To actualize these goals, Drs. Alina Suris and Carol North applied for funding from VA OPCC&CT. The grant was funded on January 25, 2013. On April 8, 2015, HMMM-V intervention became fully operational at Dallas VAMC. This program was incorporated into the Dallas VAMC's Health Care for Homeless Veterans (HCHV) program, under Ms. Tammra Wood's leadership. The frontline HMMM-V team consists of social worker, peer support specialist, program support assistant, psychiatrist, and physician assistant positions. The HMMM-V team collaborates with the VA North Texas Health Care System (VANTHCS) medical administration, pharmacy, pathology and laboratory medicine, IT, infection control, emergency management, motor pool services, Vet centers, Parkland (Dallas County's Public Hospital), and numerous other community partners.

Context

VANTHCS consists of Dallas VAMC, Sam Rayburn Memorial Veterans Center in Bonham, three Outpatient Clinics, and five CBOCs. In FY 2014, VANTHCS served 116,221 unique Veteran patients, had 1,384,554 outpatient visits, and had 227,964 total inpatient bed days. VANTHCS serves both urban and rural Veteran populations. CHCP has a total of 152 full-time equivalent employees and is part of VANTHCS Mental Health Service. In addition to homeless outreach, CHCP includes housing programs and Therapeutic and Supported Employment Services. The 2015 Point-in-Time (PIT) Veteran Homeless Count for state of Texas and VANTHCS catchment area was 2,393 and 654, respectively (PIT count is acknowledged to be an underrepresentation of the homeless count). Reaching 2,074 calls in FY 2015, CHCP had the second highest call volume in the nation from the Veteran Homeless Hotline. HMMM-V Intervention addressed the challenge of providing both social services and medical care in a non-hospital/clinic setting to reach Veterans experiencing homelessness. During CHCP's 2015 Commission on Accreditation of Rehabilitation Facilities (CARF) Survey, HMMM-V Intervention became CARF-accredited. CARF surveyors remarked favorably on HMMM-V's ability to provide care. This engagement style motivates Veterans to be more open to further care.

Practice Description

VA OPCC&CT is cultivating the metamorphosis of VA health care delivery from treating specific disease conditions to promoting whole health. The office funded VANTHCS Mental Health Services (MHS) clinicians to provide Veteran-centered care to the Veteran homeless population through the HMMM-V Intervention. This intervention brings social, medical, and mental health care to Veterans experiencing homelessness, and engages Veterans in a "What matters to you" rather than "What is the matter with you" style. It took less than two years for HMMM-V Intervention to become fully operational. During this time, HMMM-V team sought guidance from other programs familiar with mobile units, and then procured a van that is equipped with a medical examination room and associated equipment. HMMM-V team also consulted with VANTHCS IT and Infection Control Services to fit the van with electronic connectivity, and to maximize protection against infectious diseases. Additionally, the HMMM-V team tailored the Patient-Centered Care Personal Health Inventory for Veteran homeless population, conducted outreach to community partners to assist in locating Veterans experiencing homelessness, and collaborated with VANTHCS Eligibility Section to devise a process to determine Veteran eligibility for VA services. Dr. Dina Hooshyar, CHCP Medical Director, worked extensively with Parkland and VANTHCS pharmacy service to determine how to create a formulary for HMMM-V, and how to stock the HMMM-V van with medications. She also worked with VANTHCS pathology and laboratory medicine service to create a process to obtain blood or urine samples from Veterans. She is also working to secure a point-of-care lab testing capacity. With this testing capability, HMMM-V would be able to process labs in the van, and know the results within minutes.

HMMM-V Intervention was created at the local Dallas VAMC to break down access-to-care barriers in the homeless Veteran population. The impetus to create the program came from VANTHCS frontline staff and leadership. VANTHCS staff is passionate about ending Veteran homelessness. A foundational factor that made HMMM-V possible was funding from VA OPCC&CT.

Replicability

Necessary conditions for HMMM-V Intervention at other facilities include: funding, especially for a van with associated equipment; collaboration from the medical facility's departments in support of a clinic on wheels; outreach staff able to deliver care in non-traditional medical settings; staff with expertise in networking and project management; and medical knowledge to create services, such as medication formulary.

Recognition

Sharon Anderson, Robin Amirkhan, Sylvia Baack, Ruth Bechdol, Susan Best, Michael Bradley, David Breedlove, Timothy Brown, Pushpi Chaudhary, Angela Christie-Smith, Dean Cromwell, Winford Cross, Scott Foster, Jerica Goodwin, Jennifer Gunter, Yolanda Haggerty, Denise Henderson, Teresa House-Hatfield, Brenda Ingram, Laurell Jackson, Johnny Joe, Kevin Kelly, Scotty Keohaname, Rhonda Kvetko, James LePage, Heidi Michaels, Jeffery Milligan, Sheryl Poyer, Jennifer Purdy, Shirley Richardson, Jason Sluder, Patrick Smith, Susan Spalding, Sheila Wise, Linda Young, VA Office of Patient Centered Care and Cultural Transformation

Bidding Adieu to the Flu in Homeless Shelters and Transitional Living Facilities

Joan Jenkins, Homeless Outreach RN/Case Manager
Louis Stokes Cleveland VAMC, Cleveland, OH
joan.jenkins2@va.gov

"Bidding Adieu to the Flu" is a nursing outreach project designed to reduce the transmission of the influenza virus in transitional living and homeless shelters by using health promotion groups and flu clinics held at these facilities.

Introduction

"Bidding Adieu to the Seasonal Flu in Homeless Shelters, and Transitional Living Facilities" has been in use since October 2014. Since that time, this health promotional group has been established in three different counties, and at seven different facilities. It will be conducted through the 2015–2016 flu season. Data has shown that these groups are a valuable tool in getting more Veterans vaccinated. Over 100 Veterans have attended the groups and have received the influenza vaccine.

Key Information

The health promotion group "Bidding Adieu to the Flu" was implemented in the Grant and Per Diem (GPD) facilities. It was created in October 2014 in response to the request of a large number of Veterans residing at the homeless shelters, and transitional living facilities. This project was important because Veterans experiencing homelessness often have greater incidences of chronic care conditions than their civilian counterparts do. They are considered to be in the "high-risk" category for developing flu-related complications. When these individuals receive the flu vaccine they reduce the possibility of developing complications related to the flu.

Context

"Bidding Adieu to the Flu" was a shelter-based initiative sponsored by the Louis Stokes VAMC, a tertiary hospital that serves over 110,000 Veterans a year. This project was designed to improve Veterans' health outcomes, and to promote better health habits among individuals experiencing homelessness. It improved Veterans access to health care professionals and health care services, decreased wait times, reduced transportation challenges, and increased Veterans' knowledge of health practices that reduce the transmission of the influenza virus.

Practice Description

This project was implemented as a health promotion group, which educated and demonstrated to Veterans the importance of handwashing, cough etiquette, and the value of an influenza vaccination. At the conclusion of each discussion group, the flu injection was offered to those without contraindications.

Replicability

The project is currently conducted at the Grant and Per Diem sites in Northeast Ohio and is replicable anywhere. This project was made possible through the participation of shelter staff, VA staff from various disciplines, and the Veterans making the request.

Recognition

Susan Johnson, Trina Zabarsky, Dr. Konicki, the WP VAMC pharmacy staff, the WP VAMC SPD staff

Rapid Re-Housing of Veteran Families

John Kuhn, National Director, Supportive Services for Veteran Families

VACO, Washington, DC

john.kuhn2@va.gov

VA's Supportive Services for Veteran Families (SSVF) pioneered an intervention that rapidly moves Veterans and their families from homelessness into permanent housing. SSVF emphasizes a housing first approach that focuses on eliminating barriers to finding and keeping housing.

Key Information

Through the Supportive Services for Veteran Families program, VA aims to improve very low-income Veteran families' housing stability. The first core concept is that SSVF programs utilize a Housing First approach. The essential idea of Housing First is that housing is a basic need that should be met as quickly as possible, without any preconditions. To meet this goal, grantees provide eligible Veteran's with outreach, case management, and assistance in obtaining VA and other benefits, which may include health care services, daily living services, personal financial planning services, transportation services, fiduciary and payee services, legal services, childcare services, and housing counseling services.

In addition, grantees also provide time-limited payments to third parties (e.g., landlords, utility companies, moving companies, and licensed childcare providers) if these payments help Veterans' families remain in or acquire permanent housing.

Context

SSVF is designed to rapidly re-house homeless Veteran families and prevent homelessness for those at imminent risk due to a housing crisis. Funds are granted to private non-profit organizations, and consumer cooperatives that assist very low-income Veteran families by providing a range of supportive services designed to promote housing stability. SSVF is a new model of care that allows VA to serve the Veteran and their dependents, working to keep their family together. In FY 2015, SSVF served 157,416 people, including 34,636 children.

Practice Description

SSVF grantees work quickly to enroll Veteran families, and identify immediate barriers to housing placement. SSVF's approach is to treat homelessness as a crisis, using a housing first model to place Veteran families as quickly as possible. In addition to addressing participants' needs, grantees work within the community to place families in permanent housing. Developing relationships with landlords is a central element of this work. Families with poor credit histories, or other problems that surface during background checks, must negotiate with the landlord for placements to occur.

Replicability

SSVF's model of rapid re-housing is supported by research from the National Center on Homelessness among Veterans. More specifically, the model shows that Veteran households placed into permanent housing by SSVF are likely to remain housed. Two years after exit, this research found that 86 percent of families and 74 percent of individual Veterans remain housed.

Supportive Services for Veteran Families University

John Kuhn, National Director, Supportive Services for Veteran Families
VACO, Washington, DC
john.kuhn2@va.gov

Supportive Services for Veteran Families (SSVF) University has made training, relevant research, information about community plans to end homelessness, and critical programs available to the public. This helps providers train staff, assess local progress, and access current information about evidence-based practices.

Introduction

Supportive Services for Veteran Families University was created as a web-based tool, to disseminate evidence-based practices. This on-demand service makes program information, outcomes, research, and training available to providers around the country as well as to interested stakeholders and members of the public. An important function is to help SSVF grantees train staff on a variety of topics related to SSVF service delivery, helping establish baseline competencies for practice. It is also a resource for ongoing community planning facilitated by SSVF grantees and VA partners to create locally responsive plans designed to end Veteran homelessness. The site can be found at www.va.gov/homeless/ssvf/index.asp.

Key Information

There are approximately 400 SSVF grantees located in all 50 states, Puerto Rico, the District of Columbia, Guam, and the Virgin Islands. Approximately $400 million in FY funding support these grantees. Because grantees are widely dispersed, virtual training and resource sharing are utilized to support evidence-based practices in each location. Furthermore, sharing outcome and research information fosters the development of rapid re-housing as well as prevention practices throughout the country.

Context

SSVF's approach to ending homelessness utilizes a crisis response system of rapid re-housing and prevention services, relatively new in the field of homeless services. As a result, staff expertise is limited. In fact, much of the knowledge base about rapid re-housing and prevention services are currently drawn from SSVF's experiences. Given its national scope, SSVF has a unique opportunity to help shape promising, cost-effective interventions by sharing what it has learned.

Practice Description

SSVF University is easily navigated through access to the Internet by any commercially available web browser. Users can access materials sorted under several program tabs.

Replicability

SSVF University was created to address the needs of a widely dispersed audience looking to access materials and information about this pioneering, national effort launched by VA. The design and support of the website was made possible by local staff who saw the value of the initiative, along with contractors who helped develop materials. SSVF University is regularly updated to include recent research, outcomes, training materials, and community plans.

Recognition

Tricia Donelan, Joshua Tuscher

Homeless PACTs: Providing Veteran-centered Care to Our Homeless Veterans

Thomas O'Toole, MD, Director, National Center on Homelessness among Veterans

VACO, Washington, DC

thomas.otoole@va.gov

Homeless Patient Aligned Care Team (H-PACT) is a multi-disciplinary, population-based medical home, designed to meet the unique challenges homeless Veterans face when engaging care. H-PACT addresses medical and social needs in one setting by incorporating social determinates of health, distinguishing it from traditional PC models.

Introduction

My name is Michael Marshall. I am a 49-year-old US Air Force Veteran who has been diagnosed with PTSD. I had a promising career with the Air Force until an unfortunate incident occurred, one in which I was too embarrassed to ever speak of again. So, I self-medicated. That proved to be the beginning of a series of extremely bad choices, and a downward spiral that eventually led me to prison. I went on using and selling all types of drugs for almost 20 years of my life.

I come from a very close-knit family that is very involved in the church. One day, in a moment of clarity, I saw my family and myself deteriorating to the point of certain death. I had lost my brother and father to the disease of addiction, yet I self-medicated even more than they did, just to cover up how I felt about what was going on within me. I got to the point where I found myself on the streets of Chicago, without a home for roughly ten years. I found myself living in and out of abandoned houses just to stay warm on winter nights.

When I came to the Jesse Brown VA, I was told about the H-PACT clinic. Although I had heard about the services available at VA, I was too embarrassed to tell anyone just how far I had fallen, and what had happened to me. The H-PACT PCP was my initial contact with the homeless program. From there, I was linked with dental care, transitional housing, treatment for my addiction, and therapy for my PTSD. Cognitive Processing Therapy was the most important component of all because it renewed my self-esteem and self-worth. I was also referred to the HUD-VASH program, and currently have a three-bedroom apartment. I was also referred to the Compensated Work Therapy Program (CWT), which further gave me the opportunity to re-equip myself with the tools necessary to become a productive member of society. I currently work in recreation therapy services through the CWT program. Working with other Veterans and employees of Jesse Brown VA has raised my spiritual awareness and given me a whole new perspective on life. All of the treatment I received enables me to confront life—not as a giant of my dreams nor a dwarf of my fears, but as a man. I am truly grateful to have walked into the H-PACT clinic and to have followed the suggestions of the H-PACT team. Now, I am humbly at the doorstep of a promising career and a renewed quality life.

Key Information

The Homeless Medical Home initiative, known within VHA as the Homeless Patient Aligned Care Team program, was launched in 2011 as part of the pilot programs initiative within the National Center on Homelessness among Veterans. The model is now present in 60 VA medical facilities, and serves over 18,000 homeless Veterans each year. The H-PACT is comprised of an integrated care team drawn from homeless programs, PC, mental health service lines, and local community partners. The intent is to improve the integration of health and social services for homeless Veterans, with a focus on high-risk populations. The goal is to facilitate access and engagement in care, stabilize them clinically, provide them with needed social services and programs, and expedite placement in housing.

Evaluation of the program to date has identified the following outcomes:

- Twenty-five percent (25 percent) reduction in both ED and inpatient admissions following enrollment in the H-PACTs, as compared with care use in the six months prior to enrollment.

- Improvements in chronic disease management outcomes among homeless Veterans.

- Cost savings in health care use averaging $9,500 per H-PACT-enrolled Veteran per year, as compared with costs when enrolled in other VA care programs. This translates to an estimated savings of $235 million per year nationally.

- Expedited housing placements with more Veterans placed in stable housing, occurring at a rate of 86 days faster among H-PACT enrolled Veterans.

Context

Homeless Veterans have a disproportionately high disease burden, mortality rates 3–4 times higher than their housed counterparts, and an average age of death in their mid-50s. They also utilize high levels of care, often in costly acute care settings: over 40 percent used the ED at least once in the previous year, and over 25 percent were hospitalized. However, homeless Veterans face multiple barriers in access to care, including transportation, limited availability, fragmentation of services, difficulty scheduling and keeping appointments, perceived or actual stigma, lack of trust, social isolation, and competing sustenance needs. These issues challenge our capacity to engage them in care and the services they need to exit homelessness, achieve health, and re-engage in our communities.

Practice Description

There are five core elements of the H-PACT model that distinguish it from traditional PC approaches: 1) enhanced, low threshold access to care, with open-access/walk-in capacity, flexible scheduling, and clinical outreach to streets, shelters, and community locations; 2) wrap-around and integrated services: homeless programs, mental health, and co-located PC staff who are identified as core H-PACT team members, and involved in care planning; onsite competing sustenance response as part of the care package (e.g., food or food vouchers, hygiene kits, clothes, bus passes, and transportation assistance); 3) intensive, community-linked case finding, treatment engagement, and care management with an emphasis on enhancing longitudinal service use; 4) ongoing staff training and homeless care skill development; and 5) data-driven, accountable care processes. During startup, teams received itemized checklists specific to the H-PACT model and were supported with monthly community-of-practice calls and supports, performance feedback, and specialized staff.

Replicability

This program has been replicated in 60 VAMCs with several additional facilities in planning stages for the program. Local leadership awareness of the needs of this population, and appreciation that our traditional care models are not well-equipped to engage these Veterans to further address the full complement of their needs, has been critical. Further, a commitment from VACO, national program offices, and local facility leadership has been critical to realizing the downstream benefits of a population health approach for homeless Veterans. Lastly, and importantly, the availability of special purpose funding from the Homeless Program Office, and evaluation support from Health Services Research and Development (HSR&D) has been critical in conducting rigorous analyses that validated this approach. The H-PACT program office developed the start-up and technical assistance support to assist other sites interested in this program.

Recognition

Thomas Lynch, Madhu Agarwal, Lisa Pape, National Center on Homelessness among Veterans, Erin Johnson

The Department of Housing and Urban Development-VA Supportive Housing Program

Jesse Vazzano, LICSW, National Director, HUD-VASH

VACO, Washington, DC

jesse.vazzano@va.gov

The Department of Housing and Urban Development-VA Supportive Housing (HUD-VASH) program is a permanent supportive housing program targeting chronically homeless and highly vulnerable Veterans. The program uses the principles of Housing First to help ensure that the most vulnerable homeless Veterans are housed.

Key Information

The Department of Housing and Urban Development-VA Supportive Housing program is the largest permanent supportive housing program in the US, with approximately 78,300 vouchers across the country. Beginning in 1992 with 500 vouchers, the program expanded in FY 2008, and has been awarded additional HUD-VASH vouchers each year since. HUD-VASH is a collaborative program between HUD and VA. Eligible homeless Veterans receive a Housing Choice rental voucher from HUD and case management and supportive services from VA, as well as recovery from physical and mental health problems and substance use disorders resulting from homelessness. This program is offered in all 50 states, the District of Columbia, Puerto Rico, US Virgin Islands, and Guam. The HUD-VASH program demonstrates the local impact of an integrated federal approach to Veteran homelessness. Along with other VA and VHA homelessness services programs, HUD-VASH is a vital strategy in the national campaign to End Veteran Homelessness (EVH).

Over the years, the HUD-VASH program has developed numerous promising practices, including:

- HUD and VA Partnership: Through this program, HUD and VA have been able to break down silos, adjust policies and program requirements, and build a program that meets the needs of local Veterans. Each agency lends their skill and experience to develop a local system to house and support homeless Veterans. VA determines clinical eligibility and homelessness for the program, while the Public Housing Authority (PHA) determines the Veteran qualification, per HUD's regulations.

- Housing First: HUD-VASH is a Housing First program. This evidence-based practice establishes that the first and primary need of a Veteran is to obtain stable housing. By following this principle, the HUD-VASH program is able to quickly house Veterans, address other service needs, and ensure long-term stability.

- Unit Pre-Inspections: Each unit rented by a HUD-VASH participant must pass a housing quality standards inspection by the PHA, to ensure the unit is safe and habitable. To expedite the process, many communities conduct pre-inspections to ensure standards are met. This practice allows voucher holders to tour pre-approved units, and enables Veterans to sign a lease within days of the viewing. As a result, the amount of time spent in the housing search process is reduced significantly.

Context

As communities across the country move closer to EVH, it is clear that the HUD-VASH program plays a pivotal role. The HUD-VASH program targets chronic and highly vulnerable homeless Veterans who need services to obtain and sustain independent housing in their community. The program focuses on the most vulnerable homeless, and all Veterans are expected to participate in the services offered. The level of case management varies along with the Veteran wants and needs over time.

Case Management is a core principle of this program, and with the additional support, the services offered have led to great success. With no preconditions to housing placements (such as long-term sobriety, etc.), the program which aims to reach 100 percent, boasts 97 percent of their vouchers in use across the country. Additionally, 89 percent of HUD-VASH vouchers were under lease, with many more in the hands of Veterans actively looking for housing. Similarly, HUD-VASH boasts low rates of Veterans who exit the program. Case managers are able to provide individualized supports to meet the differing needs of Veterans, which allows for greater self-sufficiency and integration into communities.

Practice Description

The HUD-VASH program has been successful, due in part to the structure of the program. VA team focuses on confirming eligibility criteria, and building an individualized housing plan to ensure success for the Veteran. The PHA determines Veteran eligibility based on income limits, verifies a unit meets required standards, and processes paperwork to ensure financial support. This approach allows each agency to address their programmatic areas of expertise to move the Veteran into stable housing.

This program represents a cultural shift within VA. Previous methods argued that Veterans needed to overcome challenges and barriers to health, such as substance use, prior to receiving housing assistance. The Housing First shift, embodied in the HUD-VASH program, demonstrated to VA and community partners that assisting Veterans in obtaining stable housing, while simultaneously addressing other barriers, significantly improves their chances to succeed in permanent housing. The HUD-VASH program strongly believes in this principle, and provides wrap-around services to ensure that a Veteran's needs are met. When accepted into the program, a member of the HUD-VASH team works with the Veteran to develop an individualized plan reflecting their goals, strengths, and barriers to maintaining housing. Through this plan, the HUD-VASH team connects the Veteran to treatment programs, employment resources, medical and mental health care, legal support, and any other need that benefits housing stability. The HUD-VASH team works to foster Veteran independence and integration into the community, while also providing long-term support to the Veteran. Regular home visits, in addition to individual and group meetings, support the Veteran in their transition from homelessness into permanent housing.

Replicability

The success of the HUD-VASH program can be attributed to the continued effort and collaboration by local VA, PHA, and HUD staff, along with VACO and HUD headquarters. Their support to institutionalize HUD-VASH practices, and promote the customization of approaches within each community has been profoundly essential. Communities have established strategies to bring key decision-makers to the table, have developed referral, screening, and lease-up systems that meet their local needs, and ensure homelessness among Veterans is as brief as possible. Community partnerships have elevated the success of the program around bridge housing, landlord outreach, housing navigation and housing search, providing move-in assistance, and locating available units.

The policies and practices of this program at the federal and community level can be replicated and enhanced. The various lessons learned and promising field practices are continuously incorporated into national guidance documentation. Using available HUD and VA resources, other agencies, communities, and programs can be supported to replicate similar initiatives, or foster a similar interagency collaborative approach. Additionally, the emphasis on cross-community learning ensures local programs are continuously improving, managing their efforts to the best of their ability, and serving the Veterans and their families in reaching their own goals.

Recognition

VA and HUD offices at the local and federal levels

Home-Based Mental Health Evaluation

Mira Brancu, PhD, Site Lead for program, Deputy Director, Bridget Matarazzo, PsyD

Durham VAMC, Durham, NC

mira.brancu@va.gov

The Home-Based Mental Health Evaluation (HOME)-Rural Extension program focuses on reducing Veteran suicidality during their highest period of risk (between discharge from the inpatient unit and beginning of outpatient care), and improving re-engagement in care to support positive long-term outcomes.

Introduction

The HOME Program Clinical Demonstration project's incredible impact on Veteran well-being and safety is best described by Veteran feedback:

- "I really like this program. My clinician is really consistent, and I feel comfortable speaking with her... it gives individuals the sort of relaxed feeling, so that the next time they're at ease and they can begin to cope and understand better—to help you not harm yourself or anyone else."

- "VA should have this service all across the country. This is something Vets and mental health patients need. The phone calls picked me up when I was down. Your calls [during this transitional time period] helped me stay on track because I had someone to talk to."

- "My clinician was very instrumental in helping me have a plan. She was able to gather the information that would help me build a plan that I could use before I slipped into a crisis... She was specific about what I can do to relieve myself of stress in any situation."

- "I could not have done it without you, thank you so much. In the past, I would have just overdosed on my medications."

When asked about their satisfaction levels with HOME, the overwhelming majority of Veterans expressed appreciation for VA outreach ("someone to talk to," "knowing (someone) actually care[s]"), and the significance of having one-on-one, in-home contact after leaving the hospital ("She came to my house and made sure it was a safe place. She thoroughly made sure I was safe, even in my house, and that meant a lot to me"). While Veterans enrolled in HOME have described different personal benefits upon completion of the program, the project has had a universal impact on coping strategies during times of risk. Family members are also encouraged to participate and provide support during the home visit to improve outcomes.

Data from the initial evaluation of the HOME program demonstrate that in the first 90-days post-hospitalization, urban/local Veterans who participated were more likely to engage in care, engage more quickly, and attend more outpatient appointments than Veterans who did not receive the HOME program intervention. Their attitudes toward seeking mental health care also improved. With the addition of a new site at the Durham VAMC, where rural Veterans have also begun to receive the program, we will be able to learn more about outcomes for both urban/local as well as rural Veterans. A multi-site clinical trial of the HOME program, supported by the Military Suicide Research Consortium, is also underway.

Key Information

The weeks following psychiatric hospitalization are a particularly high-risk period for suicide. In addition, weeks following hospitalization also present a high risk for lack of post-hospitalization care. The HOME program is a clinical demonstration project focused on helping Veterans who are at risk for suicide and to increase their likelihood of outpatient care after hospitalization. In FY 2012 researcher-clinicians Bridget Matarazzo, PsyD and Melodi Billera, LCSW, along with their colleagues at the Rocky Mountain MIRECC (Denver), developed and implemented the HOME program to support Veterans after a psychiatric stay, encourage treatment engagement, and enhance coping for suicidal crises. The success of the program at Denver VAMC facilitated additional funds from mental health services and the ORH to expand the practice to urban and rural Veterans. Since the expansion to the Durham facility in FY 2015, the Mid-Atlantic MIRECC has helped 102 Veterans at risk for suicide, as they transition from the Durham VAMC inpatient unit back to their homes.

Context

The HOME program is currently being implemented at two large medical center facilities (Denver and Durham VAMCs). The Mid-Atlantic MIRECC (Durham) receives oversight from the developers at the Rocky Mountain MIRECC. The Rocky Mountain MIRECC focuses on suicide prevention and intervention, and the Mid-Atlantic MIRECC focuses on post-deployment mental health. The HOME program addresses the significant problem of needing to: 1) reduce Veteran suicide during the high-risk period between discharge from the inpatient unit and the beginning of outpatient care; and 2) improve re-engagement in care to support positive long-term outcomes. The program utilizes expertise and support from the inpatient and suicide prevention teams at each site.

Practice Description

The HOME program aims to reduce the risk of suicide after inpatient psychiatric discharge, and improve engagement in follow-up outpatient mental health visits by ensuring that rural Veterans receive additional care during that transition period. This is accomplished through intensive follow-up care, including 1) telephone contact within one business day of discharge to conduct a suicide risk assessment, review safety planning, and remind the Veteran of a scheduled home visit and other mental health appointments; 2) an in-person meeting in the Veteran's home environment within one week of discharge; and 3) ongoing safety planning and oversight until the Veteran is engaged in mental health care. The HOME program accomplishes its aims by addressing known suicide risk factors (e.g., lack of treatment engagement) and common barriers to care. The HOME program has demonstrated reduced time to outpatient care, and higher treatment engagement when implemented with suicidal Veterans living in urban environments. The program is currently evaluating how HOME can be implemented with rural Veterans, and assessing the necessary accommodations required to target risk factors and barriers specific to rural Veterans (e.g., mental health stigma, care coordination, distance, and isolation).

Currently we are evaluating in-person visits, which require available government vehicles, considerable travel, and ruling out environments that may be unsafe for provider visitation. We have preliminary evidence that HOME is working well under the current infrastructure. However, over time, we also hope to be able to evaluate options for telemedicine. This would reduce some of the visitation challenges, and increase the number of Veterans served.

Recognition

Janet Kemp, Caitlin Thompson, ORH, Rocky Mountain MIRECC, Bridget Matarazzo, Melodi Billera, Lisa Brenner, Durham VA Suicide Prevention Team, Gary Cunha, Ryan Higgins, Sonja McRae, Durham VA Inpatient Team, Tracey Holsinger, Madrianne Wong, Meredith Burger, Joy Close, Juanita Hill

Traumatic Brain Injury Interdisciplinary Fitness and Social Engagement

Shane Chanpimol, PT, DPT, Polytrauma/TBI Advanced Research Fellow
Washington DC VAMC, Washington, DC
shane.chanpimol@va.gov

Traumatic Brain Injury (TBI) Interdisciplinary Fitness and Social Engagement (InFuSE) provides a team model to improve cognitive executive function. It uses exercise as a scaffold for the promotion and maintenance of positive health behaviors in Veterans with a history of TBI.

Introduction

Traumatic Brain Injury has become the defining injury of our military over the last two decades. The difficulties following TBI can vary widely, including memory problems, sleep disturbance, weakness, poor balance, PTSD, and difficulty reintegrating to civilian life. The findings from research efforts have been pivotal in directing the care of Veterans who have suffered a TBI. A majority of these efforts have focused on the diagnosis and initial treatments of TBI. However, we know that TBI will likely have effects on our Veterans over their entire lives. Veterans with a history of TBI commonly experience significant cognitive and physical difficulties. Many persist even after they complete months or years of skilled therapies (speech-language pathology, physical therapy, and occupational therapy). These difficulties can place significant stress on the Veteran's family, friendships, employment, mental health, physical health, and overall quality of life. The VHA is charged with providing the best quality care for these Veterans for the rest of their lives.

The TBI Interdisciplinary Fitness and Social Engagement program was developed to promote physical activity, group exercise, social interactions, community engagement, and improve quality of life of Veterans with chronic TBI. InFuSE was designed to specifically address the difficulties of chronic TBI management, and to improve prevention of secondary conditions. The foundation of InFuSE is built upon the development of self-efficacy, and promotion of self-regulatory behaviors. Essentially, InFuSE provides a structured and socially rich environment to empower Veterans with TBI to manage their own physical and leisure activities.

The combined efforts of polytrauma, physical therapy, and recreation therapy departments initiated the development of TBI InFuSE in late 2014 at the Washington DC VAMC. Our interdisciplinary team collaborated alongside department chiefs to address issues of workload credit, CPRS documentation, and appropriate billing practices. Space and equipment within the physical and recreation therapy department were allocated to hold a 90-minute group intervention each week.

Key Information

Each InFuSE session includes a 30-minute patient education and group discussion followed by 60-minutes of exercise. InFuSE utilizes a semi-formal patient education curriculum. Education topics covered include goal setting, exercise programs, cognitive skills, fall prevention, and recreation opportunities, among others. Exercise programming consists of a warm-up, cardiovascular training (20–30 minutes), strengthening (15 minutes), balance/dual-task training (15 minutes), and a cool-down. InFuSE is primarily staffed by Polytrauma/TBI physical therapy fellows and a recreation therapist. However, professionals from psychiatry, speech-language pathology, occupational therapy, neuropsychology, and vocational rehabilitation have provided education and aided in InFuSE's ongoing development.

Context

Implementation of InFuSE began in January of 2015. Initially, InFuSE focused care toward Veterans with moderate to severe TBI. Participants were specifically approached because they were referred to skilled therapies on a frequent and recurring basis. These Veterans showed greater dependence on health care utilization, tended to have lower functional mobility, and generally lacked leisure or physical activity routines. Recently, InFuSE has opened its treatment paradigm to mild TBI as well.

Practice Description

Over the last year, InFuSE has provided treatment to about a dozen Veterans and has averaged two to three participants per session. Over this time, approximately 75 percent of all participants maintained or engaged in recreation therapy activities or social outings. Significant improvements were found in the Berg Balance Scale, Function in Sitting Test, self-selected walking speed, and fast walking speed in a cohort of participants with moderate to severe TBI, over a 12-week period.

We believe the strength of InFuSE comes from the collaboration of numerous disciplines and a group dynamic. The physical rehabilitation expertise provided by physical therapy is strengthened by the knowledge of adaptive sports and leisure resources familiar to recreation therapy. Yet, the knowledge provided by these disciplines must be supplemented by evidence-based practices to support positive behavior change. The utilization of cognitive aids and strategies commonly employed by speech-language pathology are vital to improve self-regulatory behaviors related to exercise, and engage in related community resources. The use of Motivational Interviewing (MI) techniques helped to promote confidence and provoke physical activity self-awareness. Similarly, appropriate goal setting and frequent review of fitness goals help to build self-efficacy and self-regulatory behaviors.

Group discussion and exercise allowed for greater socialization and enjoyment in physical activities. Generally, each week's topic becomes a group discussion and often behaves similar to a peer support group. Therapists primarily moderate the topic, keep the group focused, and provide relevant health and wellness information. Veterans are able to utilize social skills and develop friendships within the group. We believe that this is an attractive component of InFuSE, and kept Veterans interested in weekly participation. Literature shows exercising with others can increase compliance and reduce the risk of, "falling off the wagon." We found this dynamic to be particularly helpful for those engaging in new activities through recreation therapy services and community outings.

Replicability

Fortunately, InFuSE requires few resources to become implemented across multiple VA facilities. Our time and space use was modest. We were able to coordinate using recreation therapy space for the first 30 minutes and move to the physical therapy gym for the last 60 minutes. This helped reduce the load on each department. Many facilities likely already have various group sessions in each rehabilitation discipline. The primary obstacle faced by other facilities is the coordination across disciplines and potentially departments. Physical therapy and recreation therapy are the foundation of InFuSE. However, clinicians that are familiar with performing group interventions, understand exercise prescription, and are knowledgeable of local community resources that can appropriately operate a program similar to InFuSE. Currently, research has begun at the Washington, DC, VAMC to further validate the InFuSE program and evaluate measures of self-efficacy, sleep quality, psychological health, and community reintegration. In the future, we hope to diffuse InFuSE across numerous VA facilities.

Recognition

Washington, DC polytrauma rehabilitation team, Joel Scholten, Lucile Lisle, Bryant Seamon, Haniel Hernandez

Mindfulness Practices to Support Well-Being

Laura Krejci, Associate Director

VA Greater Los Angeles Healthcare System, Los Angeles, CA
laura.krejci@va.gov

Mindfulness is a way to pay attention to the present moment with compassion, acceptance, and non-judgment. This evidence-based approach has been demonstrated to improve Veterans' health and well-being, anxiety, depression, and pain. Mindfulness can rewire the brain and bring joy into the lives of those who have served.

Introduction

Mindfulness is simply paying attention in a particular way. It is learning to cultivate attention in a friendly, compassionate, and non-judgmental manner. Mindfulness training is an evidence-based practice that is resource effective as it is most easily taught in groups, has minimal to no side effects, and shifts the locus of control for health from a professional provider to self-management skills for the Veteran. Some Veterans returning from combat suffer from PTSD. Being able to practice mindfulness, to pause and focus on their breathing, can allow a person to make a better decision.

An Iraqi Combat Veteran was in the supermarket. He had a PTSD diagnosis and had been participating in a Mindfulness-Based Stress Reduction class at his local VAMC. It was 5:00 p.m., it was busy, and the shopping carts were coming from unexpected places. He was getting more and more anxious. Finally, he gets to the checkout line and the lady in front of him only has one item. He starts telling himself that she is in the wrong place. "Why is it taking so long?" She has a baby. She is talking to the checker about the baby, and it goes on and on. He is getting more and more anxious. It is all he can do to just stay there, just to breathe and track his breath. Then she hands the baby over to the checker. He finally gets up to the checker and instead of yelling at her he says, "Cute baby." The clerk says, "Oh, you think so? Thanks. That's my son. My husband was killed in Iraq last year so I have had to go back to work to support my family. My Mom just brings him in a couple of times each day and buys one thing. Just so I get to see my son."

"The ability to observe the sensations in the body and the thoughts that go through their minds helps Vets to find their way back to being at peace in their bodies again."—Greg Serpa

To help support clinicians and Veterans in the use of mindfulness, VA Office of Patient Centered Care & Cultural Transformation (OPCC&CT) partnered with VA Greater Los Angeles Healthcare System and funded the development of a series of resources related to mindfulness. These resources are supporting VA clinicians, staff, and Veterans and their loved ones by enhancing well-being so everyone can live their lives to the fullest.

Context

Veterans and the general public experience a lot of chronic pain and diseases that show up as people age, including cancers, heart disease, arthritis, Multiple Sclerosis (MS), and diabetes. Veterans often have other specific health concerns related to their service, such as PTSD, Traumatic Brain Injury (TBI), physical injuries like loss of limbs, impaired mobility, and scarring of the body. Another major concern Veterans face is drugs and alcohol addiction. They also have the stressors of daily life, including adapting back into civilian life. Clinicians who work with Veterans are unique, because they spend their time listening to patients' traumatic experiences and stories. Many Veterans are dealing with the devastation of body and mind that result from wartime combat. Mindfulness can address three components for VA community. First, it can help Veterans with coping skills. Second, it can help the clinician with stress reduction, and better self-care. Third, it can help the clinician to be a better care provider for the Veteran. It helps the clinicians relate to the stress and challenging stories that they have to hear on a daily basis. Mindfulness can help Veterans, and the clinicians who work with the Veterans, make peace with things as they are. Mindfulness allows people to cope better with what their circumstances are, without losing hope.

Practice Description

To help support clinicians and Veterans in the use of mindfulness, VA OPCC&CT, VA Greater Los Angeles Healthcare System, and VA Evidence Synthesis program developed a series of resources to support VA Clinicians, staff, and Veterans and their loved ones.

Replicability

There is vast literature that supports the use of mindfulness for leaders who are building programs to better serve Veterans. The mindfulness videos and toolkit can be used to train staff and Veterans about the power of mindfulness practices. The podcasts can be used to expand mindfulness practices anywhere. The Greater Los Angeles VA Healthcare System is offering virtual mindfulness training for clinicians in both the Blackboard (independent study with a weekly live call) and video telehealth platforms. The Mindfulness Facilitator Certification program is a hybrid model that includes both in-person and virtual training elements.

Recognition

Sandra Robertson, J. Greg Serpa, Christiane Wolf, Joan Cohen, Wendy Schmelzer, Paloma Cain, Linda Good, Captain Peter Lisowski, Krystal Rains, Manuel Negrete, Paul Shekelle, Susanne Hempel, Paul Shekelle, Stephanie Taylor, Nell Marshall, Michele Solloway, Isomi Miake-Lye, Jessica Beroes, Roberta Shanman, VHA OPCC&CT

Veteran "X" Program

David Shaw, PhD, Clinical Psychologist; Thomas Pratt, CPSS, Peer Support Specialist; N. Sarah Magnes, LCSW, PhD, Deputy Chief Mental Health Officer

Hampton VAMC, Hampton, VA
david.shaw3@va.gov

Veteran "X" is a peer-led program in which group members collaborate as a treatment team. The team empowers Veteran "X" in his recovery efforts by helping him navigate obstacles on the recovery path through role-play, brainstorming, information-gathering, and facilitator-led group exercises.

Introduction

When recovering from a mental illness, Veterans are often challenged by feelings of powerlessness and dependence on VA system. A primary element of person-centered-care is the involvement of the individual in defining what is important in their care. The Veteran "X" program empowers individuals to navigate many challenging obstacles on the path of recovery in a supportive, collaborative environment with peers through role-play, brainstorming, information-gathering, and facilitator-led group activities. Veteran "X" is a peer-led mental health recovery program in which the participants serve as the treatment team for a fictitious Veteran "X." Veteran "X" has a number of social barriers that are similar to those encountered by the group's participants. While empowering Veteran "X" to solve issues, the participants are also gaining valuable recovery skills, and factual information to resolve their own concerns.

The following comments from some of the more than 1,900 Veterans participating in Veteran "X" demonstrate the impact of this program:

- "Veteran 'X' is a very powerful group."
- "A lot of knowledge and understanding."
- "Very serious and informative."
- "Issues get discussed, not presented."
- "Great camaraderie!"
- "The program has motivated my action to not 'just do it, but do it now.'"
- "This is a necessary ingredient to the soup of our recovery."
- "Helped me advocate for my needs."

In a study completed in 2015, Veteran "X" participants reported significantly greater improvement in symptoms and functioning as compared to "treatment as usual" on the following measures:

- Overall symptoms and functioning, including:
  - Depression
  - Interpersonal functioning
  - Psychotic symptoms

- Emotional lability
- Substance use risk factors
- Substance use protective factors
- Recovery well-being

Key Information

Veteran "X" was developed at the Hampton VAMC by Thomas Pratt, CPSS, in 2009. Veteran "X" provides a unique manualized program developed in VA by and for peer specialists to empower Veterans to participate in their own recovery.

Context

Veteran "X" was developed in the Mental Health Rehabilitation and Recovery program, a 169-bed facility that houses two homeless programs, a PTSD program, and a substance abuse program. Veteran "X" was developed to meet the needs of Veterans with multiple psychosocial issues, including homelessness, substance use, mental health, financial, legal, and social barriers that impede independent living.

Practice Description

Veteran "X" programs are based on a fictitious Veteran scenario with characteristics and social barriers that are similar to the program's participants. The scenario is developed in collaboration with the program facilitator, Veterans, and clinical staff to enhance identification with the scenario. Program participants work in a team-spirited fashion to empower Veteran "X" to achieve his/her goals through the activities previously noted.

Replicability

Veteran "X" was adopted to fill a void in the implementation of the Mental Health Recovery Model at the medical center. The success of the program is best credited to the Veterans who have advocated for themselves in their own recovery. Veteran "X" is the recipient of a 2012 VHA Innovation Award. The VACI has supported the development of a Veteran "X" Facilitator Training Curriculum, which resulted in expansion of the Veteran "X" model to 22 VAMCs nationwide in FY 2015. A team of trainers is available for sites that are interested in hosting the minimum 36-hour face-to-face training program. Training is followed up with six months of consultation.

Recognition

David Carroll, Harold Kudler, Jeffrey Burke, Dan O'Brien-Mazza, Peggy Henderson, the VACI staff, David Buyck, Michael Dunfee, Deanne Seekins, Priscilla Hankins

Healthy Teaching Kitchens

Anne Utech, Deputy National Director, Nutrition and Food Services; Ellen Bosley, National Director, Nutrition and Food Services

VACO, Washington, DC

anne.utech@va.gov

Healthy Teaching Kitchens (HTK) teaches Veterans and their families how to select healthier food options and learn healthy cooking skills. Over 120 facilities around the country have implemented the program.

Introduction

Over 120 facilities around the country have implemented Healthy Teaching Kitchens to empower Veterans to make healthy choices when cooking at home. For example, in Oklahoma City, where HTK has a 12-week program, a Veteran returned to VA for care after three years with a new diagnosis of diabetes, along with high blood pressure and hyperlipidemia. Throughout the 12-week program, the Veteran lost over 50 pounds, his A1C dropped from almost seven mg/dL to under six mg/dL, and his triglycerides drastically changed from 240 mg/dL to 130 mg/dL. At the end of this class, the Veteran was a new man, and no longer needed blood pressure medications.

This is just one of the many stories reflecting the positive impact these classes have on Veterans, both clinically and personally. Veterans are always excited to come to HTK classes to learn a new recipe; some even test their cooking skills. All the classes discuss how to make the recipes and healthier choices in the home. If a dietitian nutritionist suggests trying brown rice or quinoa, and a Veteran has never tried it or doesn't know how to cook it, the chance of that Veteran buying that healthy whole grain is small, and the odds of the Veteran cooking and trying the food is even smaller. However, when the HTK instructors provide these foods and recipes, Veterans state, "I did not think healthy food could taste that good."

Key Information

The Nutrition and Food Services (NFS) program office in Specialty Care Services established the Healthy Teaching Kitchens as a way to teach Veterans and their families how to select healthier food options, and learn healthy cooking skills. Ellen Bosley, Director, NFS and Anne Utech, Deputy Director, NFS led the collaboration to implement these programs nationwide. The goal of these programs is to provide effective nutrition education and counseling, support wellness and disease prevention by promoting healthy food choices, and improve Veteran satisfaction. Research has shown that nutrition instruction is critical in addressing the diabetes and obesity epidemics plaguing our Veteran population. Additionally, hands-on nutrition and wellness education programs have been shown to improve weight management for certain chronic diseases.

Context

To date, 120 facilities nationwide have implemented HTK in their facilities. The frequency of the programs ranges from quarterly to weekly classes. A select group of 40 facilities is collecting

Hemoglobin A1C, Body Mass Index (BMI), and weight changes to track Veterans' clinical outcomes. As a result of participating in these classes, a few facilities now collect Veterans' lipid measurements. The goal of the HTK is to have a positive impact on Veterans' clinical outcomes through cooking demonstrations, or hands-on cooking classes.

Practice Description

Two HTK co-chairs, four VISN consultants, and 138 dietitian nutritionist Subject Matter Experts (SMEs) worked to implement the model nationwide. This group of experts worked to create HTK kitchens throughout the country. The most basic classes are quarterly cooking demonstrations, and the most advanced classes are hands-on weekend or evening classes that include grocery store tours, and gardening classes. In order for these classes to be created, funding for equipment, food, and staffing needed to be acquired by each facility. Facilities collaborated with Nutrition Food Services, National Center for Health Promotion Disease and Prevention, Canteen Services, and Voluntary Services just to name a few. These collaborations have resulted in HTK programs that have shown a positive impact on Veterans' A1C, BMI, and weight.

Replicability

Support and funding from specialty care services allowed 15 VAMCs to implement level three or above HTKs. There are five total levels for HTK. To reach these higher levels, facilities must incorporate hands-on cooking, night and weekend classes, workload credit, hot and cold items, and a set curriculum. Nutrition and Food Services VACO developed HTK strategic goals from 2013 to present.

The HTK subcommittee co-chairs provide national monthly calls that aid in implementing or advancing a HTK. These calls also assist in creating best practices in the HTK programs, along with the NFS SharePoint site resources that offer a plethora of information. Our NFS SharePoint includes a HTK toolkit, a manual providing specific details on the steps and considerations taken to create a HTK. Facilities find that HTKs are in high demand, require little advertising, and provide positive clinical outcomes.

Recognition

VA NFS Field Advisory Committee, Healthy Teaching Kitchen Subcommittee, Jessica Mooney, Sean Walsh, Gail Schechter, Joan Ramirez, Carrie Gibson-Sanchez, Kathryn Shanahan

Academic Detailing Impacting Implementation of Opioid Overdose Education & Naloxone Distribution

Melissa Christopher, PharmD, National Director PBM Academic Detailing Services; Elizabeth Oliva, PhD, National Coordinator, Opioid Overdose Education and Naloxone Distribution
VACO, Washington, DC
melissa.christopher@va.gov

VA academic detailing provides clinician education outreach to increase the use of evidence-based practices to improve Veteran outcomes. VA is impacting opioid overdoses through increasing provider and patient awareness of overdose prevention education and treatment with naloxone.

Introduction

"Here's something that I struggle with that you guys don't even know about because I haven't shared it and it's something that I live with every day… [my friend] died from the first shot of heroin I gave… Didn't have a kit, couldn't save him. If I had a kit, he might be here… So… that's why I'll take [a naloxone kit]. I hope it collects dust, and that's my goal is for it to collect dust."

In light of promising evidence supporting the effectiveness of training laypersons to administer naloxone, and to reduce Veterans' risk for opioid-related death, VA launched a national Opioid Overdose Education and Naloxone Distribution (OEND) program in 2014—the first and only integrated health care system in the US to do so.

Key Information

The OEND program is a harm reduction and risk mitigation initiative that aims to decrease opioid-related overdose deaths among VA patients by providing education on opioid overdose prevention, recognition of opioid overdose, and training on the rescue response, including provision of naloxone. The first VA OEND program, a pilot program, began in Cleveland (VISN 10) in August 2013, and then spread to other VAs across the country. In January 2014, VA OEND National Support & Development Workgroup convened, comprised of representatives from different VA program offices (e.g., Pharmacy Benefits Management Services (PBM), Office of Mental Health Operations (OMHO), Mental Health Services, National Pain Management), and developed an implementation and evaluation plan for OEND. PBM and VA Consolidated Mail Outpatient Pharmacy standardized naloxone kits for national use and added naloxone kits to the national formulary so that Veterans could access this life-saving medication. To support implementation of OEND, PBM launched a "Free-to-Facilities" Naloxone Kit Initiative that began in July 2014. The initiative allows naloxone kits to be dispensed to Veterans without the medical center incurring the cost of the kits. Since implementation of the national OEND program, every VA facility provides naloxone, and Veterans received more than 20,300 kits. The success of the initiative resulted in 172 reported opioid overdose reversals. The success of VA OEND program demonstrates the powerful impact that can be achieved when VA program offices work together to improve care for Veterans.

Context

VA OEND program seeks to reduce the risk of opioid-related death among our nation's Veterans. From an implementation perspective, there are three main areas that need to be addressed to maximize the impact of OEND in saving lives: 1) logistics (e.g., kit availability), 2) patient education, and 3) provider education. PBM addressed a number of the logistical issues to ensure access to naloxone kits (e.g., standardized kits, added kits to national formulary, made kits "Free-to-Facilities"). VA academic detailing also provided support to address logistical issues that arise (e.g., naloxone kit ordering), and OMHO provided ongoing general technical assistance. VA National Support & Development Workgroup supported the development of patient and provider education. Regarding patient education, the national workgroup identified and tailored patient education to two target patient populations for OEND: 1) patients with opioid use disorders and 2) patients prescribed opioids. The training brochures include links to "How To" YouTube videos on the different VA naloxone kits and are available in Spanish. With regard to provider education, the national workgroup developed accredited provider training on OEND, which includes the "How To" videos (funded by VA academic detailing) demonstrating introduction of OEND to the two targeted patient populations as well as the naloxone kit videos. PBM also has a "Recommendation For Use" document, an important pharmacy policy document, which includes recommendations for issuing naloxone kits, including how to identify patients who may be candidates for OEND.

Practice Description

OEND is a one-time, proven life-saving training that requires providers to educate patients about opioid overdose prevention, recognition of opioid overdose, and training on the rescue response, including provision of naloxone. Although a prescription is required for a naloxone kit, most of the patient education can be carried out by other providers (e.g., nurses, pharmacists, or other licensed providers). Training can be done individually or in group settings, and significant others are encouraged to attend (as they may be the ones to administer naloxone to the patient in the event of an opioid overdose). To assist in providing OEND education, the OEND workgroup provided patient educational brochures and instructional videos on YouTube and DVD. Models for how to train groups of patients are included on VA National OEND SharePoint site's "Program Models" page. OMHO and VA have developed many informatics tools to help evaluate and track OEND implementation. These tools are available to the field and have been important in tracking implementation of OEND and identifying facilities that may need support for OEND implementation. These tools were critical in expediting OEND implementation nationwide, and ensuring naloxone distribution from every VA facility.

National implementation of the OEND program required a coordinated effort between stakeholders, such as PBM and OMHO. Key steps involved in implementation of this program included academic detailing pharmacists so they could train staff and patients on how to identify patients at risk for an overdose, how to recognize and respond to an overdose, and how to administer naloxone; developing and compiling OEND educational materials and resources for staff; and collecting data, such as number of kits dispensed and location of dispensing. VA PBM Academic Detailing Service along with Elizabeth Oliva (OMHO) provided education and training to VA staff across the country on various OEND-related issues, including the importance of the program, identifying Veterans at risk, recommendations for implementation, and resources available.

Replicability

VA OEND National Support & Development Workgroup has developed standardized patient education brochures, provider TMS training courses, and "How To" videos to ensure that best practices can be replicated. VA National OEND and Academic Detailing OEND SharePoint sites include these and other tools to enhance replicability. Example implementation plans, note templates, ordering procedures, policies for vulnerable populations (e.g., homeless Veterans), and many other examples are available on these sites. Key stakeholders have been socialized and trained in OEND through national presentations and trainings, and academic detailing has provided local, in-person training to assist with partnerships between clinicians (e.g., prescribers, patient educators) in support of implementation.

OMHO and VA have worked together to ensure that consistent messages are shared with the field to enhance replicability. They have emphasized OEND as one component among many (e.g., Opioid Agonist Treatment, risk-benefit discussion of prescription opioids), with an overall emphasis on providing effective treatments that minimize risk of adverse events.

Recognition

Robert Jesse, Carolyn Clancy, Thomas Lynch, Maureen McCarthy, Phillip Coffin, Sharon Stancliff, Alexander Walley, Eliza Wheeler, Andrew McAuley, Eric Konicki, Jesse Burgard, VA OEND National Support & Development Workgroup, VHA staff

Enhancing Transgender Veteran Care: Training and Support for Providers

Michael Kauth, PhD, Director; Jillian Shipherd, PhD, Director
VACO, Washington, DC
lgbtprogram@va.gov

The practice is providing training and clinical support to VHA providers so that they can deliver responsive and culturally appropriate care to transgender Veterans.

Introduction

"I think a lot of people have prejudice against us, and that stems over into the medical profession as well. Some people, I don't know whether they think they are going to catch something, but they don't really want to treat somebody who is transsexual. We're people, just like anyone else. We're different, yes, but we're still human beings, just like everyone else." —Testimonial from web-based VHA staff training program "An Introduction to Transgender Veteran Health Care"

Despite DoD's former ban on transgender Service Members, Veterans who identify as transgender served—and serve today—the nation with distinction. Transgender Veterans, and non-Veterans, frequently experience social discrimination, harassment, and prejudice, including difficulty accessing appropriate care, which contributes to poor health outcomes. In addition, transgender people have unique health issues related to gender transitioning. Unfortunately, many health care providers get little training in transgender care, and few providers have much experience with transgender patients.

In 2011, VHA issued a national policy mandating clinical services for transgender Veterans. These services included gender counseling, evaluation for and provision of cross-sex hormone therapy, evaluations for transition-related surgeries (but not provision of surgeries), postsurgical care, and support letters for legal name and gender change. Because VHA had few providers experienced in transgender care, clinical capacity to provide appropriate transgender care needed to increase. Many providers needed basic information on transgender care (e.g., using Veterans' preferred pronouns per VHA policy), while others needed training and access to experts for consultation.

We developed levels of information and training for staff to meet a variety of needs. First, we created an internal website (SharePoint) to host resources on transgender Veteran care, such as archived presentations, journal articles, links to policies, links to professional society guidelines, information about support groups for Veterans, and awareness campaign posters. This site is the one-stop shop for information on transgender Veteran care and is regularly updated. We also worked with Subject Matter Experts (SMEs) to create three on-demand webinars about transgender Veteran health care for the VHA online educational system. To further support providers, we established transgender e-consultation at every VHA facility. Any VHA provider can submit a clinical question through the patient's EHR (with Veteran consent), and an experienced interdisciplinary team will respond through the patient's record. For more intensive training of interdisciplinary treatment teams, we created a national training program through videoconferencing. This program has trained 35 interdisciplinary teams to date, with another 20 teams graduating in June 2016. The education and clinical support programs in place have increased VHA's capacity to provide clinically and culturally appropriate care for transgender Veterans.

Key Information

The transgender education SharePoint (launched 2012), online trainings (launched 2013–2014), e-consultation program (launched 2014), and video training/consultation (launched 2014) are national programs and are available to all VA employees and community providers who treat transgender Veterans. Any VHA provider can access transgender e-consultation through the EHR. Clinical treatment teams at any VHA facility are eligible to participate in the seven-month video training program. The Lesbian Gay Bisexual and Transgender (LGBT) program took the lead in implementing these programs with support from the Office of Specialty Care, Office of Mental Health Services, and the Employee Education System (EES). Experts in transgender care from several VHA facilities (Loma Linda, Tucson, Minneapolis, and Boston) helped design and deliver the video training and respond to e-consultation. These efforts matter because transgender Veterans have unique health care needs and experience a number of health disparities relative to cisgender (those whose gender identity aligns with what they were assigned at birth) Veterans. VHA providers and staff need training in transgender care, and need to know how to create a welcoming clinical environment for this historically marginalized and underserved population.

Context

Issuing a national policy on transgender care does not in itself change institutional culture or improve providers' understanding of transgender health care issues. The literature shows that most health care professionals have received little training in transgender health and feel uncertain how to care for them. VHA health care providers are no different. The challenge is to provide training and clinical support to VHA providers so they can deliver responsive and appropriate care to transgender Veterans.

Researchers estimate that there are at least 134,000 transgender Veterans and another 15,450-transgender individuals currently serving in the US military in silence. The need is greater than ever for VHA to increase its clinical capacity to provide appropriate care to transgender Veterans.

Practice Description

After the release of the 2011 VHA transgender health care policy, we were appointed to lead a workgroup to educate clinical staff on implementation of the policy. We presented a proposal to the Office of Patient Care Services for multiple levels of education, training, and clinical support, including a budget. Patient Care Services encouraged us to proceed and established agreements with Mental Health Services and Specialty Care Services to provide initial pilot funding for the clinical consultation projects. Given the data, discussions have begun with the ORH to determine how we can adapt and disseminate the aforementioned programs to better meet the needs of rural providers who are treating transgender Veterans. Patient Care Services also worked with the Employee Education System (EES) to gain support for development of three online programs and educational materials.

Replicability

The need to increase clinical capacity to provide transgender care and create a more welcoming clinical environment for transgender patients is not unique to VHA. The DoD will soon change their policy on transgender Service Members and will need to raise cultural awareness and train health care providers. As SMEs, we have been involved in discussions of how they might begin to meet that challenge, including potential collaborations between DoD and VHA. In addition, non-governmental health care organizations face similar issues, and there are good examples of progressive policies and health care provision in the private sector, which have been valuable resources. The lack of professional training in and experience with transgender care is not unique to VHA providers and we are hopeful that by making our VHA webinars publicly available, we can assist other organizations. Factors that have contributed to our success in VHA include a clear health care policy on transgender care; a patient non-discrimination policy that includes gender identity and expression; the dedication of organizational resources, such as funding and clinician time for training; and the time of thoughtful subject matters to lead the effort. As a large non-profit organization, VHA can block clinic time sp providers can participate in intensive training over seven months to raise their cultural awareness and increase clinical skills. The DoD is similar to VHA in this respect and may well manage providing intensive training to large numbers of health care providers. However, for-profit organizations have more difficulty taking providers away from clinic for an extended time without other compensation for lost workload. Nevertheless, the benefits of well-trained staff who can respond to complex patient care issues are greater patient satisfaction and better patient health outcomes.

Recognition

Alexis Matza, George Brown, Rajiv Jain, Maureen McCarthy, Antonette Zeiss, Harold Kudler, Susan Kirsh, and training and clinical support teams

Clinical Pharmacy's Impact on Rural Veterans

Anthony Nelson, CPS

Twin Falls Idaho Outpatient Clinic, Twin Falls, ID
anthony.nelson4@va.gov

Clinical pharmacists are important members of PACTs who improve outcomes and increase access for our rural Veterans and serve as a valuable information resource to other members of the PACT team.

Introduction

The promotion and implementation of PACTs within VA has been a key step to improving patient-centered care and outcomes for our Veterans. Clinical pharmacists are an essential part of this team due to their unique knowledge base, ability to manage patients with complex chronic disease states independently, and their willingness to provide interdisciplinary education to promote the practice of evidence-based medicine. They often utilize technology, such as telehealth, to provide convenient and effective care. At the Boise VAMC and associated CBOCs, CPSs have been integrated well into the PACT model and improved outcomes in the lives of our Veterans have been the result.

An example of how a clinical pharmacist has positively affected patient care at the rural Twin Falls CBOC relates to a pharmacist's ability to manage complex chronic disease states within a scope of practice, such as hypertension. One patient was consulted to the clinical pharmacist due to his uncontrolled resistant hypertension, treated with four different antihypertensive medications. Appointments were conducted over the phone, saving the patient time and money, as he did not have to come into the clinic for each encounter. His average blood pressure at the time of referral was 152/101mmHg. As part of the pharmacist's assessment, the patient was screened very closely for secondary causes of hypertension. Aspects of his presentation were suspect for a less common condition called hyperaldosteronism, so labs were ordered, and results were consistent with the condition.

Endocrinology was consulted for further evaluation as well as confirmatory testing, which required adjustment of blood pressure medications that interact with the confirmatory lab. After the pharmacist altered the blood pressure regimen, endocrinology was able to proceed and officially diagnose the patient with Primary Hyperaldosteronism. He was started on a medication targeted to block the effects of aldosterone, which was the cause of his hypertension. Over the course of 20 encounters, the pharmacist was able to reduce his hypertension regimen from the initial four agents down to one. At the time of discharge, his home blood pressures were normotensive, averaging around 120/80mmHg, with the most recent clinic pressure of 137/86mmHg. The patient expressed his gratitude for the help getting his blood pressures under control. The patient's provider also personally thanked the pharmacist, citing that it would have been very difficult for him to help the patient due to time constraints.

Key Information

This is just one example of how clinical pharmacy can improve outcomes. Pharmacists can be utilized within the PACT model to improve many aspects of patient-centered care. At the CBOC, non-visit consults are often placed by providers to help with clinical decision making. Questions are also fielded from nursing and non-clinical staff. Pharmacists offer evidence-based recommendations in a timely manner to respond to specific issues, such as: perioperative anticoagulation recommendations; how to taper or transition between medications; assessment of possible medication-related side effects; clarification regarding vaccine schedules; and antibiotic recommendations.

Context

With the implementation of the Opioid Safety Initiative (OSI), the clinical pharmacist worked closely with nursing staff and others to organize a day of Shared Medical Appointments (SMAs), which quickly brought the clinic into compliance with opioid monitoring measures. Alerting providers to incoming patients on chronic opioids who require further monitoring is also completed every two weeks. These combined efforts have brought the all clinic providers to greater than 90 percent compliance with urinary drug screens and iMed Consents. State prescription drug monitoring screens for all patients on greater than five morphine equivalents are also performed by pharmacy to prevent diversion and inappropriate use of opioids.

The clinical pharmacist also provided several education sessions since starting the position eight months ago, with the goal of promoting evidence-based medicine as well as addressing concerns of the clinic. Topics have included: role of clinical pharmacy; treatment of upper respiratory tract infections; a discussion of new ordering menus developed at the VAMC to improve practice; pneumococcal vaccine recommendations; and a review of antihypertensive medications to help nursing staff begin managing chronic disease states, fulfilling their PACT role as nurse care managers. Periodic reviews such as these will help align care at the clinic with current evidence-based medicine, which will likely improve outcomes over time.

Practice Description

The addition of a clinical pharmacist to the rural Twin Falls CBOC has been an effective, economical strategy to address many issues with rural health. The clinic serves 3,144 Veterans who live up to approximately 80 miles from the clinic, often in rural communities where care is limited. The clinic itself has one MD, one physician assistant, two NPs, three RNs, three clinical associates (LPN, MA), and three clerks. Clinical pharmacy provided through conducting telehealth appointments, represents a high level of care for rural Veterans without requiring extensive travel to the clinic. This secures access for consulted patients and improves care. For example, in the target population of diabetic patients with an A1C greater than 9 percent consulted to the clinical pharmacist, the average A1C reduction observed at the time of discharge was 2.7 percent. The number of patients getting care at the CBOC with an A1C greater than 9 percent was reduced by 18 percent after six months with the addition of the clinical pharmacist, using numbers from the Diabetic Registry. Utilizing telehealth as the delivery method of care, over 24,000 miles were saved for the rural Veterans served. This addresses a huge barrier to care for these patients, which is distance to quality care.

This position was initially created using a grant approved through the ORH. The pharmacist was able to integrate quickly into the team by focusing on good communication and making personal connections with the other PACT members. Due to recognized benefits with the addition, the decision was made by facility leadership to fund the position following the completion of the grant.

Replicability

The aforementioned results reflect only some of the positive outcomes that CPSs can offer the PACT team. The results may be easily replicated on any outpatient PACT team by creating a position and hiring a qualified, residency trained/board certified, CPS. Cost-saving benefits have also been demonstrated by the Pharmacists Achieve Results with Medication Documentation (PHARMD) project, which continues to analyze data within the VA setting. I would suggest incorporation of their findings to position proposals to help local leadership recognize what clinical pharmacists really bring to the table. Seeking grant funding can also be a great tool in getting services started, with the goal of seeking long-term funding through VA.

Recognition

Paul Black

ActiVets Mental and Physical Wellness for Veterans with Post-Traumatic Stress Disorder

Patricia Dubbert; Psychologist Investigator; J. Vincent Roca, Chief; Kathleen Harris, Recreational Therapist; Penelope Polluck, NP

Eugene J. Towbin Healthcare Center, Little Rock, AR
patricia.dubbert@va.gov

The ACTiVets program was designed to help rural Veterans with PTSD learn and adopt healthier eating and exercise behavior.

Introduction

The ACTiVets program was designed to help rural Veterans with PTSD learn and adopt healthier eating and exercise behavior. Veterans attend two small group classes and optional monthly larger follow-up groups for six months.

As part of the significant changes observed in the participant group as a whole, individual participants have made remarkable changes. One Veteran and his wife lost weight by using smaller plates, preparing only what they needed with no leftovers, eating more plant-based foods, and being more physically active. He and his wife also started volunteering in a community nursing home. He recently commented that his relationship with his wife had improved because he felt better and they did not argue as much. Another started to walk pushing his wheelchair and, with persistence, graduated to walking with a cane. Several have described their delight at fitting into jeans or belts that had been too small. After encouragement, some women Veterans who had been reluctant to attend groups with men decided to try the program and began interacting with the male participants. At the monthly follow-up meetings, Veterans can be observed showing each other their step counts on their smart phones and discussing healthy recipes for favorite foods.

During the first 18 months, ACTiVets distributed more than 1,000 healthy lifestyles information sheets to Veterans attending PTSD initial appointments and enrolled 120 Veterans in groups. Participants were mostly ethnic minority (65 percent), rural (76 percent), average age 57, overweight or obese (88 percent) with little or no leisure exercise, and reported an average of about 20 days per month of poor mental and physical health. Our project evaluation data revealed that ACTiVets participants significantly increased days/week walking for health and wearing an activity tracker and increased their frequency of consuming healthy foods. Although there is no focus on weight loss, medical record review confirmed weight reductions of at least five pounds in more than 40 percent of participants. Program satisfaction ratings were high and most participants reported they achieved their goals. After program development funding ended, ACTiVets transitioned to a clinically supported program in the PTSD Clinic with the support of the Associate Chief of Staff, Mental Health Service. A toolkit will be available to assist implementation in other facilities. Through its patient-centered approach, ACTiVets provides a model response to VHA's Blueprint for Excellence.

Key Information

ACTiVets was developed in collaboration with the Central Arkansas Veterans Healthcare System Outpatient (CAVHS) PTSD Clinic which has traditionally provided a holistic health approach to treatment. The Mental Health Service, the VISN 16 Geriatric Research Education and Clinical Center (GRECC), and the South Central VA Mental Illness Research Education and Clinical Center (MIRECC) were our original partners. Recently the ACTiVets team also began partnering with the CAVHS pilot implementation of VA's Whole Health transformation initiative. Funding for program development was provided by VA ORH (Project #P00861 VISN 16).

Context

Sedentary lifestyles, obesity, and chronic disease are prevalent in the rural US, especially areas like Arkansas. Mental illness, including PTSD, adds additional risk of poor physical health and early mortality. Many of the rural Veterans living in the southeastern and south central states lack basic preventive health information and have no access to community health and fitness facilities. It is believed that support of physical wellness would enhance treatment for PTSD, and improvement in PTSD symptoms in turn would free up emotional energy for making changes in health behaviors.

Practice Description

Veterans are introduced to ACTiVets when PTSD clinic staff members distribute one-page healthy lifestyle suggestions and ACTiVets invitations to all new clinic patients. From new and continuing clinic patients, a cohort of seven to ten Veterans is enrolled each month, and meets with co-leaders for two 90-minute classes two weeks apart. In the first class, participants discuss basic healthy nutrition and physical activity information based on public health recommendations and educational handouts from US government websites, learn about portion size with food models, and receive pedometers or activity trackers. The second class focuses on motivational strategies consistent with Acceptance and Commitment Therapy and leads participants through several exercises to teach ACT skills. ACTiVets participants set their own goals that often include behaviors, such as substituting water for sugary soft drinks, walking daily, increasing their step count, measuring portions and using smaller plates, and eating more fruits and green and colorful vegetables. After completing the two group classes, ACTiVets may then attend up to six monthly 90-minute follow-up groups of 20 to 30 Veterans. Activities include supportive discussions of progress and challenges, sharing healthy recipes, indoor physical activities appropriate for adults with impaired health, and reinforcement of motivational strategies. To help monitor and change health behaviors, ACTiVets receive their choice of high-tech activity trackers or low-tech pedometers, water bottles, measuring cups and spoons for portion size, and a booklet on healthy food choices. Healthy cookbook door prizes promote timely arrivals and good attendance. Leaders emphasize choosing healthy behavior change goals based on personal values while meetings emphasize a values-based positive approach and supportive interaction. At monthly meetings Veterans report on what they have been doing in the past month for wellness, their thoughts and feelings when taking these actions, what thoughts and feelings helped them continue their actions in spite of barriers, and how they choose to continue these actions although they have discouraging thoughts and feelings. Participating Veterans often share highly emotional experiences at the monthly meetings and receive support from other Veterans as well as the leaders.

Replicability

Key ingredients in the success of ACTiVets at our facility included the supportive whole health-oriented environment of the PTSD Clinic and Mental Health Services and the availability of experienced group leaders with expertise in ACT and health promotion. Leaders must be able to present public health wellness behavior recommendations in a brief and simple manner and help participants choose goals that are appropriate for their readiness to change, even when the goals seem very limited, such as drinking more water. In our experience, initial success with very small goals has led to more challenging goals like walking regularly or changing food choices. We encouraged Veterans who were attending or considering intensive weight management to complete their obesity treatment program before joining ACTiVets. Veterans who need physical therapy or other supervised exercise or specialized nutrition counseling are not included until they are ready for a more wellness-oriented intervention. Veterans' organizations can be asked to help with funding for the cookbooks and other incentive items we distributed at monthly meetings. ACTiVets program manuals, with educational materials and suggested program evaluation instruments, are available from the leaders.

Recognition

Amanda Hubbard, Traci Abraham, LaNissa Gilmore, the staff of the PTSD Clinic at Central Arkansas Veterans Healthcare System, administrative support staff of the VISN 16 GRECC

Chaplain-Led Post-Traumatic Stress Disorder and Moral Injury Groups

Kerry Haynes, DMin, BCC/MH, Mental Health Chaplain
South Texas Veterans Health Care System, San Antonio, TX
kerry.haynes@va.gov

Some Veterans with PTSD also battle moral injury, a searing wound of the conscience. As faith leaders, Chaplains specialize in morally injurious subjects such as guilt, shame, and forgiveness. I formed both an open PTSD group and a closed moral injury group to help Veterans heal.

Introduction

Even though PTSD has been around since the earliest wars, we only recently gave it a name. So, it is with moral injury, a new name for a timeless ailment of war: A searing wound of the conscience. Recently, mental health providers' efforts have led to helping Veterans find healing. Yet chaplains, as faith leaders, specialize in morally injurious subjects like guilt, shame, and forgiveness. As a result, we formed a specialized, closed group for Veterans who desired to combat their own moral injury.

One Vietnam Veteran in the group recalled carrying out a personal, unsanctioned revenge mission to atone for his buddy's death. Afterwards, the Veteran lacked the fulfillment he sought and feared recriminations for his actions. He redeployed from Vietnam and left the service as soon as possible, immersing himself in work for 40 years to forget his deeds. However, retirement brought plenty of time for thinking. His mental health provider referred him to my group. After six sessions of faith-based stories, evidence-based forgiveness models, and personal sharing of failures and searches for forgiveness, the Veteran commented, "I wish this had been offered when I first got home!"

That proved to be true for all the Veterans in the group. Each Veteran worked through his or her issues and moved toward healing. Each Veteran was administered the "State Self-Forgiveness Scale" (Wohl, 2008) at the beginning and end of our series of six meetings; everyone improved and the group, as a whole, reflected a 26 percent increase in self-forgiveness.

Key Information

In the spring of 2015, the South Texas VA Health Care System implemented the first Moral Injury Group. Mental health providers referred Veterans struggling with moral injury. The group used developed materials and worked with ongoing PTSD spirituality groups started in our PTSD Clinic in coordination with a psychologist there. Staff participated in a national yearlong Mental Health and Chaplaincy Collaboration along with teams from other VA and DoD centers. We worked on goals to increase collaboration between disciplines. The Moral Injury Group and PTSD Group flowed out of this collaborative effort. As a team psychologist stated, "Prior to the Collaborative, we were missing out on treating a very important part of the Veteran - his or her spirituality. But now we are providing truly holistic, integrated care."

Context

The South Texas Veterans Health Care System consists of two hospitals and 13 outpatient clinics. The System serves some 80,000 distinct Veterans, with over one million outpatient visits a year. The Moral Injury and PTSD Groups sought to provide another avenue of healing for those Veterans open to a faith-based construct.

Practice Description

As a new endeavor, the Moral Injury Group required curriculum, advertising among providers, and implementation by Chaplain Service. The ongoing PTSD spirituality group included the same, with integration of the Mental Health Chaplain into the PTSD clinical team, participating in weekly interdisciplinary team meetings, leading groups, opening individual outpatient clinics, and collaborating individually, as needed, with mental health providers.

Replicability

Mental health and chaplaincy integration succeeded at our facility due to several factors. Our leadership was committed to the process, including the hospital director, chief of staff, associate director for patient care services, associate chief of staff for mental health, and chief of chaplain service. Similarly, staffs were self-driven to pursue integration and more holistic care. The staff recognized a need for the Moral Injury Group, developed the curriculum for it, sought referrals, and facilitated the group. Support from our chaplain and mental health providers proved key. The group's success, along with that of the ongoing PTSD spirituality group, is in large part due to interdisciplinary relationships that lead to referral. The group also requires chaplain leadership that is both non-judgmental and non-anxious.

Several other VA facilities have started chaplain-led PTSD groups. Chaplains are networking now, to share curriculum ideas and integration success stories.

Recognition

Nicole Braida, Sharon Millican, Uma Kasinath, Juliana Lesher, Anushka Pai

Post-Traumatic Stress Disorder Consultation Program

Sonya Norman, PhD, Director

White River Junction VAMC, White River Junction, VT

sonya.norman@va.gov

Expert clinicians consult with any provider, in or outside of VA, who has questions about treating a Veteran with PTSD. Consultation can be about treatment, assessment, resources, or anything PTSD-related. The goal is to help health care professionals provide the best possible PTSD care to Veterans.

Introduction

Dr. A, a psychologist who worked in a rural VA, was concerned about how to proceed in treating a Veteran with PTSD who was drinking frequently and heavily. The Veteran was willing to engage in an evidence-based psychotherapy for PTSD, but the therapist was concerned that talking about his trauma during this psychotherapy would make the Veteran's drinking and symptoms worse. Dr. A. contacted the PTSD Consultation Program by email and asked to speak with a consultant before his next session with the patient. Within two days of contacting the Consultation Program, he spoke with a consultant by phone. The consultant asked questions to understand the specifics of the care of this particular Veteran and Dr. A's concerns. She shared with Dr. A. the VA/DoD Clinical Practice Guidelines (CPGs) regarding treating co-occurring PTSD and problem alcohol use and recent research findings on effective treatment strategies for individuals with these co-occurring problems. The consultant also shared her own experience treating Veterans with PTSD and problem alcohol use. Dr. A. and the consultant discussed what local resources were available to help treat this Veteran. Dr. A. stated at the end of the call that he now had a plan for how to proceed with treating this Veteran. Because of consultation, Dr. A. decided to initiate Prolonged Exposure Therapy (PET) for PTSD, an evidence- based treatment that has helped many Veterans recover from PTSD. He expressed gratitude to the consultant for being available so quickly and for helping him think through next steps in the care of this Veteran. He has since contacted the PTSD Consultation Program on several occasions with other questions about treating Veterans with PTSD.

Key Information

The PTSD Consultation Program is a national VA program whose goal is to help providers deliver excellent care to Veterans with PTSD. In 2011, the executive branch of the National Center for PTSD in White River Junction, Vermont, launched the PTSD Consultation Program. The program was initially implemented such that consultation was available to VA providers nationally, but over time, it became clear that a large number of Veterans were seeking some or all of their care outside VA. In early 2015, the PTSD Consultation Program began to offer consultation to any provider treating Veterans, whether in private practice, community treatment centers, or any other setting. Free Continuing Education Credits (CEUs) for participating in the PTSD Consultation Program's monthly lecture series, which covers topics relevant to treating Veterans with PTSD, also became available to providers outside of VA in 2015. Since 2011, the PTSD Consultation Program has consulted on over 4,000 questions from providers treating Veterans with PTSD. Since launching to community providers in 2015, the team has consulted with over 400 providers who treat Veterans outside VA. The PTSD Consultation Program has been used by providers in over 45 states.

Context

There are approximately 21 million Veterans in the US and more than 3.7 million have trauma-related mental health problems, such as PTSD. Approximately 10 percent of all VHA users have PTSD (25 percent among OEF/OIF Veterans) and as many as 30 to 56 percent of Veterans receive at least some care outside of VA facilities. These statistics suggest that providers both within and outside of VA are likely to encounter Veterans in their practices. Assessing and treating PTSD can be complicated. As many as 80 percent of Veterans who have PTSD also have other problems, such as depression, anxiety, and substance use. Guilt, grief, aggression, and dissociation are examples of issues that can further complicate assessment and treatment. Providers will at times need consultation to help them treat PTSD effectively, help them with particular issues that come up in treatment, and to stay current on important new developments in assessing and treating PTSD. The PTSD Consultation Program addresses these needs by providing consultation to providers when such questions arise. Through the monthly PTSD Consultation Program lecture series, providers can learn evidence-based clinical strategies to help them treat Veterans with PTSD.

Practice Description

The PTSD Consultation Program offers consultation to providers who treat Veterans with PTSD on clinical questions, questions that arise in the treatment of a particular Veteran, or about assessing and treating PTSD in general. Consultants assist providers with questions about clinical practice, resources for PTSD care, administration and programmatic issues, and improving care for Veterans. Consultation is over phone or email, based on the provider's preference, and, if by phone, is scheduled at the provider's convenience. The consultants are senior VA psychologists, psychiatrists, and other mental health professionals who have many years of experience in treating PTSD, leading clinical programs, and conducting PTSD-related research. The Program is utilized by a variety of professionals, including psychologists, social workers, physicians, nurses, administrators, pharmacists, researchers, and others. Health professionals in a number of care settings use the PTSD Consultation Program. Within VA, these include PTSD outpatient clinics, outpatient mental health clinics, residential treatment programs, homelessness programs, substance use disorder (SUD) clinics, and the Veterans Justice Outreach program. Outside of VA, these have included private practice, community mental health, and hospice.

Replicability

The evidence that the PTSD Consultation Program has been successful is seen through steady growth in the number of consultation requests over time and a high number of repeat users (39 percent in FY 2015). Success was made possible by identifying a topic area (PTSD) that is not only highly relevant to Veteran care, but also challenging; having a strong and diverse team of expert consultants; a program coordinator who is able to receive consultation requests and triage them to the best suited consultant quickly; and ongoing efforts to market the program and disseminate information that PTSD consultation is available to providers treating Veterans. Feedback from providers who have used the program is critical to continuously improving processes. Meeting these conditions makes it possible for others to reproduce or replicate similar practices. For example, this practice has been adopted by other health care groups within VHA such that now there is a Suicide

Risk Management Consultation Program and a Military Sexual Trauma Consultation Program. These new programs worked with the PTSD Consultation Program leadership to develop and launch their consultation programs.

Recognition

Sonya Norman, Todd McKee, Jessica Hamblen, Nancy Bernardy, Matthew Friedman, Matthew Yoder, Carie Rodgers

Getting Veterans the Job They Want, With Evidence-Based Supported Employment

Lance Goetz, MD, Staff Physician, SCI&D, and Co-Principal Investigator, Predictive Outcome Model Over Time for Employment (PrOMOTE)

Richmond Vet Center, Richmond, VA
lance.goetz@va.gov

This VA-funded research demonstrated success with an evidence-based approach to help Veterans with significant spinal cord injuries obtain the job of their choice. Other groups of Veterans with disabilities are now being helped by this approach, as well.

Introduction

Mr. X is a Veteran who became spinal cord injured as a result of a motor vehicle collision. At the time of injury, he was intoxicated and using illegal drugs. After his rehab, he enrolled in the Supported Employment (SE) program. His SE specialist helped him get a job at a local deli, where his personality blossomed. He loves his job, was named employee of the month, and is even referred to as the "mayor" of the deli. He has stopped using illegal drugs, is active in adaptive sports, has extra spending money, and a new lease on life.

Many other Veterans with Spinal Cord Injuries (SCIs) of all levels and severity have been helped by Supported Employment programs at their centers. Some of these Vets can walk, but most need power or manual wheelchairs to get around. One SCI Veteran, hired as a sous chef, stated, "Being in the...program has changed my life. I love getting up in the mornings and I look forward to going to work." Another, who got a job as a tutor, said, "This job has been life changing for me." Yet another, now working as a computer technician, stated, "This job is awesome." Finally, another SCI Veteran, who obtained an office position, stated that he planned to work at the position, "Until I retire. I see myself moving up…"

These programs have resulted in 142 new jobs for Veterans with SCI, over a million dollars in income, and more importantly, significant improvements in life satisfaction for Veterans.

Key Information

Interventional research using evidenced-based supported employment for spinal cord injuries was initially implemented starting in 2005 at the Dallas VA SCI Center and several other VA SCI centers, and in partnership with their local Compensated Work Therapy (CWT) services, under the leadership of Lisa Ottomanelli, PhD Meeting with success, it expanded to more centers through 2015. Dr. Ottomanelli and her colleagues in SCI collaborated with leaders from VA Mental Health's Therapeutic and Supported Employment Services. The success was significant because it showed that even persons with severe physical disabilities, such as SCI, could reap the social, psychological, and financial rewards of work.

Context

The VHA has a network of 24 SCI centers which provide rehabilitation and medical care to Veterans with spinal cord injury and disorders. Despite the fact that many Veterans with SCI express a desire for employment, employment rates among Veterans with SCI are very low, around 35 percent. In the past, vocational services have largely been provided outside of the center, through state or other agencies. However, this was inconvenient and cumbersome for Veterans, who often found themselves working with people unfamiliar with their challenges. An approach was needed that would help Veterans with SCI in their SCI centers as well as in their communities.

Practice Description

The Individual Placement and Support (IPS) model of "best practices" Supported Employment (SE) is an integrated, person-centered, zero exclusion approach to help persons gain competitive employment of their choice in their community. Benefits counseling is also integrated into this model to help Veterans understand the economics of getting a job. The model has been repeatedly demonstrated to be highly effective in many studies for helping people with serious mental illness return to competitive work. However, it had never been tried with people with physical disabilities like spinal cord injury.

Using this model, Lisa Ottomanelli—Tampa VA Health Services Research and Development (HSR&D) Center of Innovation on Disability and Rehabilitation Research—and her colleagues found that using this approach was better for gaining competitive employment for Veterans with SCI. Veterans also reported improvements in their quality of life and were very satisfied with their participation. The cost per Veteran was very low, less than the cost of two days in the hospital. Dr. Ottomanelli and colleagues repeated their program with another, larger group of spinal cord injured Veterans, with even better success this time. Because of this approach's success in these areas, clinician researchers, such as Lori Davis at the Tuscaloosa VA and her colleagues, are now studying this promising model for Veterans with PTSD.

Replicability

Successful adoption of IPS SE at the facilities required integrating vocational services alongside ongoing SCI health care by using a team-based model. Specific factors that made this possible included: outlining clear expectations for evidence-based IPS practices, monitoring adherence, and providing feedback for program improvement; cultivating active and obvious leadership support at both the service and upper management level; and promoting seamless collaborative care by broad education about IPS-supported employment that included sharing outcomes with staff. A guide for implementing IPS-supported employment in SCI care is currently under development and will be available for other facilities who are interested in replicating this practice in their centers.

Recognition

Lisa A. Ottomanelli, Virginia Keleher, Rich Toscano, Sunil Sabharwal, Maggie Budd, Melissa Amick, Mary Ann Richmond, Tom Dixon, Jim LePage, Fides Pacheco, Sally Ann Holmes, Herb Ames, Tony Kerrigan, Doug Ota, Jenny Kiratli, Scott McDonald, Kevin White, Kirsten Fisher, Catherine Wilson, the CWT program managers, each Vocational Rehabilitation Specialist, Charles McGeough

Universal Military Sexual Trauma Screening

Susan McCutcheon, RN, EdD, National Mental Health Director

VACO, Washington, DC

susan.mccutcheon@va.gov

In 2000, national policy was established that all Veterans seen at VHA are screened for experiences of Military Sexual Trauma (MST). Based on the growing literature on trauma-sensitive care and the evolving grassroots clinical knowledge from our skilled staff in the field, the MST Clinical Reminder was revised in 2015.

Introduction

The following recent clinical examples illustrate the power of sensitive screening to promote Veteran-centric care characterized by respect and integrity:

- A Veteran declined to answer the Military Sexual Trauma questions, unwilling to share something so private with a doctor he had never met before. A year later, the doctor was re-prompted to rescreen the Veteran. After a year of forming a close relationship, the Veteran was ready to ask for more information on MST and talk to someone about MST groups for male survivors.

- A Veteran answered "Yes" to the screening questions but did not want to talk more. The staff completing the screening was trained in this scenario and was supportive and warm with the Veteran, offering a brochure and her contact information if the Veteran would like to talk to someone in the future. Two days later, the Veteran called back to ask for help and was seen the same day by the local MST coordinator and the psychiatrist.

MST is the term used by VA to refer to sexual assault or repeated, threatening sexual harassment experienced by a Veteran during military service. Recognizing that many survivors of sexual trauma do not disclose their experiences unless asked directly, VA established in 2000 a universal screening policy whereby every Veteran seen for VA health care is asked by a provider whether he/she had experienced MST. In 2015, 4,900,694 Veterans (98.7 percent) seen in VHA had been screened for military sexual trauma, and 145,632 had disclosed an experience of MST.

Universal screening is a critical mechanism to provide all Veterans with information on MST and offer a clear referral path for MST survivors who would like to access free MST-related care available through VHA. For Veterans who experienced MST, universal MST screening and the documentation of the MST experience in the medical record also helps ensure that their trauma history is considered in provision of care. Finally, detection of trauma history via MST screening is associated with a twofold increase in mental health care utilization, suggesting that MST screening is a powerful method to begin the conversation that helps connect Veterans with needed care (Kimerling, Street, Gima, & Smith, 2008)

Key Information

In 2000, VHA established a national policy that all Veterans seen for health care services are screened for experiences of MST. This is an important way to ensure that Veterans are aware of and offered the free MST-related care available through VHA. For Veterans who experienced MST, it also helps ensure that their trauma history is considered in provision of care. Over the past 15 years, sensitive screening efforts have been refined to reflect both the growing empirical literature on trauma-sensitive care and the evolving grassroots clinical knowledge from our skilled staff in the field. These empirical developments and on-the-ground clinical insights led to the recent revision of the MST Clinical Reminder and intensified screening training efforts.

Context

As with any trauma, the impact of MST varies tremendously. Some Veterans show remarkable resilience and may function quite well despite their experiences of MST. Among users of VA health care, the mental health diagnoses most commonly associated with MST are PTSD, depressive disorders, anxiety disorders, bipolar disorders, drug and alcohol disorders, and schizophrenia and psychoses. Other mental health diagnoses more common among sexual trauma survivors as opposed to other trauma survivors include eating disorders, dissociative disorders, and somatization disorder. MST is also associated with a range of physical health conditions, such as chronic fatigue, chronic pain, gastrointestinal problems, and fibromyalgia.

MST often occurs when survivors are young, in unfamiliar environments, and far from friends and family (Bell & Reardon, 2011). MST survivors may be forced to live and work with or for the perpetrators, making escape difficult or impossible and increasing the risks of repeated victimization, isolation, and helplessness. Further, those who disclose to family, friends, or other potential sources of support often encounter negative reactions, including blame or rationalization of perpetrator actions. Such victim-blaming messages may further compound feelings of self-blame, shame, and guilt (Bell & Reardon, 2011).

Many survivors of sexual trauma want to be asked about trauma histories in health care contexts (e.g., Friedman, Samet, Roberts, Hudlin, & Hans, 1992; Havig, 2008), as long as it is done sensitively (Campbell, Adams, Wasco, Ahrens, & Sefl, 2009), but they may not disclose their experiences unless asked directly. The universal MST screening program is an efficient method to promote access to specialty mental health care (Kimerling, Street, Gima, & Smith, 2008).

Practice Description

All Veterans seen for VA health care are asked whether they have experienced MST. Screening is conducted in a private setting by qualified providers (typically in PC) who have been trained in sensitive screening practices and supportive responses to disclosure.

A Clinical Reminder in the EHR alerts providers of the need to screen a given Veteran, provides language to use in asking the Veteran about MST, and documents the Veteran's response to the screen. In 2015, the MST Clinical Reminder was updated, containing several important changes. First, the screening language was revised to make the questions more readily understandable to Veterans. Second, an explicit option to "decline" screening was added, allowing Veterans to choose when and with whom they would prefer to disclose their experiences. Veterans who decline are automatically rescreened in a year. Third, the EHR reminder now includes an option to initiate a referral for services. This provides more streamlined access for Veterans and facilitates improved monitoring of screening and follow-up at the national level. In conjunction with the rollout of the revised Reminder, VHA has engaged in efforts to provide staff with additional training on how to screen and respond sensitively to disclosures of MST.

Replicability

Universal one-time MST screening via the revised MST Clinical Reminder is implemented in each VA facility nationwide. Similar sensitive trauma screening practices could be implemented in private health care systems by developing a trauma screening prompt in the medical record, which includes a recommended script. Suggested components of the script include: 1) an introduction to the screening questions to provide a rationale; 2) screening questions with behaviorally specific language and examples; 3) brief education and resources following disclosure; and 4) a clear referral pathway for trauma survivors who are interested in additional information or mental health care. Staff education should include role plays to increase provider comfort with screening script and emphasize authentic, compassionate responding to trauma disclosure.

Recognition

Program offices, including Women's Health, PC, and Primary Care-Mental Health Integration; local staff, including MST coordinators and Clinical Application Coordinators (CACs); and clinical staff

Emerging Consciousness Program: Polytrauma System of Care

Risa Richardson, MD, Neuropsychologist, Micaela Cornis-Pop, MD, Manager
James A. Haley Veterans' Hospital, Tampa, FL
risa.richardson@va.gov

This novel, inpatient, rehabilitation program for catastrophically brain-injured persons has evolved from emerging science created during the recent war-related conflicts. The treatment framework addresses unique health care and family needs and serves as a model for the international community.

Introduction

They are fathers, husbands, and sons. Some are wives, mothers, and daughters. Their families receive the news that no one wants to hear. Suffering a catastrophic brain injury under any circumstance, including war, motor-accidents, or falls, has a lifelong impact on patients, family members, and VA personnel who take care of all of them. Within the five VA Polytrauma Rehabilitation Centers, a specialized rehabilitation program exists that is virtually non-existent within civilian health care settings. Veterans and Service Members who suffer severe brain injury resulting in prolonged disorders of consciousness (coma, vegetative state, or minimally conscious state) have the opportunity to receive specialized brain injury medical care and rehabilitation to improve their outcome. Most of the families entering this program have been told that their loved one would not survive the first few days of injury and have a poor to non-existent chance of improved outcome. Most of this information is based on information from decades ago. Faced with these facts, families are ill-prepared to make the decisions that they have had to face without their loved one's input.

For families who hope for a better outcome, the uniquely positioned VA Emerging Consciousness Program is an option. This specialized rehabilitation program treated a record number of catastrophically injured brain injury survivors during the recent OEF/OIF/Operation New Dawn (OND) conflicts. VA clinical investigators published their experiences treating this unique group of survivors and led collaborations with civilian investigators to publish the largest studies of rehabilitation outcome for this patient group in the research literature. Because of this work, clinicians now can inform families that 60 to 70 percent regain consciousness during rehabilitation, approximately 20 percent regain the ability to live independently or be employed again within the first five years' post-injury, and that approximately 70 percent of the relatively younger survivors become independent in their ability to take care of their basic needs such as eating, walking, going to the bathroom, and others. With the clinical science created by VA, families can make decisions that are more informed with the help of specialists trained to guide them in their lifelong journey. The journey is slow and it takes its toll on patients, family members, and the providers. Even the small victories are cherished. The academic work of VA investigators has helped lead the way to define the rehabilitation outcome and improve the information that family members receive to make better health care decisions for them and their loved ones. These efforts have had an international impact.

Key Information

VA program for rehabilitation of disorders of consciousness (Emerging Consciousness Program) was formalized during the OEF/OIF conflicts in response to the record number catastrophic brain injuries being treated in VA Polytrauma Rehabilitation Centers. VA physicians, neuropsychologists, and rehabilitation therapists came together to formalize the program and initiate infrastructure for research. The program created across the five VA rehabilitation specialty hospitals provided a framework from which other rehabilitation programs, including the private sector, could follow. Scientific publications describing the program and rehabilitation outcomes were published in leading academic journals. Formal research programs in VA Polytrauma Rehabilitation Centers followed to characterize outcomes and inform the health care system of future needs. These findings are being used in guidelines and position statements about minimal needs of rehabilitation programs treating severe brain injury.

Context

VA's Polytrauma System of Care (PSC) with its over 110 coordinated programs across the nation that specialize in polytrauma and Traumatic Brain Injury (TBI) rehabilitation has provided the framework and opportunity for the development of best practice models and the emergence of creative solutions to the health problems affecting the recovery from brain injury. PSC was created in 2005 to address the extraordinary needs of severely injured Veterans and Service members, many of whom served in combat in Iraq and Afghanistan. Subsequently, the PSC has developed and matured to extend services to those Veterans who continue to suffer from chronic symptoms and problems secondary to their injuries. PSC unites a diverse team of medical professionals offering coordinated rehabilitative services to severely injured Veterans to achieve maximum health potential and well-being. Through PSC programs, Veterans once sidelined from society due to devastating injuries, can achieve their personal best—provide for their own livelihood, have families, and once again serve their country as contributing members of their communities.

Practice Description

Rehabilitation has been described as a black box due to poorly defined practices that are unique to providers. VA clinical investigators in VA Emerging Consciousness Rehabilitation program have participated in national guidelines and position statements being developed by the American Academy of Neurology, American Congress of Rehabilitation, and National Institute on Disability, Independent Living, Rehabilitation Research TBI Model Systems Research Program in efforts to standardize delivery of care for the catastrophically brain-injured persons entering rehabilitation. These guidelines and position statements will provide a framework for rehabilitation that includes 1) specialized brain injury medical management of co-morbidities that hinder recovery and functional potential, 2) expertise and framework for accurate diagnostic assessment of disorder of consciousness and evidence-based prognostication, 3) defining critical members of the interdisciplinary team and accessible consultants, 4) ongoing educational needs of providers, 5) requirement for defined protocols for trying evidence-based and off-label medications to promote recovery, 6) training caregivers to manage day-to-day with their loved ones and their regained abilities, 7) promoting activities that integrate them into communities and home settings, 8) facilitating smooth transitions to next settings, and 9) addressing ethical issues that arise.

Publications describing these efforts are forthcoming from the American Academy of Neurology, American Congress of Rehabilitation Medicine, and National Institute on Independent Living, Disability, and Rehabilitation Research TBI Model Systems Program.

Replicability

At a time when the influx of severe brain injury was at a peak during OEF/OIF, the need to standardize rehabilitation practices for this patient group was critical. Given the lack of existing guidelines to inform clinical practice, the Polytrauma Rehabilitation Centers invited academic and clinical experts to help formalize the program. In 2008, experts met with the Polytrauma Rehabilitation Center clinical teams to accomplish new goals in establishing best clinical practices and research infrastructure. Those goals have been accomplished with high visibility in the media and academia. The Polytrauma Rehabilitation Centers continue to meet monthly and work toward ongoing improvement in clinical programming. VA's experience and expertise continues to be evident through academic publications in high profile research journals and invitations to speak at national and international meetings on the topic of rehabilitation for severe brain injuries. Collectively, the impact of VA experience has forever changed the health care environment for severe TBI in the VA, DoD, and civilian health care systems.

Enhancing Tobacco Cessation Treatments Through Training

Timothy Chen, PharmD, BCACP, CGP, Director, Clinical Pharmacist Specialist
VA San Diego Healthcare System, San Diego, CA
timothy.chen@va.gov

The Tobacco Cessation Trainings were designed to train all health care professionals of various disciplines to be able to provide effective tobacco cessation treatments as well as to implement programs into practice.

Introduction

In 2010, the VHA "Smoking and Tobacco Use Survey Report" identified some potential barriers to tobacco cessation treatment within VA, which included lack of training and knowledge for programs to provide effective behavioral treatment and pharmacotherapy.

Cigarette smoking is the single most preventable cause of death and cessation treatment is a very cost-effective initiative. With this in mind and as a priority, Tobacco & Health: Policy and Programs in the then VHA Office of Public Health and its field-based Tobacco Cessation Clinical Resource Center (TCCRC) at VA San Diego, developed several mechanisms to enhance practice, one of which was clinical training/implementation of tobacco cessation programs.

Given the high costs for national conferences and training, a plan was devised to employ site-specific training at a low cost. This involved having two faculty members travel to a site and train more than 100 individuals per visit. The cost of the site-based training, which included travel expenses for two faculty members, was significantly lower than attendance at a national conference and provided the opportunity for more health care professionals to be trained since travel was not required. Training sites were identified based on lower prescribing rates, areas with high smoking prevalence, and sites interested in initiating evidenced-based practices. This model used a "train-the-team" approach to training and implementation. In contrast to a national conference, this model allows an entire team of providers to participate and work together to enhance tobacco cessation treatment at all points of care. It also provides the face-to-face training needed for instruction in the behavioral skills required for effective counseling. Academic detailing is provided to give feedback to the sites on how their facility compares with others on rates of utilization of FDA-approved smoking cessation medications, as a marker of evidence-based care. To encourage health care professionals from diverse disciplines to attend training, the training program obtained continuing education accreditation from multiple professional organizations.

Training was first conducted at the Puerto Rico and West Palm Beach VAs and had immediate impact. Prescribing rates for all their smokers increased significantly (~20 percent) post-training. In addition, both facilities have stayed involved in enhancing tobacco cessation treatment programs, such as increasing tobacco cessation groups. Both sites have several tobacco cessation experts, actively participating in national calls and programs to better enhance tobacco treatment for Veterans.

Key Information

A committee of seven clinical experts representing medicine, nursing, pharmacy, and psychology designed and ensured that the training objectives met knowledge and skills criteria for each discipline. A four-hour curriculum was developed and has met continuing education accreditation requirements for the following: Accreditation Council for Continuing Medical Education (ACCME), ACCME—NP (Non-Physician), American Psychological Association, American Nurses Credentialing Center, Accreditation Council for Pharmacy Education, and California Board of Registered Nursing (CA BRN). Accreditations were coordinated by VHA Employee Education Service and expansion to other disciplines, such as dentists and social workers, has been added. Since implementation in 2011, over 30 sites and 15 VISNs have received this training. Results show increased self-rated abilities to provide tobacco cessation treatment by health care professionals who attended the training, an increase in evidenced-based tobacco cessation programs at training sites, as well as increased prescribing and elimination of potential prescribing barriers. Feedback has been positive from all the sites and this model has been highly successful. The effectiveness of this training model has been described in a peer-reviewed journal article.

Context

Tobacco & Health: Policy and Programs in VHA Mental Health Services and its field-based Tobacco Cessation Clinical Resource Center (TCCRC) at VA San Diego work to increase Veterans' access to evidence-based tobacco cessation treatment nationally.

Practice Description

The first three hours of training were adapted from the existing Rx for Change curriculum. One to two core objectives for behavioral intervention retained from the Rx for Change focused on the "five As" (Ask, Advise, Assess, Assist, Arrange) and the "five Rs" (Relevance, Risks, Rewards, Roadblocks, and Repetition). Pharmacotherapies were a key component of the training program. Adaptations focused on incorporating special considerations in patients with co-morbid Mental Health (MH) and Substance Use Disorders (SUDs), such as co-managing MH/PTSD/SUDs while quitting tobacco, drug interactions with tobacco smoke and dose adjustments for antipsychotic medications, conditions that may worsen MH while quitting, potential need for more behavioral treatment in certain Veteran groups, nicotine as a stimulant and its relationship with stress, and behavioral coping strategies. Adaptations to the existing curriculum also included specific tobacco cessation information related to women.

VHA facilities were chosen to receive tobacco cessation training based on analysis of internal data sources to indicate a need for increased tobacco treatment programs and for greater prescribing of tobacco cessation medications, in addition to considering logistics and scheduling. Faculty consisted of two tobacco cessation experts, both clinical pharmacists' specialists. Training attendees were recruited by Health Promotion Disease Prevention (HPDP) health care personnel and the Smoking Cessation Lead Clinician at each respective facility. Local personnel may have also arranged for video teleconferences to permit participation by offsite providers. All on site attendees who registered received educational credits and their responses were included in the evaluation of the training program.

Replicability

The training was successful because participants demonstrated improvement in 1) self-rated overall ability to deliver tobacco cessation treatment, 2) each of the five components of comprehensive counseling for cessation (the 5As), and 3) self-efficacy for cessation counseling. In addition, prescribing increased to above the national average in these sites after the training. The training curriculum also met the rigorous continuing education requirements of the respective accrediting bodies for multiple care disciplines, further supporting the validity of the program. This program has been replicated since 2010 and has been a valued asset.

Recognition

Dana Christofferson, Jennifer Javors, Julianne Himstreet, Kim Hamlett-Berry, Mark Myers, Pam Belperio, Mercedes Dashefsky, Linda Allen. Kristie Short, Lorraine Bem, Madelyn Phillips, HBC, HPDP, and tobacco lead clinicians at each VA training site

VA Fisher House Program

Jennifer Koget, MS, LCSW, BCD, National VA Fisher House and Family Hospitality Program Manager
VACO, Washington, DC
jennifer.koget@va.gov

This program offers a home away from home for families of Veterans while receiving care at VA facilities. Fisher Houses enable a loved one's presence at the Veteran's bedside as the result of a successful Public-Private Partnership between VA and Fisher House Foundation.

Introduction

There are many great examples of Veterans and their family members who have been helped by VA's Fisher House program. Here is a great recent example. A Veteran was diagnosed with stage II Lung Cancer. He was informed that treatment would require a stay in VA facility over 120 miles from his small hometown. Unfortunately, there were no facilities close to the Veteran's home that offered the extensive treatment he needed to fight his cancer. The Veteran's primary support system was his wife and daughter, and he made it very clear to his treatment team that he needed his family by his side through his course of treatment. The Veteran indicated to his treatment team he would not travel away from home, even if it meant he would not receive the life-saving treatment unless his wife and daughter could stay with him. Community hotel accommodations nearby VA facility were costly, and the Veteran could not afford this out of pocket expense. The Veteran explained to his treatment team that he was ready to accept the fate of his illness and remain at home, even though the Veterans' chances of recovery were good if treatment was initiated.

The treatment team informed the Veteran that a VA Fisher House was available on the grounds of the facility and could accommodate his wife and daughter at no cost while he received treatment for his cancer. The Veteran was skeptical and wanted to see the facility before he would agree to treatment and allow his wife and daughter to stay. When the Veteran arrived at the Fisher House, he was overwhelmed and became very tearful. The immediate comfort of the home provided a feeling of relief knowing that his wife and daughter would be safe, comfortable, and staying close by the hospital. The Veteran agreed to move forward with his cancer treatment and was an inpatient at VA facility for over three months. The wife and daughter were at the Veteran's bedside every day and surrounded by the support of other families staying at the house.

About one year following treatment, the Veteran returned for an outpatient appointment with his Oncologist and received the news that he was now cancer free. Following the appointment, the Veteran visited the Fisher House to thank the Fisher House Manager and express his gratitude to the staff for caring for his family while the hospital staff cared for him. The Veteran stated, "The Fisher House saved my life! Without a place for my family to stay, I would not have agreed to come so far away from home to treat my cancer, and I would have died as a result. Thank you Fisher House!" This is a familiar story shared by over 100,000 Veterans, active duty Service Members, their family members and caregivers since the first VA Fisher House opened its doors in 1994. "A family's love is good medicine."

Key Information

VA Fisher Houses provide a "home away from home" for the family members and caregivers of hospitalized Veterans and Active Duty Service Members. VA Fisher Houses are constructed by Fisher House Foundation on the grounds of VA facilities and gifted to VA. These comfort homes allow families to stay at no cost so they can be at the bedside of their loved one. VA Fisher Houses foster a healing environment where guests form a support network, sharing their experiences and offering comfort to one another through life's most challenging times. The first VA Fisher House was constructed by Fisher House Foundation in 1994 on the campus of the Albany VAMC, Albany, NY. To date, the successful public-private partnership between Fisher House Foundation and the VA resulted in the construction of 30 VA Fisher Houses located at 28 VA facilities. As this successful partnership continues, VA and Fisher House Foundation plan to expand the number of VA Fisher Houses to at least 46 by 2020. The success of VA Fisher House is led at the national level through VA and Fisher House Foundation partnership. This partnership extends to the local level in which VA facilities and communities establish partnerships for Fisher House construction, operations, and ongoing support for Fisher House families. VA Fisher Houses become a conduit for enhanced community engagement and support for the Veteran/military community.

Context

VA Fisher Houses have up to 21 suites, with private bedrooms and baths. Families share a common kitchen, laundry facilities, a warm dining room, and an inviting living room. VA Fisher Houses serve Veterans from all eras of service. No time limitations exist on VA Fisher House stays. VA Fisher Houses support the invaluable involvement of an individual's support system during treatment of a serious illness or injury. Active involvement and support from loved ones make a tremendous difference in the Veterans' adjustment and engagement in treatment, which impacts treatment outcomes. Also, VA Fisher Houses promote access to VA care for those traveling long distances who cannot afford costs hotel lodging during treatment. Fisher Houses eliminate the burden of community lodging costs. Also, more Veterans travel to receive care at VA Facilities once informed that their loved one will receive accommodations and support in a VA Fisher House.

Practice Description

VA and Fisher House Foundation partnership was established with input and guidance from VA and Fisher House Foundation leaders. The partnership was formalized though the establishment of federal regulations to support the construction of Fisher Houses on VA property by Fisher House Foundation. Section 221(a) of the Veterans Benefits and Health Care Improvement Act of 2000 (Public Law 106–419) (codified at 38 USC 1708) authorizes VA to operate Fisher Houses donated by the Fisher House Foundation. Federal Regulations (38 CFR 60) were finalized and published in the Federal Register (77 FR 59089 on September 26, 2012). One of the keys to successful program implementation is the consistency of collaboration and involvement with the Fisher House Foundation and national VA leaders. Successful construction and operation of each VA Fisher House involve extensive planning and collaboration from local communities, federal, state, and local governing bodies. Every project involves engagement of site-specific local, state, and federal partners.

Replicability

The National VA Fisher House program, in collaboration with VACO, regularly initiates a formal call for VA Fisher House Applications to VA facilities. The facility makes a determination whether a Fisher House is needed to support Veterans, Active Duty Service Members, and their families/caregivers traveling long distances for care. Facilities servicing large catchment areas offering specialty care programs or serving as Centers of Excellence consistently report that Veterans and their loved ones receive great benefit from the addition of a VA Fisher House. Veteran access to care enhanced the Veteran experience and inclusion/support of the Veteran's support system contribute to improved treatment outcomes. The availability of family members/caregivers to stay at the Fisher House supports consistent caregiver training and improves the opportunity for a successful transition to the home upon discharge.

The National VA Fisher House program created a Fisher House Toolkit and a Fisher House program TMS (Talent Management System) web-based training for facilities to reference when considering the addition of a local Fisher House. VA facilities also receive extensive support and guidance with Fisher House planning, construction, activation, and operations. The level of support offered and VA Fisher House program impact on the care of Veterans while supporting their loved ones allows for successful replication of the program by other VA facilities.

Recognition

Ken Fisher, the Fisher family, Fisher House board of trustees, Fisher House Foundation staff, VA community partners, the American public

MOVE! Grocery Store Tours

Lori Carlson, MOVE! Program Coordinator and Registered Dietitian

VA Illiana Health Care System, Danville, IL

laura.carlson@va.gov

This interactive group visit advances health care value by engaging Veterans' first line of defense in preventing and treating chronic disease through practical, patient-centered nutrition education to increase food selection knowledge and confidence.

Introduction

Mr. X weighed 300 pounds when he started the MOVE! Weight Management program at VA Illiana Health Care System in Danville, IL, in 2013. He lost 30 pounds (10 percent loss) in six months but had difficulty maintaining motivation and lifestyle changes to keep the weight off. After a break from the program, he ended up regaining the weight plus five additional pounds. He decided to refocus and get more involved with MOVE! at the end of 2014. He attended MOVE! Healthy Cooking Classes and MOVE! Grocery Store Tours with his wife. He has since returned to a weight in the 270s and successfully maintained this loss for the past four months. Both Veterans and staff provide rave reviews after participating in the classes, and the outings have been included in VA Illiana's marketing efforts using social media.

"It was interesting to learn about things we buy and new items we buy now; we started buying acorn squash. We read the labels on everything. It was surprising to see some of the numbers on those things, the high numbers," remarked Mr. X.

"Grocery store tours are a great way for clinicians to better relate to the Veterans they serve. This experience was great to use hands-on practice to teach the Veterans about the foods they select. I also took from the experience an understanding of how to better meet the Veteran's needs, when it comes to nutrition education and grocery shopping," stated dietitian Angie Sebree, MS, RDN, LDN.

Key Information

VA Illiana's MOVE! grocery store tours offer interactive, hands-on group nutrition education. An important skill to learn when planning healthy meals is how to shop. One can design the best meal in the world, but if the food isn't in the house, that meal has no chance of turning into reality.

The pilot store tour was offered to MOVE! weight management program participants from the main medical facility in June 2014. The program gradually expanded to two CBOCs in fall 2014 with continued growth to three additional CBOCs in spring 2015. MOVE! Registered dietitian nutritionists have formed partnerships with Meijer, Aldi, and Hy-Vee to allow Veterans to learn in their store of choice. Each 60 to 90-minute class of about eight Veterans and spouses explores the grocery store following a scavenger-hunt style worksheet, focusing on comparing nutrition facts labels and prices to make budget-savvy purchases that meet their individual health needs. Veterans leave with the completed worksheet along with educational handouts on how to read a nutrition label and grocery store shopping guidelines.

While registered dietitians can instruct on label reading using nutrition facts samples in the clinic setting, offering in-person interactive classes that get clients engaged in hands-on experiences of making healthy choices lets them be in the driver's seat of their health care. Learning how to select, prepare, and enjoy cooking foods follows the same principles of the Cone of Learning or Cone of Experience. After weeks, we tend to remember 10 percent of what we read and 20 percent of what we hear but 90 percent of what we say and do. Therefore, providing knowledge alone may be ineffective in altering eating behavior, whereas offering of hands-on demonstration appears to be more encouraging.

Context

The National Center for Health Promotion Disease Prevention (NCP) estimates that 77 percent of Veterans in the US are overweight or obese and could potentially benefit from prevention services. (VHA Handbook 1120.01). VAIHCS MOVE! program started in July 2006 and had tremendous growth, expanding to meet the needs of our Veteran population using technology and innovation. The program currently has a penetration of 15.8 percent with 5,217 patients seen out of 32,949 unique PC patients (MOVE! Pyramid, September 2015). 30.2 percent of participants achieved clinically relevant weight loss (≥5 percent weight loss).

Practice Description

The MOVE! coordinator contacted retail dietitians within her professional network to identify grocery stores that would allow outside organizations to host grocery store tours at their location. Tours were piloted at the Meijer in Danville, IL, with staff from the main medical facility before expanding to CBOC locations near Meijer stores. Each participant received a calculator obtained with Health Promotion Disease Prevention (HPDP) funds to use during class, a written summary of healthful shopping tips and nutrition label education, and a tour worksheet that the class completed together to help guide them through the store. Some CBOCs were not located by the Meijer store, and Veterans started requesting tours at additional store chains, so the MOVE! Coordinator reached out to Aldi's retail dietitian who directed her to a corporate contact. Before scheduling each tour, the MOVE! Coordinator sends a request to each corporate contact person who then obtains approval from local district managers or store directors. Stores prefer to limit tours to eight Veterans during non-peak days and hours. With the addition of Aldi stores, each of the six sites within VA Illiana Health Care System achieved the ability to host grocery store tours locally for MOVE! Veteran participants. The Springfield CBOC dietitian scheduled a tour with the Hy-Vee dietitian in January 2016 to add a third store chain to the list. We now plan to expand tour availability to additional programs, such as the Psychosocial Residential Rehabilitation Treatment program.

Replicability

MOVE! grocery store tours was a low-cost program to implement. It was successful because each CBOC along with the medical facility has registered dietitians onsite along with one to two dietetic interns who can travel to assist, as needed. As a team, we shared tour curriculum and materials, so startup required low staff time as well. The MOVE! coordinator used existing contacts and relationships from involvement in professional organizations. Tours have worked thus far because they have been offered as an outpatient program, so Veterans provide their transportation to a designated grocery store. VA and the store benefit from the community partnership.

Recognition

VA Illiana's dietitians, Meijer, ALDI Inc., Hy-Vee

Women's MOVE! Program

Julie Harmon, Registered Dietitian and MOVE! Weight Management Program Coordinator
James A. Haley, Veterans Hospital, Tampa, FL
julie.harmon2@va.gov

Female Veterans endure unique challenges regarding weight management. A female-only group fosters sensitivity toward social pressures, prior weight loss attempts, and body image issues prevalent in the female population.

Introduction

The prevalence of obesity among Veterans continues to rise at an alarming rate. According to VA Office of Research & Development, more than seven in ten Veterans who receive VA care are either overweight or obese. In 2013, estimates from the James A. Haley Veterans Hospital and Clinics (JAHVH) in Tampa, Florida suggested that 84.3 percent of male and 80.4 percent of female Veterans seen via PC clinics were overweight or obese. The MOVE! Weight Management program, supported by VA's National Center for Health Promotion and Disease Prevention (NCP), is designed to assist Veterans in achieving clinically significant weight loss via an intensive 16-week lifestyle intervention involving nutrition, physical activity, and behavioral modification elements.

Key Information

JAHVH served as a pilot site for the MOVE! program in 2004. However, multi-disciplinary weight loss efforts have existed there since the 1980s. JAHVH MOVE! program has a reputation for innovative change and consistent quality improvement. The Bright Spot Award from VA National Center for Health Promotion and Disease Prevention is awarded to health programs that showcase the use of standardized improvement processes with evidence of data review and collaboration that is consistent with evidence-based practice. JAHVH MOVE! received this recognition to honor our redesign, including the implementation of Women's MOVE! and the addition of supervised exercise sessions.

Context

In 2013, JAHVH MOVE! program utilized systems redesign tools to define challenges, areas for improvement and improve program access. Focus groups revealed expansion to specialty populations was warranted. In July 2013, Women's MOVE! was implemented. This program has the same structure as MOVE! but is specifically tailored to women Veterans and led by female health care providers. Weight loss is not a one-size fits all approach and women often endure unique challenges regarding weight management. While weight loss principles are comparable for both genders, Women's MOVE! provides an environment that fosters sensitivity toward social pressures and prior weight loss attempts, as well as body image concerns prevalent in the female population.

According to the VISN 8 Annual Report, 92,950 Veterans were treated last year at JAHVH, and, on average, 3,446 Veterans visited our outpatient clinics daily in 2015. Women Veterans represent 11.2 percent (about 10,500 Veterans) of the population served at JAHVH. Before Women's MOVE!

the percentage of women Veterans enrolled in the program was very low, and attrition rate was greater than 50 percent. Our implementation of the program has greatly improved women Veteran engagement and satisfaction.

Practice Description

Since 2013, 103 Veterans have enrolled in Women's MOVE! and 62 have completed the program (60 percent retention). The average change is 6.72 percent weight loss. Of the 62 women who completed the 16-week program, 16 percent achieved between 5 and 10 percent weight loss and 8 percent achieved greater than 10 percent weight loss. For women Veterans who began the program with an elevated Hemoglobin A1C (greater than or equal to 6.5), the average reduction was 1.52. For women Veterans who began the program with an "at-risk" Hemoglobin A1C (between 5.7 to 6.4), the average reduction was 0.3. Additional outcome measures are tracked, and on average, Glucose, Total Cholesterol, LDL Cholesterol and Triglycerides decreased, and HDL Cholesterol increased.

During the implementation of Women's MOVE!, our team attended weekly PC meetings to educate VA staff. We also reviewed Motivational Interviewing (MI) strategies to help engage women Veterans in a conversation about weight reduction. Our Women's Center Clinic Dietitian offered a review of the anthropometric screening provided to women Veterans to showcase the individual treatment of each participant. We collaborated with the Women Center Clinic Program Coordinator, Physicians, Nurses and Program Support staff to recruit interested women Veterans. Finally, we attended VA health fairs to promote the program to women Veterans.

Replicability

While JAHVH was the first facility to offer a Women's MOVE!, the concept was adopted by other facilities nationally. The program fosters a positive environment for women to share their weight struggles and develop friendships with fellow women Veterans. To enhance the Veteran experience, it is important to take steps to ensure a "women-only" environment is respected: 1)seek female staff members only and 2) if women ask to bring a male guest, respectfully decline their request and explain the rationale for maintaining the "women-only" environment.

Recognition

Melody Chavez, Julie Harmon, Vanessa Milsom, Andrew Philip Tara Tyler, Mike Rohr, Racheal Samec, Nadine Skelton-Khouzam, Chelsea Skillman

MOVE!: VHA's Evidence-Based, Population Approach to Weight Management

Susan Raffa, PhD, National Program Director for Weight Management
VACO, Washington, DC
susan.raffa@va.gov

This evidence-based, Veteran-centered approach to weight management provides a variety of options for participating, including in-person, telephone, and home telehealth modalities as well as the MOVE! Coach mobile app.

Introduction

Much like the general population, the prevalence of overweight and obesity in the population of Veterans seen in VHA has continued to increase over the past several decades. Overweight and obesity are associated with a number of chronic health conditions that are common in Veterans treated in VHA. MOVE! is VHA's evidence-based, population-focused weight management program available to Veterans at every VA medical facility across the country. Since national implementation in 2006, more than 650,000 Veterans have participated in MOVE! The impact of MOVE! can be seen and felt through more than 100 Veteran MOVE! Success Stories featured on VHA's MOVE! website. Following are a few excerpts:

"I'm 66-years-old, but I feel like I'm 50. I look better, feel better, and I enjoy life much more than I used to. I plan to keep on doing what I've learned through MOVE!"

"With the help of two MOVE! programs, I've lost 170 pounds and no longer require insulin," she says. "My most recent A1C was 5.2 percent—a normal value and a drastic improvement from 9.0 percent in 2006."

"The most important thing was learning that MOVE! isn't a "diet," because all diets end. To be able to get the weight off and keep it off it requires a total lifestyle change." The same Veteran also said, "I tell other Veterans never to give up. When I talk to a class, I like to end my session by saying, 'If you are tired of starting over, just stop quitting!' I love being able to 'pay it forward.'"

Key Information

In collaboration with other key program offices (including Nutrition and Food Services) and VHA leaders, MOVE! was developed by the National Center for Health Promotion and Disease Prevention (NCP) and implemented nationally in 2006. Initially, MOVE! was primarily delivered through in-person group sessions. Alternative MOVE! delivery methods have been developed to provide increased access to care as well as options to participate in weight management based on individual needs and preferences. The expansion of MOVE! options reflect collaborations across VHA to develop Veteran-centered solutions to increasing access to care. For example, MOVE! Telephone Lifestyle Coaching (TLC) was piloted in collaboration with VISN 2 and the Center for Integrated Health before national implementation. Also, as a result of collaborations with the Office of Connected Care, Veterans may choose to participate in TeleMOVE!, supported self-management through in-home messaging devices, or MOVE! Coach, a mobile app that Veterans may download and use on their own or in conjunction with care. Be Active and MOVE!, physical activity programming delivered as an adjunct to MOVE!, is the result of a collaboration of NCP, the Office of Connected Care, and Physical Medicine and Rehabilitation.

Context

The VHA National Center for Health Promotion and Disease Prevention (NCP; 10P4N) is a VACO Program Office within Patient Care Services (10P4). NCP is VA's primary source for healthy living, prevention and health education. It provides evidence-based programs, resources, and policy guidance to engage Veterans in healthy living. NCP programs and resources work to empower health, reduce chronic disease and improve VA health care. MOVE! is NCP's flagship clinical program to address overweight and obesity among Veterans receiving care in VHA.

Practice Description

MOVE! is VHA's comprehensive, interdisciplinary approach to weight management in VHA. With the implementation of MOVE!, regular screening for overweight and obesity has become the standard of care; more than 90 percent of Veterans receiving care in VHA are screened annually for overweight and obesity. Veterans are referred to MOVE! through a process of shared decision making that includes assessment of factors related to overweight and obesity. MOVE! provides an infrastructure for weight management programming at every facility through the designation of a local MOVE! Coordinator and MOVE! Physician Champion. MOVE! is an evidence-based intervention developed by NCP and adapted for delivery through multiple modalities.

Replicability

MOVE! programming is highly replicable; it has been implemented at every VAMC across all 19 VISNs. As a result of the infrastructure and support for MOVE! provided by NCP, program office partners, and local facilities, VHA has disseminated a comprehensive behavioral weight management program on a scale not achieved by others in the world. MOVE! has been adapted by the US Army and implemented as Army MOVE! program evaluation and sharing of field-based best practices will inform improvements and opportunities to expand MOVE! options of care.

Recognition

Field-based MOVE! teams

The Arts and Humanities Heal the Wounds of War

Laura Krejci, Associate Director
VACO, Washington, DC
laura.krejci@va.gov

The VA Arts, Health, and Well-being pilot project expands community partnerships to promote Veteran healing, wellness, and engagement through participation in the Arts and Humanities.

Introduction

David Jones was a medic in the Army and Air Force and served six tours of duty in Iraq and Afghanistan. He came back with the wounds of war but did not fully understand the effect these experiences had on his mind and his soul. It was not until he began working with his art therapist that he began discovering all of the feelings that were impacting his life. David credits this work with his art therapist as saving his life as four of David's comrades committed suicide after returning from their service. Today, David is not only surviving; he is thriving.

Key Information

In March 2015, the VA Office of Patient Centered Care and Cultural Transformation (OPCC&CT) worked with Americans for the Arts, the National Center for Creative Aging and Johnson & Johnson to coordinate a pilot project that provided information and education on how to develop and/or expand local VA/Community Arts Partnerships to support Arts in Healing. A major goal of the VA Arts, Health, and Well-being pilot project was to build the capacity of the VHA health care workforce to enhance and expand their current creative arts therapies and arts programming in their medical centers through strong community partnerships.

Context

The pilot project provided the opportunity for VA art therapists, providers, artists, and Veterans to come together with teams of art experts who served as consultants. VA OPCC&CT Field Implementation team coach partnered with the art consultants to support and assist VA teams in applying the knowledge, skills, and ideas presented in a two-day Arts, Health, and Well-being Symposium. Specifically, they are strengthening the Arts and Humanities Programming for Veterans with these primary goals:

- To build the capacity of the multi-disciplinary health care team to integrate evidence-based Arts and Humanities Programming for Veterans, beyond—but inclusive and supportive of—the formal therapeutic setting.

- To improve the health, well-being, and quality of life for Veterans with a special focus on those affected by combat injuries.

- To improve the health, well-being, and quality of life for the Veteran family members, caregivers, and significant others.

Practice Description

The three steps are: 1) planning and coordinating the conference, 2) hosting the conference, and 3) site visits.

Outcomes:

- Leisure interest assessment developed and utilized to link staff with Veterans with similar interests
- Family inclusion in arts planning
- Activity carts created and utilized for spontaneous engagement
- Experiential lunch-and-learns held for staff to expand knowledge of the arts in healing
- Professional development (Journal club)
- Patient Art Display areas and protocols
- Clear instructions for volunteers and staff
- Continuous internship programs
- Develop unit arts champions
- Community partners present proposals to arts team
- Creation of Gardening program
- Use of evaluation tools to measure outcomes

Replicability

Americans for the Arts and Johnson & Johnson were so pleased with the results of the first pilot project that they wanted to sponsor additional forums. In March 2016, a new VHA Memorandum of Agreement was drafted and has been signed in support of this effort. Johnson & Johnson is providing a grant to support this expanded effort in 2016.

The practice is highly replicable and in fact, this partnership has resulted in two additional VHA conferences with 12 teams participating from across the country. The group has utilized the lessons learned from the first pilot to enhance the ongoing work and to develop a Guidebook for Expanding the Arts and Humanities through Community Partnerships.

Recognition

Ashley Atkins, Donna Faraone, Mary Therese Hankinson, Gay Hannah, Laura Krejci, Larry Long, Ken Mizrach, Judy Rollins, Marete Wester, Cindi Wilson, Kim Decataldo, Laurie Tomaino, Ilysa Michelson, Susan Pisano, Rosemarie Rogers, Julia Anderson, Tenisha Ruffin, Sara Stein, Rachel Yahes

Headache Care: A Proactive, Patient-Driven, and Personalized Approach

Karen Williams, MSN, CRNP

Olin E. Teague Veterans Medical Center, Temple, TX
karen.williams1@va.gov

This patient-centered approach to headache management uses a holistic approach and multiple modalities to reduce the headache burden and improve the quality of life for the Veteran.

Introduction

Imagine having a 51-year-old Veteran with a 23-year history of refractory headaches walk into your clinic for a consult. The Veteran has a defeated-looking demeanor, wearing sunglasses and a baseball hat, slumped over in the shoulders, slow gait, with a quiet and sad tone to his voice. He has a current headache rated as 6/10 and anxiety rated as an 8/10. These headaches have been occurring about 2–4 times per month, lasting 3–6 days, described as throbbing, pain to the left temple with stabbing pain behind his eyes, associated with such light sensitivity that he needed to use sunglasses even inside, sensitivity to noise, nausea, and vomiting, and worse with movement. His pain would range from 6/10 to 10/10. He has had trials of five different medications to prevent his headaches and an additional four to stop them, with little relief. The medications are the usual migraine preventive and abortive medications that are recommended for treatment by headache experts. He has been evaluated by multiple providers, to include PC and neurology. What would the average clinician be able to do for this Veteran? More medications, which have not worked for the last 23 years?

Would you believe that this Veteran walked out of his consult appointment 90 minutes later without a headache and a reduction in his back pain and his anxiety? He had a plan of care that made sense; he understood why he had these headaches and what to do for them, what the provider could do for him, and he had something that he had given up on...HOPE.

This particular Veteran had a complicated headache, which started after his head injury during a parachute jump and worsened after further deployment-related head injuries. His co-occurring PTSD, insomnia, and chronic back pain increased his headaches and complicated his care. During his consult appointment, he was treated with an occipital block (local numbing agent to nerves at the back of the neck) and acupuncture. He was instructed on what to do when headaches occurred. Over the course of two months, his headaches became more manageable. Within six months, he no longer needed to wear sunglasses and a year later his life was restored. "I do not feel broken anymore." While his individual story is unique to him, his complex headaches and co-occurring issues are common findings in the Headache Clinic population.

Key Information

In November 2013, the Headache clinic was established at the Temple Texas VA. This VA is the closest to Ft Hood, the largest US Army Base and home to many of the Veterans who retire out of Ft Hood. This clinic was established to help with the overflow of complex headaches and was approved to use alternative therapies of BOTOX and Occipital blocks by Supervisor of Neurology,

Dr. Guttikonda; ACOS, Dr. Hussain; and COS, Dr. Harper. Karen Williams, the NP who was hired to set up and run the Headache Clinic, utilizes these therapies and implemented the use of acupuncture, alpha-stim, a 90-minute consult, a follow-up in one to two weeks, patient education (covering their headache, home treatments, relaxation techniques and, if needed, healthy dietary recommendations/smoking cessation techniques). The treatments are administered in a calm, soothing, comfortable environment (reduced lighting, soothing scenes of nature streaming on a photo frame, pictures with words of encouragement hanging on the wall, and curtains shading the bright sunlight). The combination of these alternative modalities administered in a calming environment, the increased time for the consult, the scheduled follow-up appointment, and attention to patient education and a chart review before the appointment have shown significant improvement in patients with complicated headaches. These outcomes include reduced and, in a few cases, resolution of the headaches, reduced use of medication, reduced or eliminated need for ER/Urgent care, improved quality of life, and reduced frustrations for both patient and provider.

Context

The Headache Clinic is in the outpatient department of the hospital. There is a single treatment room dedicated to the Headache Clinic and the provider shares nursing support. Headaches are one of the top ten service-connected injuries and are very disabling, especially when combined with PTSD, anxiety, chronic pain, and/or sleep disorders. About 75 percent of the Veterans cared for in the Headache Clinic have the co-occurring diagnoses, a long list of medications and need treatments that are safe, effective, do not cause additional complications with possible organ damage, require laboratory monitoring or interfere with their other needed medications. Despite the challenge of one room and the complex patient issues, the therapies offered in the Headache Clinic reduce the headaches, often reduce the anxiety, and improve sleep. This one room acts as a haven for the Veterans as they find it safe, relaxing, and a place of healing.

Practice Description

A time commitment up front is needed to set the stage for proactive, patient-driven, and personalized care. In this particular clinic, a chart search prior to the Veteran's initial appointment is completed by the provider with an eye on a holistic approach to the issue. This chart search is essential in establishing a possible cause for the headaches, identifying any and all past treatments that have been tried, and understanding additional factors that are affecting the Veteran's life. Having a chart search already completed and a 90-minute consult allows the provider to maximize the time of the appointment to do an exam, educate the Veteran on the findings and treatment options, and to administer a procedure. This extra time at the first visit allows the provider the opportunity to ask open-ended questions, establish a relationship with the Veteran, and establish an individualized plan of care and to treat at the time of the initial appointment. Treatment at the time of the initial appointment is essential as it establishes a sense of hope in a set of patients who often have no hope left in getting help from their chronic pain.

The Veteran needs to have time to discuss what their real issues and concerns are and to feel they are being heard in order to trust the provider. If they do not trust the provider, they will not speak up, are less likely to follow recommendations and care will be compromised.

Replicability

Leadership recognized that these complex headache patients were not responding to traditional western medication-driven treatments and were feeling hopeless. Initiative was taken to hire a NP to focus specifically on this patient population. Karen Williams arrived with skill sets in neurology, acupuncture, occipital blocks, BOTOX, and a vast history of treating Service Members with Traumatic Brain Injury (TBI) and PTSD. Ms. Williams was given the leeway to establish her clinic based on her experience and sound medical judgment.

To replicate this initiative, leadership support is essential for successful development and implementation of this program. Provider(s) should be trained and credentialed in BOTOX, occipital blocks and, at a minimum, auricular acupuncture. Providers require dedicated space, support staffing, medical equipment, and some leeway to set up the treatment room conducive to a safe, calming, and environmentally appropriate patient-centered state. Leadership support for template management is needed to allow for extensive chart reviews, 90-minute consults, 60-minute BOTOX appointments, and 30-minute follow-ups. The schedule for new patients will have to be adjusted as the clinic fills up. There needs to be adequate room to see the patients in follow-up within one to two weeks of their initial consult. Additional follow-ups every one to two weeks for several appointments may be needed to provide additional treatments or to make adjustments to the treatment plan and to reinforce the home treatments. Once a headache is under good control, the follow-up appointments can be spaced out. At a minimum, those who are treated with BOTOX will need to be seen every 12 weeks for repeat administrations of the medication.

Recognition

Nasir Hussain, Gopal Guttikonda, Padma Kumar, Dr. Harper, Dave Williams

The Maternity Care Coordinator Telephone Care Program

Kristina Cordasco, MD, MPH, MSHS, Core Investigator, Internal Medicine Physician
VA Greater Los Angeles Healthcare System, Los Angeles, CA
kristina.cordasco@va.gov

This program supports telephone-based care coordination for pregnant Veterans, aiming to improve pregnant Veterans' experience with maternity care by providing Veterans with education, screening, coordination with VA services, and referral for community (non-VA) services.

Introduction

Pregnant women Veterans are a vulnerable and high-risk patient population, with a high prevalence of mental health and medical co-morbidities, as well as socioeconomic concerns. VA arranges for non-VA health care providers to deliver maternity care while continuing to care for Veterans' mental health and medical co-morbidities, as well as to provide social services support through VA. This arrangement of simultaneous VA and non-VA care results in many care coordination challenges. Communication and coordination between non-VA obstetricians and VA providers are often lacking as information about what is happening with Veterans' maternity care is absent from VA medical records, and non-VA providers have limited information about VA care. Further, although professional maternity services are rendered outside of VA, Veterans need to obtain maternity-related medications and supplies through VA. Therefore, in the midst of dealing with the stress of pregnancy, and needing to obtain timely care that has been proven to be associated with improved health outcomes for both mother and baby, Veterans are faced with navigating a complicated interface between VA and non-VA providers and systems.

Key Information

A multi-disciplinary workgroup at the Greater Los Angeles (GLA) health care system initiated the development of The Maternity Care Coordinator (MCC) Telephone Care program by first identifying potential informational and screening needs of pregnant Veterans. The workgroup performed a literature scan and augmented this scan with knowledge from their professional experiences. Then, using Plan-Do-Study-Act quality improvement methods, the workgroup formulated and iteratively tested and revised materials. The following year, the program expanded to three additional VA health care systems, and materials were again modified to account for variations in resources and processes across VA health care systems as well as differences in patient needs related to geography (e.g., rural vs. urban patients). In the third year, the program again expanded to include a total of 11 VA health care systems, serving nearly 1,000 Veterans nationally, and a formative evaluation of the materials was conducted and further refined. In 2015, the developed materials were distributed to 102 VA health care systems nationally.

Context

In 2012, VHA Handbook 1330.03 established that each VA health care system must have an MCC who has regular contact with pregnant Veterans. However, the content of this position was not specified. Therefore, The GLA VA Healthcare System, with funding from the ORH and Women's Health Services, took on the challenge of defining content for a series of seven scheduled phone calls to pregnant and post-partum Veterans. Other VISN 22 health care systems, and VA health care systems across the nation in states with sizeable numbers of rural Veterans, then collaborated with the GLA team to make the materials usable and applicable across diverse VA settings and patient populations.

Practice Description

The developed MCC Telephone Care program consists of seven scheduled phone calls from the time that pregnancy is confirmed by VA through six-weeks post-partum (at initiation of maternity benefits; 12-weeks gestation; 20-weeks gestation; 28-weeks gestation; 36-weeks gestation; one-week post-partum; six-weeks post-partum). Topics and sub-topics vary by call, timed to match the Veteran's anticipated needs. Call topics include aiding a pregnant Veteran in navigating the non-VA care process, making sure she understands the full range of VA maternity benefits and services, assisting her in obtaining needed medications and supplies (e.g., prenatal vitamins, breastfeeding supplies), screening her for targeted health and social needs for which VA directly provides services during pregnancy (e.g., smoking cessation, post-partum depression, interpersonal violence), facilitating her obtaining VA care when needed, and transitioning her back to VA PC post-partum. Between scheduled phone calls, the MCC is available to the Veteran, as needed, and makes additional phone calls to follow up on problems identified during the scheduled calls. Each topic has suggested scripts, with additional scripts available for potential interventions or care coordination when needed (e.g., positive depression or interpersonal violence screen). The MCC additionally uses clinical judgment and knowledge of local resources to triage and respond to identified issues. Topics and sub-topics for each call are outlined in worksheets to facilitate fidelity to the program content.

The workgroup developed additional resources to support the phone calls, including a workbook to assist MCCs in compiling information on local resources relevant to maternity care coordination, and note templates to assist with documentation, and a spreadsheet tool for tracking completed and upcoming care coordination calls and activities. Recorded educational webinars and a resource guide to web-based educational materials provide MCCs with needed background information on topics addressed by calls. Web-based tutorials were also developed to demonstrate how to use program materials.

Replicability

This program has been very successful with women Veterans residing in urban and rural areas, providing them with Veteran-centric care throughout their pregnancies, coordinating their non-VA obstetric services with any VA medical, mental health, or social services they may be receiving, and helping them seamlessly transition back to VA PC post-partum. Logs reveal that over 60 percent of the scheduled phone calls are completed, indicating that the Veterans are engaged in this program. MCCs report that the program is highly valuable in serving Veterans. In a survey with open-ended questions assessing MCC perceptions about the program, one MCC wrote, "I appreciate being a part of the customer service we provide. I think the patients also appreciate that they have someone to contact to help them through a situation." Another MCC wrote, "I love connecting with these women and providing them the resources they need. They are truly appreciative of all we can do for them."

Recognition

Judith Katzburg, Elaine Maxwell, Fatma Batuman, Callie Wight, Lakisha Swindell, Robin Moyer, Nichole Erb, Zeny Velasco, Carolyne Corpas, Lisa Roybal, Katie Westanmo, Kathleen Blashko, Erin Krebs, Holli McDonald, Mary (Betty) Dillon, Catherine Shackleford, Jonna Brenton, Ana Holcombe, Tammy Story, Ishita Thakar, Carlissa Brooks-Ashley, Beth Holt Wright, Faith Good-Cole, Colleen Butler, Joann Frampton, Lynn Webster, Catherine Nadal, Laurie Zephyrin

Improving the Health Care Experience of Women Veterans

Sherrill Hooke, MEd, RN, CGRN, CCCTM, VANAP Nurse Faculty
VA Portland Health Care System, Portland, OR
sherrill.hooke@va.gov

This initiative by the Portland, OR VA Nursing Academic Partnership (VANAP) began by holding focus groups for local women Veterans to identify their health care concerns. Faculty, nursing students, and VA staff worked together on resulting projects: e.g., a women-only reception area remodel at an outpatient clinic.

Introduction

Ms. X, a young woman who has served in the US military, walks into a major VAMC to seek health care. She is confronted with crowded public areas filled with male Veterans and others, but she is most often in the minority due to her gender. She may or may not be recognized as a Veteran by staff or other Veterans. She is not fully aware of the resources and services available to her and wonders if VA offers contraception, mammography, or pregnancy care. She would like to see a counselor but finds it hard to admit she needs help. As she looks around, she thinks, "Some of these guys have had it so rough, my problems don't seem nearly as bad as theirs." She is nervous and apprehensive, but hopeful.

Key Information

Nationally, VA has identified the care of women Veterans as one of its priority initiatives. Women comprise the fastest growing demographic within the Veteran population, and there are known care disparities between male and female Veterans. Discovering the top issues female Veterans report at the local level will lead to identifying the best ideas for improving their care and satisfaction.

Context

VA Portland Health Care System (VAPORHCS) in Portland, OR serves more than 17,000 women Veterans. Within the last six years, a Women Veteran PC Clinic was added, and each of the other outpatient clinics now has a designated women's health team. The women Veterans program manager at the facility conducts regular audits to assure adherence to VA directives regarding women Veteran care.

Practice Description

Improving women Veterans' health care experiences at VAPORHCS is an identified practice improvement initiative for VA Nursing Academic Partnership (VANAP), partnering VAPORHCS and Oregon Health & Sciences University School of Nursing to promote Veteran care. As part of this initiative, three undergraduate VANAP VA Scholar nursing students studied women Veterans specifically in a population health course. They identified military sexual trauma (MST) as the most compelling issue facing women Veterans after interviewing many of the local VA providers and reviewing the literature. Three focus groups targeting women Veterans were conducted in July 2015. The list of questions used was developed by the workgroup with input from the women Veterans program manager. The women Veterans were not required to be enrolled at VA to participate. The one-hour focus groups were held at different sites within the VA health care system. Over the course of the three focus groups, a total of 11 women Veterans participated. The largest group was at an outlying campus (n=7) comprising women Veterans who stayed after an already scheduled therapy group. The other two groups had two attendees each. The women were very willing to share stories of their experiences and make suggestions that could improve their health care. Three main themes emerged: 1) discomfort with the preponderance of men in waiting areas at VA; 2) lack of female providers and women-only groups and services; and 3) problems accessing information about coverage and available services for women Veterans. The topic areas expressed by the women confirmed those identified nationally throughout VA. Several intervention ideas grew from this information, and plans for addressing the concerns are driving new initiatives. VANAP faculty, VA staff, and nursing students are working collaboratively to develop women Veteran care improvement projects. Examples of such projects include the addition of a women-only reception/lactation area at a Community-Based Outpatient Clinic, and revamping of the local Women Veteran Health Program SharePoint page to inform/educate staff about current resources for women Veterans. Through this work, Veteran care is improved, and foundational Veteran care competencies are further integrated into the nursing school curriculum. Care continuity is enhanced over time, and the academic-practice partnership is strengthened.

Replicability

Wherever women Veterans are served within VA, steps can be taken to gather feedback about how to improve their health care. At the Portland facility, VANAP students and faculty increased staff awareness and involved both VA staff and women Veterans in quality improvement. Even in facilities that do not have academic partners, focus groups, and other experience indicators can and should be used by staff to identify specific local improvements for the care of women Veterans. These types of activities uphold VA's organizational value of Veteran-centric care.

Recognition

Michele Cooper, Paula Gubrud-Howe, Lisa Oken, Layla Guerrigas, Nancy Sloan, West Linn, Sonya Howland-Paul, Brooke Misley, Jolea Hollyfield, Jooae Park

HONORABLE MENTION

When asking VHA employees to submit promising practices, we never anticipated we would receive so many qualified responses—far more than could be included in one volume. We would like to thank each of the employees listed in the following pages for their commitment to providing excellent, innovative care to our nation's Veterans.

Joy Adeola, *Veterans Experience*
Chillicothe VA Medical Center (Chillicothe, OH)

Julie Alban, *Promoting a Positive Culture of
Service Through Honoring the Wishes of Veterans*
North Florida/South Georgia Veterans
Health System (Gainesville, FL)

Sumana Alex, *Clinical Pharmacist
Specialist, Internal Medicine*
Washington DC VA Medical Center (Washington, DC)

Ayse Aytaman, *Creation of a VISN wide
Liver Cancer Team/SCAN—ECHO Tumor
Board and National Spread of the Practice*
Brooklyn Campus of the VA NY Harbor
Healthcare System (Brooklyn, NY)

Mark Bauer, *VA National Bipolar
Telehealth Program*
VA Boston Healthcare System, Brockton
Campus (Brockton, MA)

Alyssa Beebe, *Same Day Access Practices*
Aleda E. Lutz VA Medical Center (Saginaw, MI)

Curt Behlow, *Encouraging
Employers to "Hire MI Vet"*
VA Ann Arbor Healthcare System (Ann Arbor, MI)

Shirley Berry, *Improving Orthopedic Clinic Flow*
North Florida/South Georgia Veterans
Health System (Gainesville, FL)

Heather Bingham, *Delivery of Effective,
Collaborative Interdisciplinary and Interagency
Care for Veterans Living with ALS*
Iowa City VA Health Care System (Iowa City, IA)

Sterling Bird, *BISL reporting tool*
William Jennings Bryan Dorn VA
Medical Center (Columbia, SC)

Suprina Bolton, *Critical Care Drips-
Quick Access for Emergent Initiation*
North Florida/South Georgia Veterans
Health System (Gainesville, FL)

Lori Butler, *VISN 8 Employee Help Desks*
VISN 8: Sunshine Health Care
Network (Saint Petersburg, FL)

Sandra Calenda, *Hypoglycemia Safety
Initiative – VISN 12 Pilot*
VA Great Lakes Health Care System (Westchester, IL)

Joseph Canzolino, *VA ADERS – Safe
Medication Use Enhancements through
Adverse Drug Event Report Review*
VA Central Office (Washington, DC)

Brianno Carbo, *Pharmacist-run
New Veteran Orientation Clinic*
Coatesville VA Medical Center (Coatesville, PA)

Laura (Lori) Carlson, *Multi-site Be Active
and MOVE! (BAM) CVT Program*
VA Illiana Health Care System (Danville, IL)

Jody Cherniak, *The Careplan Improvement Project*
Durham VA Medical Center (Durham, NC)

Michele Clements-Thompson, *System
Redesign-Integrated Tobacco Cessation Program*
South Texas Veterans Health Care
System (San Antonio, TX)

Cathleen Colon-Emeric, *Rural Osteoporosis
Evaluation Services (ROPES)*
Durham VA Medical Center (Durham, NC)

Debra Corbin, *Use of laptops
for field documentation*
Richmond Vet Center (Richmond, VA)

Jennifer Cournoyer, *Using Patient
Registries to Fight Diabetes*
New Mexico VA Health Care
System (Albuquerque, NM)

Nicole Cupples, *Improved Access for Patients
Discharged from Inpatient Psychiatry*
South Texas Veterans Health Care
System (San Antonio, TX)

Stuti Dang, *Providing Dementia Consultations
to Veterans Using Clinical Video Telehealth Set
up and Evaluation of a Remote Memory Clinic*
Miami VA Healthcare System (Miami, FL)

Judith Davagnino, *Caring for Older Adults
and Caregivers at Home (COACH)*
Durham VA Medical Center (Durham, NC)

Kathryn DeSilva, *Using Clinical Pharmacy Specialists to Improve Access & Treatment of Veterans with Hepatitis C Virus Infection*
Atlanta VA Health Care System (Decatur, GA)

Tina Dorman, *Primary Care-Mental Health Integration (PCMHI) e-Consult Service*
South Texas Veterans Health Care System (San Antonio, TX)

Karen Drexler, *Providing Life-Saving Medication Assisted Treatment for Opioid Use Disorder*
VA Central Office (Washington, DC)

Jane Driver, *Pharmacological Intervention in Late Life (PILL) Program*
VA Boston Healthcare System (Jamaica Plain, MA)

Jane Driver, *Pharmacological Intervention in Late Life (PILL) Program*
VA Boston Healthcare System (Jamaica Plain, MA)

Connie Eddy, *BAM! Body & Mind for Residents Living on a Community Living Center with Dementia*
VA Western New York Healthcare System at Batavia (Batavia, NY)

Derek Elofson, *Facility COR Team*
William Jennings Bryan Dorn VA Medical Center (Columbia, SC)

Mandi Evanson, *Utilization of contingency management and health outreach programming to promote 1-855-QUIT-VET and SmokefreeVET for homeless Veterans*
Edward Hines Jr. VA Hospital (Hines, IL)

Eileen Farrell, *Implementation of VHA Directive 1005, Informed Consent for Long-Term Opioid Therapy for Pain, through Shared Medical Appointments*
North Florida/South Georgia Veterans Health System (Gainesville, FL)

Kim Fisher, *Using Huddle Boards to Engage Frontline Employees in Improvement*
North Florida/South Georgia Veterans Health System (Gainesville, FL)

Sheila Ford, *The e-Huddle*
Oakland Outpatient Clinic (Oakland, CA)

Andrew Franck, *Pharmacy-cardiology collaborative antiarrhythmic drug management (AAD)*
North Florida/South Georgia Veterans Health System (Gainesville, FL)

Julie Gagnon, *Addressing Unscheduled Walk-ins: A PI Project using the DMAIC Method (Define, Measure, Analyze, Control)*
William V. Chappell, Jr., VA OPC (Daytona Beach, FL)

Chris Geronimo, *SFVAHCS Veterans Strength and Wellness Program*
San Francisco VA Health Care System (San Francisco, CA)

Chad Gladden, *Teleaudiology*
VA Central Office (Washington, DC)

Timothy "Sebastian" Godbey, *SICU in "75 seconds"*
Louis Stokes Cleveland VA Medical Center (Cleveland, OH)

Adam Gold, *Embracing VA Secure Messaging to Drive Diabetes Self-Care and Increase Veteran Access, Improve Outcomes, Lower Costs, and Keep Veterans Healthy and Working*
Martinsburg VA Medical Center (Martinsburg, WV)

Michael Goldstein, *Clinician Training and Coaching to Enhance PACT Clinicians' Use of Veteran-Centered Communication Skills*
VA Central Office (Washington, DC)

Theresa Hancock, *The Root of Success: It's all about the Employees*
VA Central Office (Washington, DC)

Carma Heitzmann, *Community Employment Coordinators*
VA Central Office (Washington, DC)

Blake Henderson, *REVAMP: Remote Apnea Management Platform*
VA Central Office (Washington, DC)

Johann Herberth, *Transformation to Sustainable Access to Primary Care Services*
Ralph H. Johnson Medical Center (Charleston, SC)

Dina Hooshyar, *Universal Homeless Housing Screening (UHHS)*
Dallas VA Medical Center (Dallas, TX)

Michal Kalli Hose, *Creation of primary care musculoskeletal clinics within the VA system: an effective method for providing comprehensive and timely musculoskeletal care*
VA San Diego Healthcare System (San Diego, CA)

Rob Hough, *24-hour Ambulatory Blood Pressure Monitoring Clinic*
West Palm Beach VA Medical Center (West Palm Beach, FL)

Marcia Insley, *Improving Access: Making Key Resources Available Across VA*
VA Central Office (Washington, DC)

Rene Jacob, *MOVE! Leaderbook Improves Consistency and Coordination of Care*
South Texas Veterans Health Care System (San Antonio, TX)

Joan Jenkins, *Bullseye Targeting Chronic Care Issues amongst Homeless Veterans*
Louis Stokes Cleveland VA Medical Center (Cleveland, OH)

Diane Johnstone, *The Journey for NICHE (Nurses Improving Care for the Healthsystem Elder) Designation*
C.W. Bill Young VA Medical Center (Bay Pines, FL)

Rochelle Jones, *FTEE request*
William Jennings Bryan Dorn VA Medical Center (Columbia, SC)

Jenna Kawamoto, *Essential Role of the Pharmacist in Hepatitis Care*
VA Greater Los Angeles Healthcare System (Los Angeles, CA)

Megan Kelly, *Increasing Access to Tobacco Cessation Treatment for Veterans Using a Multi-Clinic Model*
Edith Nourse Rogers Memorial Veterans Hospital (Bedford, MA)

Forrest Kirk, *Moral Injury Grand Rounds for Clinicians*
Vinita Outpatient Clinic (Vinita, OK)

Laura Krejci, *Healthy Communities— Greenhouse Project*
VA Palo Alto Health Care System (Palo Alto, CA)

Laura Krejci, *Veteran Family Advisor Programs*
VA Palo Alto Health Care System (Palo Alto, CA)

John Kuhn, *Community Planning*
VA Central Office (Washington, DC)

John Kuhn, *Online Grants Management System*
VA Central Office (Washington, DC)

Clinton Latimer, *Perceptive Reach*
VA Central Office (Washington, DC)

Lisa Lehmann, *iMedConsent*™
VA Central Office (Washington, DC)

Lorry Luscri, *The Wellness Workshop Series (WWS) for Veterans*
Edward Hines Jr. VA Hospital (Hines, IL)

John Lynch, A *Measurement Informed Approach to Structured Group Therapy for Veterans with Combat Related PTSD: The PTSD Recovery Series*
Hunter Holmes McGuire VA Medical Center (Richmond, VA)

April Maa, *Technology-based Eye Care Services (TECS): A Remote Care Initiative to Provide Better Access to Eye Care Screening for Veterans*
Atlanta VA Health Care System (Decatur, GA)

Anne Marie Mahoney, *Improving Patient Care Outcomes in Rural Community-Based Outpatient Clinics*
William S. Middleton Memorial Veterans Hospital (Madison, WI)

Victory Marasigan, *Veteran Engagement in Usability Quick Studies for the My HealtheVet Portal Redesign*
VA Central Office (Washington, DC)

Kathleen Matthews, *Behavioral Recovery Outreach (BRO) Team*
VA Central Iowa Health Care System (Des Moines, IA)

Shawn McFarland, *Clinical Pharmacist Decentralization (Acute Care Clinical Pharmacist) to include clinical pharmacist on the healthcare system's medical teams*
Tennessee Valley Healthcare System (Nashville, TN)

Shane McNamee, *Joint Legacy Viewer's Impact on Patient and User Experience*
VA Central Office (Washington, DC)

Penny Melder, *New to the VA: Patient Orientation*
Lewiston VA CBOC (Lewiston, ID)

Emily Melin, *CHAMPIONS (Comprehensive Home Based Acute Care Medical Program Initiative for Older Noncritical Surgical Patients)*
VA Connecticut Healthcare System (West Haven, CT)

Troy Moore, *Opioid Overdose Education and Naloxone Dispensing (OEND)*
South Texas Veterans Health Care System (San Antonio, TX)

Tera Moore, *Reducing Heart Failure Readmissions and Mortality*
South Texas Veterans Health Care System (San Antonio, TX)

Kevin Morton, *GOD 100 Day Challenge/Sustainability Project*
Washington DC VA Medical Center (Washington, DC)

Nicole Najar, *Healthier Living with Chronic Conditions*
Battle Creek VA Medical Center (Battle Creek, MI)

Lisa Nashton, *Improving Data Quality in SAIL - Complications and PSIs*
William Jennings Bryan Dorn VA Medical Center (Columbia, SC)

Lynn Novorska, *MOVE!® Coach mobile application*
VA Central Office (Washington, DC)

Michael Ohl, *HIV Telehealth Collaborative Care*
Veterans Rural Health Resource Center (Iowa City, IA)

David Omura, *Leveraging Technology to Improve Access and Streamline Scheduling*
William Jennings Bryan Dorn VA Medical Center (Columbia, SC)

Kalpana Padala, *Geriatric Walking Clinic: Meeting Rural Veterans Where They Are*
Eugene J. Towbin Healthcare Center (Little Rock, AR)

Jung Hyun Park, *Utilizing a Share Point site with Medicine Admission Log*
Michael E. DeBakey VA Medical Center (Houston, TX)

Jason Petti, *Same Day Access Audiology*
Minneapolis VA Health Care System (Eagan, MN)

Patricia Pitkin, *Clinical Daily Worksheet, AKA: "Who gets the view alert?"*
VA Connecticut Healthcare System, Newington Campus (Newington, CT)

Dee Ramsel, *Civility, Respect, and Engagement in the Workplace (CREW) Initiative*
VA Central Office (Washington, DC)

Dee Ramsel, *National Center for Organization Development — Internal Resource*
VA Central Office (Washington, DC)

Dee Ramsel, *Participating in 360 assessments advances employee interactions with Veterans*
VA Central Office (Washington, DC)

Donna Rasin-Waters, *Psychosocial Distress Monitoring and Navigation in Oncology*
Brooklyn Campus of the VA NY Harbor Healthcare System (Brooklyn, NY)

Pamela Reeves, *Population Health management risk stratification tool*
John D. Dingell VA Medical Center (Detroit, MI)

Kimberly Reno-Ly, *Increasing Hepatitis C Treatment Access through a Group Clinic Model*
Orlando VA Medical Center (Orlando, FL)

Kelsey Rife, *Maximizing Capacity with Hepatitis C Group Clinics*
Louis Stokes Cleveland VA Medical Center (Cleveland, OH)

Jane Robbins, *Human-Centered Design for Colorectal Cancer Screening Templates in CPRS*
VA Central Office (Washington, DC)

Michelle Rossi, *Tele Dementia Clinic*
VA Pittsburgh Healthcare System (Pittsburgh, PA)

Rebecca Rottman-Sagebiel, *Geriatric Medication Education on Discharge (GMED)*
South Texas Veterans Health Care System (San Antonio, TX)

Karine Rozenberg-Ben-Dror, *HCV care: Built for Safety AND for Speed — one story of VA's transformation to cure Hepatitis C*
VISN 12: VA Great Lakes Health Care System (Westchester, IL)

Karen Rubenstein, *Controlled Substance Oversight Board*
Alexandria VA Health Care System (Alexandria, LA)

Steven Sayers, *Coaching Into Care family member call center*
Corporal Michael Cresenz VA Medical Center (Philadelphia, PA)

Kimberly Schnacky, *Improving Access in Specialty Care, the Orlando VA Pharmacy Rheumatology Clinic*
William V. Chappell, Jr., VA OPC (Daytona Beach, FL)

Kimberly Schnacky, *OVUM Pharmacy Rheumatology Clinic*
William V. Chappell, Jr., VA OPC (Daytona Beach, FL)

Cathy Schubert, *Mobile Acute Care for Elders (ACE) Consultation*
Richard L. Roudebush VA Medical Center (Indianapolis, IN)

Donnie Seay, *Improving your VAMC Credentialing Program*
Mountain Home VA Medical Center (Mountain Home, TN)

Raj Sehgal, *Paracentesis Clinic*
South Texas Veterans Health Care System (San Antonio, TX)

Monica Sharma, *Access to excellent healthcare when needed*
Edith Nourse Rogers Memorial Veterans Hospital (Bedford, MA)

Kenneth Shay, *Geriatric Evaluation*
VA Central Office (Washington, DC)

Barbara Snyder, *Veteran-Centered Health Education Workbook*
VA Central Office (Washington, DC)

Jeff Soots, *Dorn VAMC Facility Acquisition Team*
William Jennings Bryan Dorn VA Medical Center (Columbia, SC)

Brian Stevenson, *Creative Arts in Mental Health Wellness*
VA Central Office (Washington, DC)

Sam (John) Sum-Ping, *Optimal Anesthesia Scheduling Non-OR cases*
VA North Texas Health Care System (Dallas, TX)

Kristopher Teague, *Advanced Environmental Controls for Veterans with Severe Disabilities*
VA Central Office (Washington, DC)

Anne Utech, *Expanding Nutrition Services to Veterans without a Home and/or Experiencing Food Insecurity, Special Populations*
VA Central Office (Washington, DC)

Anne Utech, *Procuring Meat, Poultry, and Seafood Produced According to Responsible Antibiotic Use*
VA Central Office (Washington, DC)

Sharon Valente, *Evidence Based Fact Sheets Help Nurses Improve Quality Patient Care*
VA Greater Los Angeles Healthcare System (Los Angeles, CA)

Kristie Van Gaalen, *Establishment of the Nursing Data Dashboard*
C.W. Bill Young VA Medical Center (Bay Pines, FL)

Laura Veet, *Women's Health Mini-Residencies, Quality and Safety*
VA Central Office (Washington, DC)

Alan Villiers, *Veterans Indicated Preference Project*
Harry S. Truman Memorial Veterans' Hospital (Columbia, TX)

Bonnie Wakefield, *Remote, Telephone-Based Delivery of Cardiac Rehabilitation*
Veterans Rural Health Resource Center (Iowa City, IA)

Mitchell Wallin, *Using Clinical Video Telehealth to Provide Comprehensive Care to Rural Veterans with Multiple Sclerosis*
VA Central Office (Washington, DC)

Tessa Walters, *Perioperative Surgical Home*
VA Palo Alto Health Care System (Palo Alto, CA)

Sharon Watts, *Diabetes Shared Medical Appointments: Improving Glucose Control*
Louis Stokes Cleveland VA Medical Center (Cleveland, OH)

Eric Weber, *Clinical Pharmacy Medication Intake Phone Calls*
Phoenix VA Health Care System (Phoenix, AZ)

Aubrey Weekes, *VHA Environment of Care (EOC)*
VA Central Office (Washington, DC)

Ian Weissman, *Breaking Down Silos and Improving Patient Care through Cross-Collaboration with Value-Based, Patient-Centered Health Care Organizations*
Clement J. Zablocki VA Medical Center (Milwaukee, WI)

Jason Wilcox, *Clinician Coaching*
VA Roseburg Healthcare System (Roseburg, OR)

Sarah Will, *The Impact of Clinical Pharmacy Specialists within the Primary Care Setting*
Kansas City Veterans Affairs Medical Center (Kansas City, MO)

Mark Wong, *Improving Antibiotic Prescribing Errors Through an Electronic Order Pop-up & Menu*
South Texas Veterans Health Care System (San Antonio, TX)